Mitral Valve Transesophageal Echocardiography

Dedication

Clare, Eleanor Isabelle, Eugenie Alice

Christina Marie, Jennifer Ann, Jacqueline Michelle, Alycia Yvonne, Dan, Laura Nicole, Alan III, Maria

Mitral Valve Transesophageal Echocardiography

MARTIN G ST JOHN SUTTON, MB, FRCP, FACC, FASE
John W Bryfogle Professor of Cardiac Imaging
University of Pennsylvania Medical Centre
Philadelphia, PA
USA

ALAN R MANIET, DO, FAAIM
St Louis University Medical Center
St Louis, MO
USA

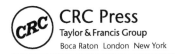

CRC Press
Taylor & Francis Group
Boca Raton London New York

CRC Press is an imprint of the
Taylor & Francis Group, an **informa** business

First published in 2006 by the Taylor & Francis Group.
This edition published in 2011 by Informa Healthcare

First published 2011 by Informa Healthcare

Published 2019 by CRC Press
Taylor & Francis Group
6000 Broken Sound Parkway NW, Suite 300
Boca Raton, FL 33487-2742

© 2011 by Taylor & Francis Group, LLC (except as otherwise indicated)
CRC Press is an imprint of Taylor & Francis Group, an Informa business

First issued in paperback 2019

No claim to original U.S. Government works

ISBN 13: 978-0-367-44642-0 (pbk)
ISBN 13: 978-1-84184-608-8 (hbk)

Visit the Taylor & Francis Web site at
http://www.taylorandfrancis.com

and the CRC Press Web site at
http://www.crcpress.com

A CIP record for this book is available from the British Library.

Library of Congress Cataloging-in-Publication Data available on application

Table of Contents

Preface

Over the past few years transesophageal echocardiography has become one of the most exciting imaging modalities available today in modern clinical cardiology. Transesophageal echocardiography and MRI imaging has substantially improved our understanding of mitral valve anatomy and physiology with multiplane transesophageal echocardiography having a true advantage through its portability, relatively inexpensive equipment and seminoninvasive nature. Multiplane transesophageal echocardiography provides high resolution cardiac images in an infinite number of planes. When combined with conventional and color Doppler modalities, this offers a superlative diagnostic tool for evaluating cardiac structure and function. Multiplane transesophageal echocardiography provides a three-dimensional perspective, especially of the mitral valve, that cannot be appreciated even by the cardiac pathologist. This point is illustrated by multiple carefully prepared anatomic sections, matched with diagrams and multiplane transesophageal images. After finishing our original text, the *Atlas of Multiplane Transesophageal Echocardiography*, we were approached by many physicians to provide a smaller concise reference just on the mitral valve, as the importance of mitral regurgitation has blossomed in modern cardiology. The aim of this atlas is to provide medical students, anesthesiologists, cardiac surgeons and cardiologists with an in-depth analysis of the mitral valve from an experience of over 15,000 transesophageal echocardiograms performed by the authors, with over 15 years in the operative arena studying mitral repair techniques. This atlas may also serve as a reference for diagnostic examples of mitral pathology for physicians who practice transesophageal echocardiography. The text is not meant to be a complete or authoritative reference for the mitral valve, but to serve as a starting point or "how-to" reference for studying the mitral valve structure and function. With the new emphasis on the possibility of replacing or repairing mitral valves when patients are asymptomatic, it is extremely important for echocardiographers to possess a clear understanding of mitral valve abnormalities in order to address surgical decision-making properly with our surgical colleagues. The format begins with normal mitral valve structure and function, followed by abnormalities of the mitral valve unit. Chapters include evaluation of prostheses, interventional cardiology techniques, and intraoperative transesophageal echocardiography, especially how it relates to mitral valve repair. A concise explanation of measurements of cardiac chamber sizes and function and Doppler are provided only for transesophageal echocardiographic applications. As in the original atlas, transesophageal echocardiographic images are juxtaposed with correlative anatomic specimens to provide a graphical understanding of normal and abnormal mitral valve anatomy.

Martin G St John Sutton
Alan R Maniet

Acknowledgements

The authors are indebted to the sonographers, cardiology fellows and secretaries of the laboratories of Thomas Jefferson University Hospital, Hospital of the University of Pennsylvania and the Episcopal Hospital for their assistance in the preparation of this textbook. It is hoped that the readers of this book will obtain as much enjoyment and knowledge as went into its preparation.

Technical expertise, Norman (Ali) Alexander, Harry Kuttner, Florence Orsini, Maureen McDonald, Lois Nitka.
Photographic assistance Frederick Ross.
Editorial assistance Alan Burgess, Tim Koder.
Surgical assistance Richard N. Edie, MD, John Mannion, MD, James T. Diehl, MD.
Echocardiographic expertise Joel S. Raichlen, MD.
Pathology assistance Theodore D. Krouse, MD.
With special thanks to Ted Plappert.

1

Introduction

Mitral valve repair • Mechanical valves • Biological valves • Further developments in mitral valve repair • The impact of echocardiography

The mitral valve, with its unique and delicate structure, has intrigued physicians and scientists for centuries. Indeed, the quest to understand the function of the mitral valve is a thread that runs through the entire history of modern cardiology.

Some of the earliest descriptions of the mitral valve were made in the 16th century by Leonardo da Vinci. His drawings and notes, based on dissected bovine and human hearts, highlighted the complex architecture of the valve and alluded to the unknown function of the individual elements of the subvalvular apparatus.[1–3] The mitral valve was named for its resemblance to a bishop's mitre, as depicted in da Vinci's drawings.

In 1543 the first complete textbook of human anatomy by Andreas Vesalius released the study of human anatomy from the restrictions of Galenic doctrine.[4] Vesalius described the heart as the center of the vascular network, and proposed that the pulmonary veins carried air from the lungs to the left atrium. Vesalius' and da Vinci's historic theories opened the doors to further study and discovery.

In the 19th century Prussian physiologists attempted to explore the form and function of the mitral valve apparatus *in vitro* using primitive organ baths. Based on simple geometric principles, Woods was the first to propose a pivotal role for the papillary muscles and mitral subvalvular apparatus in left ventricular systolic function.[5]

MITRAL VALVE REPAIR

Attention turned to the clinical recognition of mitral valve disease in the late 1800s, when Samways[6] and Brunton[7] proposed that mitral stenosis could be treated by performing a transventricular valvotomy. This was of particular importance because, at the time, operating on the heart was in direct violation of common thought and practice. Samways hypothesized that "the severest cases of mitral stenosis will be relieved by slightly notching the mitral orifice and trusting to the auricle to continue its defence." Brunton had carried out preliminary experiments on diseased cadaveric mitral valves and healthy feline valves, and believed that mitral stenosis could be corrected despite the risks of surgery. He suggested "elongating the natural opening, cutting through the thickened edge of the commissures along their natural openings or incising the leaflets in the middle through a ventricular approach", considering that the thicker wall of the left ventricle would be less prone to bleeding than the thinner left atrium. With the exception of the ventriculotomy, this description closely resembles modern-day surgical techniques. Nevertheless, Brunton was severely criticized by his peers for even proposing cardiac surgery.[8,9]

Mitral valve surgery lay dormant until the 1920s when the first valvotomies were performed by Cutler and Levine at the Peter Bent Brigham Hospital in Boston,[10] and by Souttar at The London Hospital.[11] Cutler attempted surgery from the auricular approach, since the difficulty with the transventricular approach "lay in locating the mitral valve so that the valve could be engaged between the cutting edges of the instrument." Despite choosing the safer atrial route, Cutler soon discovered that those patients who had parts of their mitral valve accidentally excised by the cardiovalvulotome had almost a 100% mortality; only one patient, whose mitral valve was left intact, survived. Henry Souttar circumvented this problem by performing the first finger dilation on mitral valve stenosis through a transatrial approach. He stated that, "the information given by the finger is exceedingly clear, and personally I felt an appreciation of the mechanical reality of stenosis and regurgitation which I never felt before." Souttar's technique of finger dilation of mitral stenosis ultimately led to more successful surgeries and fewer mortalities in a time before direct visualization was possible. However, the number of failed cases in the 1920s was high enough to discourage mitral valvotomies despite many new proponents for heart surgery.

Mitral valvotomy for mitral stenosis was redefined during the late 1940s and early 1950s by Bailey[12,13] and Harken[14–16] in the USA, and by Brock[17] and Tubbs in the UK. Harken (who continued the work of Cutler) and Bailey had accumulated a wealth of surgical experience prior to performing their first valvotomies. Harken's experience had come during World War II repairing hearts injured during battle, while Bailey's was gained through laboratory surgeries on canine mitral valves. Both men believed that "palpation of the valve [was] critical to ensuring an equilibrium between stenosis and regurgitation and [that] selecting patients with stenosis and no complications was most important". In 1948 Bailey and Harken performed their first transatrial commissurotomies, on June 10th and June 16th respectively. Bailey had to endure four surgical mortalities before his first success at Philadelphia's Episcopal Hospital, where he used a hooked knife guided by his index finger to perform the procedure. By 1956, Bailey had performed over 1000 commissurotomies with an operative mortality of 7.9%. Harken performed over 1000 valvulotomies over a 20 year period, including a large percentage in patients under the age of 40 with mostly noncalcified valves. Although these patients had improved long-term survival rates, he was quick to point out that the results were palliative rather than curative.

Enthusiasm for mitral valve surgery continued to grow in the 1950s. The development of the heart–lung machine and mechanical oxygenation allowed Gibbon[18] to perform the first successful open-heart operation with direct visualization of the heart in a bloodless field at the Thomas Jefferson University Hospital. Bigelow[19] used hypothermia to reduce oxygen usage during heart surgery, an approach that Lewis[20] used in conjunction with caval occlusion. These technical advances played a crucial role in providing surgeons with an opportunity to look inside the heart and directly view the damaged mitral valve, thereby enabling more extensive mitral valve surgeries.

Meanwhile, other physicians were investigating mitral insufficiency. Griffith[21] and Hall[22] in 1903 proposed that an apical late systolic murmur might denote mitral regurgitation. In 1937, White[23] suggested that mid-systolic sounds might sometimes arise from abnormal chordae tendineae. This theory was revived by Reid[24] in 1961, who postulated that clicks and late systolic murmurs were of mitral valvular origin. The clicks arose from the chordae, and Reid used the terms "chordal snap" and "nonejection systolic click" in order to differentiate them from aortic and pulmonary ejection sounds. The physiologists Rushmer, a bioengineer at the University of Washington, and Tsakiris, working at the Mayo Clinic, further defined chordae tendineae. In 1956, Lillehei[25,26] in Minnesota attempted to repair leaky valves under direct vision, and McGoon[27] at the Mayo Clinic introduced "repair of mitral regurgitation for ruptured chordae tendineae by performing a triangular resection of the prolapsing leaflet segment."

MECHANICAL VALVES

Although initial surgical repairs of regurgitant and stenotic mitral valves were now being commonly performed, the long term success rate was unsatisfactory. The search for alternative, more successful treatment strategies led to the development of prosthetic valves.

The first steps towards valvular replacement came with the selective mechanical replacement of specific parts of the mitral valve. These included Gott's replacement of the posterior mitral leaflet, and King's replacement of the chordae tendineae.[24] While these procedures looked promising theoretically the results were disappointing; either the replacement parts failed to achieve full function or the rigidity of the prosthetic parts worsened mitral valve function by causing stenosis. The first mitral valve replacement was performed by Chesterman[28] in England on July 22nd 1955.

The design of the valve used by Chesterman closely resembled that of the first successful mitral valve replacement – the Starr-Edwards ball-and-cage valve. The original idea for the Starr-Edwards valve came from a bottle stopper patented in 1858. The design was modified and refined based on data from canine experiments. Starr used strict selection criteria to maximize the success rate of the procedure, focusing on patients whose mitral valves had been damaged beyond repair and who needed surgery quickly. The Starr-Edwards valve led to the first ever published report of survival beyond three months for patients with total valvular replacement. Following the success of the Starr-Edwards valve, mitral valve mechanical replacement flourished in the 1960s under Starr, Braunwald and Harken, even though initial mitral valve replacement mortality rates were 30% and higher.[29-33] New prosthetic mitral

valve designs proliferated, using a range of synthetic materials (from Teflon to Mylar and Dacron) and shapes (depending on the designer's understanding of how normal physiology could be maintained).

BIOLOGICAL VALVES

The high rate of thrombosis experienced with the mechanical valves available at the time led to the idea of using biological valves (bioprostheses). Homografts (transplants from human cadavers) were introduced by Ross and Barratt-Boyes in the 1960s.[34,35] Binet and associates developed tissue valves from formaldehyde-fixed xenografts.[36,37] The initial results were promising, but within a few years these valves began to fail because of degeneration and calcification of the tissues. Carpentier and associates studied the valves of various animal species and found that porcine valves closely resembled human valves.[38] In 1966 Carpentier began working with porcine valves fixed in glutaraldehyde rather than formaldehyde and mounting them on a stent, allowing the valve to be placed in the mitral position. He found that although the use of gluteraldehyde almost eliminated the inflammatory reaction, the implants had to be replaced within five years due to calcification and cuspal tearing. Further research built on this early work and led to the development of the Carpentier-Edwards, Hancock and Angell-Shiley bioprostheses.

Mitral valve replacement, whether mechanical or biologic, was associated with an unacceptably high surgical mortality, due to the removal of the leaflets and subvalvular apparatus. In 1972, Kirklin remarked that "we should expect to see a lower LV ejection fraction after mitral valve replacement for mitral regurgitation due to elimination of the 'systolic pop-off' mechanism, resulting in higher left ventricular systolic wall stress (or afterload)".[39] In the 1980s, David, Hagl and surgeons at Stanford found that preserving the mitral subvalvular apparatus improved clinical outcome, preserved LV shape and systolic function and reduced mortality.[40]

FURTHER DEVELOPMENTS IN MITRAL VALVE REPAIR

Mitral valve repair continued into the late 1950s, but it was technically challenging and infrequently performed, and most surgeons chose to use prosthetic valves. However, Wooler, Reed and Kaye refined the techniques for mitral annuloplasty, allowing some surgeons to continue repairing stenotic and regurgitant valves. [41–44]

At about this time the epidemiology of mitral valve pathologies began to change. Rheumatic mitral valve disease declined, due largely to the introduction of penicillin and a general improvement in socioeconomic conditions.[45,46] Degenerative diseases of the mitral valve thus became more prominent, with mitral valve prolapse taking center stage as the most important cause of mitral regurgitation.

In 1963 Barlow and associates[47–50] identified late systolic murmurs as an indicator of billowing mitral leaflets or mitral valve prolapse allowing regurgitation of the mitral valve (a condition now known as Barlow's syndrome). During the 1970s the cardiology literature experienced an "information explosion" relating to mitral valve prolapse syndrome.[51] The frequency of mitral valve prolapse and regurgitation as defined with echocardiographic reports ranged between 4% and 21% of the normal population. As far back as 1953, McKenzie and Lewis had stated that systolic murmurs were harmless in the absence of the evidence of myocardial disease. Nevertheless, it soon became clear that a differentiation would have to be made between patients with severe mitral regurgitation, and patients with trivial or mitral valve reflux, as detected by echocardiographic and Doppler techniques. Over the next decade the etiology, diagnosis, prognosis and management of patients with mitral valve prolapse and regurgitation was defined. In the early 1980s, Carpentier redefined the essential and important differences between "prolapse" and billowing by careful analysis of mitral valve pathology during mitral valve repair.

During the 1980s mitral repair continued to flourish under the direction of Carpentier[52–54] and Duran,[55–57] both of whom introduced several reparative techniques using annuloplasty rings determined by the functional classification of the specific mitral valve lesion. Using these techniques mitral valve repairs were performed with: lower operative and late mortality rates; improved hemodynamics; fewer thromboembolic complications with a reduced risk of anticoagulant-related hemorrhage; a reduced risk of infective endocarditis. These factors combined to make mitral valve repair especially appealing to developing countries.

Although mitral valve reparative techniques were initially largely used for cases of mitral regurgitation, they were also employed in the treatment of mitral stenosis. With the expansion of the field of interventional techniques in the cardiac catheterization laboratory, Inoue[58] and Lock[59] pioneered balloon catheters to dilate stenotic mitral valves in 1984, avoiding the risks associated with thoracotomy. Long-term studies at three and five years showed that balloon valvuloplasty and open-heart surgical commissurotomy had similar survival and restenosis rates.[60,61]

THE IMPACT OF ECHOCARDIOGRAPHY

Over the last decades, echocardiography has played an important role in understanding mitral valvular disease. In the early days of M-Mode echocardiography, the mitral valve was frequently the only discernible cardiac structure, allowing mitral stenosis to be diagnosed noninvasively.[62] With the development of two-dimensional echocardiography a spatial evaluation of the mitral valve could be obtained, and the importance of the mitral subvalvular apparatus, the valve leaflets and their motion was recognized for the first time, eliminating many of the misconceptions about the mitral valve[63–68]. The mitral valve prolapse syndrome was highlighted by echocardiography. Doppler echocardiography in conjunction with two-dimensional imaging has provided a method of quantifying the degree of stenosis and regurgitation in mitral valvular disease.

In surgical repair of mitral valvular disease,[69] transesophageal echocardiography gives the precise assessment of mitral valvular structural abnormalities that is necessary to direct appropriate treatment.

Prior to the mid-1990s, the decision to intervene in mitral valvular disease was based on the presence of severe stenosis or regurgitation, and was followed by replacement of the valve with a prosthesis. This strategy frequently resulted in an imperfect functional result, substituting one disease process for another, and led to disconcertingly high morbidity and mortality.[70] A better appreciation of mitral valvular disease has evolved, largely due to the improvement in imaging techniques. The ability to define specific structural abnormalities of the valve leaflets and subvalvular apparatus has allowed the development of reparative surgical techniques that overcome the shortcomings prosthetic valves. The success of managing and surgical techniques have improved the longevity of patients with mitral valve disease.[70–72]

It is essential that the physician performing transesophageal echocardiographic studies has a complete and thorough understanding of normal mitral valvular anatomy, in order to recognize abnormalities. The physician must be able to evaluate the motion of the valve leaflets as well as the subvalvular apparatus, to describe anatomical abnormalities due to the disease process.[73–75] The physician must be well versed in the principles and practice of Doppler methodology in order to identify abnormalities. Finally the echocardiographer must possess the technical ability to obtain all of the views necessary to evaluate the whole structure and function of the mitral valve, which are uniquely acquired with multiplane transesophageal echocardiography, in order to provide a complete assessment.

REFERENCES

1. Kemp M. Dissection and divinity in Leonardo's late anatomy. J Warbug Courtauld Inst 1972;35:200–225.

2. Kemp M. Leonardo da Vinci: The Marvellous Works of Nature and Man. Dent & Son, London, 1989.

3. Keele K, Pedretti C. Leonardo da Vinci. Corpus of anatomical studies in the collection of Her Majesty the Queen at Windsor Castle. Harcourt Brace Jovanovich, New York, 1979.

4. Vesalius A. De Humani Corporis Fabrica. Basel, 1543.

5. Snellen HA. History of cardiology: a brief outline of the 350 years' prelude to an explosive growth. Netherlands: Donker Academic Publications, 19–26.

6. Samways DW. Cardiac peristalsis: its nature and effects. Lancet 1898;1:927.

7. Brunton L. Preliminary note on the possibility of treating mitral stenosis by surgical methods. Lancet 1902;1:352.

8. Harken DE. The emergence of cardiac surgery. I. Personal recollections of the 1940s and 1950s. J Thorac Cardiovasc Surg 1989;98:805–813.

9. Editorial. Surgical operation for mitral stenosis. Lancet 1902;1:461–462.

10. Cutler EC, Beck CS. The present status of the surgical procedures in chronic valvular disease of the heart. Arch Surg 1929;18:403–416.

11. Souttar HS. The surgical treatment of mitral stenosis. Br Med J 1925;2:603–606.

12. Bailey CP. The surgical treatment of mitral stenosis (mitral commissurotomy). Dis Chest 1949;15:377–397.

13. Bailey CP, Bolton HE. Criteria for and results of surgery for mitral stenosis. Part II. Results of mitral commissurotomy. N Y State J Med 1956;56:825–839.

14. Harken DE, Ellis LB, Ware PF, Norman LR. The surgical treatment of mitral stenosis. I. Valvuloplasty. N Engl J Med 1948;239:801–809.

15. Collins JJ Jr. Dwight Harken: the legacy of mitral valvuloplasty. J Card Surg 1994;9(2 Suppl):210–212.

16. Ellis LB, Singh JB, Morales DD, Harken DE. Fifteen- to twenty-year study of one thousand patients undergoing closed mitral valvuloplasty. Circulation 1973;48:357–364.

17. Baker C, Brock RC, Campbell M. Valvulotomy for mitral stenosis. Report of six successful cases. Br Med J 1950;1:1283–1293.

18. Gibbon JH Jr. The development of heart-lung apparatus. Am J Surg 1978;135:608–619.

19. Bigelow WG, Callaghan JC, Hopps JA. General hypothermia for experimental intracardiac surgery. Ann Surg 1950;132:531–539.

20. Acierno LJ. The history of cardiology. New York: Parthenon Publishing Group, 1994:597–697.

21. Griffith JPC. Midsystolic and late systolic mitral murmurs. Am J Med Sci 1892;104:285.

22. Hall JN. Late systolic mitral murmurs. Am J Med Sci 1903;125:663–666.

23. White PD. Heart Disease, ed 2. Macmillan, New York, 1937;211.

24. Reid JVO. Mid-systolic clicks. S AFR Med J 1961;35:353–355.

25. Lillehei CW, Cohen M, Warden HE, Varco RL. The direct-vision intracardiac correction of congenital anomalies by controlled cross circulation. Surgery 1955;38:11–29.

26. Lillehei CW, Gott VL, DeWall RA, et al. Surgical correction of pure mitral insufficiency by annuloplasty under direct vision. Lancet 1957;77:446–449.

27. McGoon DC. Repair of mitral insufficiency due to ruptured chordae tendineae. J Thorac Cardiovasc Surg 1960;39:357–362.

28. Norman AF. The first mitral valve replacement [letter]. Ann Thorac Surg 1991;51:525–526.

29. Cooley DA. Recollections of early development and later trends in cardiac surgery. J Thorac Cardiovasc Surg 1989;98:817–822.

30. Braunwald NS, Cooper T, Morrow AG. Complete replacement of the mitral valve: successful clinical application of a flexible polyurethane prosthesis. J Thorac Cardiovasc Surg 1960;40:1–11.

31. Starr A, Edwards ML. Mitral replacement: clinical experience with a ball-valve prosthesis. Ann Surg 1961;154:726–740.

32. Pluth JR. The Starr valve revisited. Ann Thorac Surg 1991;51:333–334.

33. Hufnagel CA, Vilkgas PD, Nahas H. Experiences with new types of aortic valvular prostheses. Ann Surg 1958;147:636–645.

34. Adebo OA, Ross JK. Surgical treatment of ruptured mitral valve chordae. A comparison between valve replacement and valve repair. J Thorac Cardiovasc Surg 1984;32:139–142.

35. Ross DN. Homograft replacement of the aortic valve. Lancet 1962;2:487.

36. Binet JP, Carpentier A, Langlois J, et al. Implantation de valves heterogenes dans le traitment des cardiopathies aortiques. C R Acad Sci Paris 1965;261:5733.

37. Binet JP, Planche C, Weiss M. Heterograft replacement of the aortic valve in Ionescu MI, Ross DN, Wooler GH (eds) Biological Tissue in Heart Valve Replacement. London, Butterworth, 1971, p 409.

38. Carpentier A. Principles of tissue valve transplantation in Ionescu MI, Ross DN, Wooler GH (eds) Biological Tissue in Heart Valve Replacement. London, Butterworth, 1971, p 49.

39. 2002 William W.L. Glenn Lecture, "Ode to the Mitral Valve", D. Craig Miller, MD, Thelma & Henry Doegler Prof. of CV Surgery, Stanford University School of Medicine.

40. David TE, Burns RJ, Bacchus CM, et al. Mitral valve replacement for mitral regurgitation with and without preservation of chordae tendineae. J Thorac Cardiovasc Surg 1984;88:718–725.

41. Wooler GH, Nixon PG, Grimshaw VA, et al. Experiences with the repair of the mitral valve in mitral incompetence. Thorax 1962;17:49.

42. Reed GE, Tice DA, Clause RH. A symmetric, exaggerated mitral annuloplasty: Repair of mitral insufficiency with hemodynamic predictability. J Thorax Cardiovasc Surg 1965;49:752.

43. Kay JH, Zubiate T, Mendez MA, et al. Mitral valve repair for significant mitral insufficiency. Am Heart J 1978;96:243.Oliveira DBG, Dawkins KD, Kay PH, et al. Chordal rupture II. Comparison between repair and replacement. B Heart J 1983;50:318–324.

44. Reed GE, Pooley RW, Moggio R. Durability of measured mitral annuloplasty. J Thorac Cardiovasc Surg 1980;79:321–325.

45. Sellers TF. An epidemiologic view of rheumatic fever. Prog Cardiovasc Dis 1973;16:303.

46. Bland EF, Jones TD. Rheumatic fever and rheumatic heart disease. Circulation 1951;4:836.

47. Barlow JV, Pocock WA, Marchand P, Denny M. The significance of late systolic murmurs. Am Heart J 1963;66:443–452

48. Pocock WA, Barlow JB. Etiology and electrocardiographic features of the billowing posterior mitral leaflet syndrome. Am J Med 1971;51:731–739.

49. Barlow JB, Pocock WA. The mitral valve prolapse enigma – two decades later. Mod Concepts Cardiovasc Dis 1984;3:13–17.

50. Barlow JB, Pocock WA. Billowing, floppy, prolapsed or flail mitral valves? Am J Cardiol 1985;55:501–502.

51. Devereux RB, Perloff JK, Reichek N, Josephson ME. Mitral valve prolapse. Circulation 1976;54(1):3–14.

52. Carpentier A. Cardiac valve surgery: the "French Correction." J Thorac Cardiovasc Surg 1983;86:323–337.

53. Carpentier A, Deloche A, Dauptain J. A new reconstructive operation for correction of mitral and tricuspid insufficiency. J Thorac Cardiovasc Surg 1971;61:1.

54. Carpentier A, Chauvand S, Fabiani JN, et al. Reconstructive surgery of mitral valve incompetence. Ten-year appraisal. J Thorac Cardiovasc Surg 1980;79:338–348.

55. Duran CMG, Pomar JL, Revuelta JM, et al. Conservative operation for mitral insufficiency. Critical analysis supported by postoperative hemodynamic studies of 72 patients. J Thorac Cardiovasc Surg 1980;79:326–337.

56. Duran DMG, Revuelta JM, Gaite L, et al. Stability of mitral reconstructive surgery at 10–12 years with predominantly rheumatic valvular disease. Circulation 1988;78(Suppl I):91–95.

57. Duran DMG, Gometza B, Balasundaram S, et al. A feasibility study of valve repair in rheumatic mitral regurgitation. Eur Heart J 1991;12 (Suppl B):34–38.

58. Inoue K, Owaki T, Nakamura T, et al. Clinical application of transvenous mitral commissurotomy by a new balloon catheter. J Thorac Cardiovasc Surg 1984;87: 394–402.

59. Lock JE, Khalilullah M, Shrivastava S, et al. Percutaneous catheter commissurotomy in rheumatic mitral stenosis. N Engl J Med 1985;313:1515–1518.

60. Reyes VP, Raju BS, Wynne J, et al. Percutaneous balloon valvuloplasty compared with open surgical commissurotomy for mitral stenosis. N Engl J Med 1994;331:961–967.

61. Bittl JA. Mitral valve balloon dilatation: long-term results. J Card Surg 1994;9(2 Suppl):213–217.

62. Edler I. Ultrasound cardiogram in mitral valve disease. Acta Chir Scand 1956;3:230.

63. Brock RC. The surgical and pathological anatomy of the mitral valve. Br Heart J 1952; 14:489.

64. Rusted IE, Scheifley CH, Edwards JE. Studies of the mitral valve. I. Anatomic features of the normal mitral valve and associated structures. Circulation 1952;6:825.

65. Chiechi MA, Lees WM, Thompson R. Functional anatomy of the normal mitral valve. J Thorac Surg 1956;32:378.

66. Van der Spuy JC. The functional and clinical anatomy of the mitral valve. Br Heart J 1958;20:471.

67. Du Plessis LA, Marchand P. The anatomy of the mitral valve and its associated structures. Thorax 1964;19:221.

68. Silverman ME, Hurst JW. The mitral complex. Interaction of the anatomy, physiology and pathology of the mitral annulus, mitral valve leaflets, chordae tendineae and papillary muscles. Am Heart J 1968;76:399–418.

69. Kinsley RH. Valve replacement. Ann Life Ins Med 1980;6:185.

70. Bonchek LI. Correction of mitral valve disease without valve replacement. Am Heart J 1982;104:865–868.

71. Antunes MJ, Colsen PR, Kinsley RH. Mitral valvuloplasty: a learning curve. Circulation 1983;68:II–70–5.

72. Cosgrove DM, Chavez AM, Lytle BW, et al. Results of mitral valve reconstruction. Circulation 1986;74:1–82–7.

73. Becker AE, De Wit APM. Mitral valve apparatus. A spectrum of normality relevant to mitral valve prolapse. Br Heart J 1979;42:680–689.

74. Roberts WC. Morphologic features of the normal and abnormal mitral valve. Am J Cardiol 1983;51:1005–1028.

75. Perloff JK, Roberts WC. The mitral apparatus. Functional anatomy of mitral regurgitation. Circulation 1972;46:227–239.

2

Normal Anatomy, Normal TEE, Normal Doppler

Normal mitral valve anatomy   •   Normal multiple transesophageal echocar diographic valve analysis
•   Multiplane Doppler examination of the nor mal mitral valve

NORMAL MITRAL VALVE ANATOMY

Leaflet

The mitral valve sits in the fibrous skeleton of the heart separating the left atrium from the left ventricle (Figure 2.1). The normal mitral valve has two leaflets that act in conjunction with the subvalvular apparatus as one functional unit.[1-6] The mitral leaflets are attached at their bases to the fibro-muscular ring or annulus fibrosis, and by their free edges to the subvalvular apparatus consisting of chordae tendineae and papillary muscles.

The two leaflets, anterior and posterior, differ in size and shape but share equal leaflet surface area (Figures 2.1 and 2.2). The anterior leaflet, also known as the septal or aortic leaflet, is triangular in shape, with a convex free edge. The width (base to free edge measurement) of the anterior leaflet is about one third larger than the posterior leaflet. The posterior leaflet, also known as the mural or inferolateral leaflet, is narrower, attaches to a larger portion of the annulus than the anterior leaflet, and has a concave free edge. Two natural indentations or clefts in the posterior leaflet produce three segments, which subdivide the posterior leaflet into lateral, central, and medial scallops. The lateral and medial scallops are smaller in surface area than the central scallop. The two leaflets are joined at their lateral free edges near the annulus just above the papillary muscles, to form two hinge points or commissures (Figures 2.1 and 2.3). When the mitral valve is closed during systole and viewed *en face*, the line of valve closure resembles a smile. When the mitral valve is open during diastole and viewed *en face*, it has an elliptical shape that gradually tapers like a funnel into the ventricle. When imaged sagittally the mitral valve resembles a trapdoor with the anterior to posterior leaflet length ratio being 2:1.

The leaflet tissue is thin and transparent near the annulus and the central portion (body) of the valve, gradually thickening near the free edge, becoming opaque and very thick at the opposing surface (rough zone). The rough zone is created by the points of attachment for each chorda, and permits a seal between the two leaflets when they approximate during closure. The leaflet edges fold over the chordal attachment (hooding), which somewhat protects the insertion point and provides increased surface area for approximation.

The posterior leaflet, with its narrow height, serves as a valance for the anterior leaflet to swing up and close against, providing a seal during closure. This leads to the concept [7] of

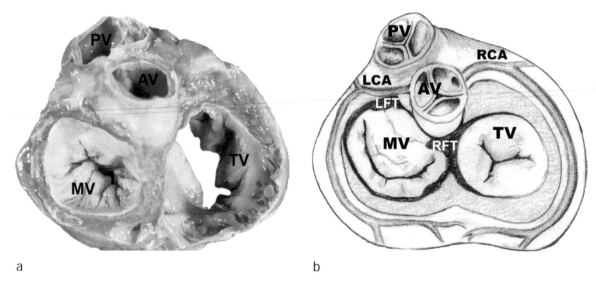

a   b

Fig. 2.1 Normal mitral valve anatomy. (a) Anatomical section at the base of the hear t illustrating the position of the four car diac valves. The mitral valve (MV) is seated posterior to the semilunar valves and is lateral and to the left of the tricuspid valve (TV). The anterior leaflet of the mitral valve is contiguous and opposite the lef and non-coronar y cusps of the aor tic valve. The posterior medial commissur e of the mitral valve lies opposite the septal leaflet of the tricuspid valve. The posterior position of the mitral valve allows optimal examination b multiplane transesophageal echocar diography. PV, pulmonar y valve; AV, aortic valve. (b) Cor responding drawing of the fib ous skeleton of the hear t. The anterior mitral leaflet is f mly attached to the aor tic annulus by dense fib ous connective tissue for ming the mitral cur tain or mitral-aor tic fib ous continuity. Two fib ous trigones situated near each commissur e represent fixation points for the fi ous skeleton pr oviding stability for car diac contraction and the valve annulus. The right fib ous trigone (RFT) is centrally located between the aor tic valve (AV), the mitral valve (MV) and the tricuspid valve (TV). The left fib ous trigone (LFT) extends superiorly and blends into the aor tic root. Both trigones pr oject connective tissue fibers laterally and posteriorly to enci cle the mitral annulus. In the most posterior por tion of the annulus the fibers p ogressively diminish leaving the central posterior annulus devoid of dense collagen fibers and only composed of loose connective tissue. Thi composition of the mitral annulus allows for annular dilatation to occur lar gely in the posterior aspect of the valve. The left cor onary artery (LCA) courses superiorly and laterally ar ound the mitral annulus and the circumflex artery wraps ar ound the posterior aspect of the valve to the cr ux of the hear t. RCA, right cor onary artery; PV, pulmonar y valve.

the anterior leaflet being the active "velocity leaflet", largely responsible for the dynamics of opening and closing of the mitral orifice. The posterior leaflet is the "passive leaflet" and is the buttress that the anterior leaflet closes against to absorb the strain transmitted to the valve from the pressure generated in the ventricle during systole. The smaller height of the posterior leaflet also defines the orientation of the inflow tract, directing the flow of blood to the posterior aspect of the left ventricle.

Annulus

The two mitral leaflets are attached at their bases to a ring of fibromuscular tissue in the fibrous skeleton of the heart, called the annulus fibrosus (see Figure 2.1).[8,9] The fibrous trigones are the major components of the annulus fibrosus and sit adjacent to the commissures. The right fibrous trigone (central fibrous body) is the more prominent of the two and is centered between the tricuspid, mitral, and aortic valves. The left fibrous trigone is seated

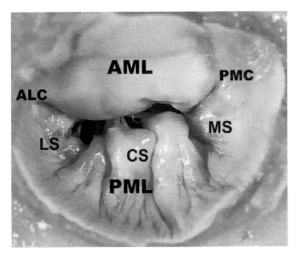

c

Fig. 2.1 (contd.) (c) Anatomic specimen of the mitral valve leaflets. The posterior mitral leaflet (PM is divided by pr ominent indentations in the leafle margin into thr ee scallops: the lateral scallop (LS); the central scallop (CS), usually the lar gest; and the medial scallop (MS). Note that the anterior mitral leaflet (AML) is fr ee of these indentations or scallops. The anterior leaflet is rather triangular in shape. Th posterior leaflet is mo e rectangular in shape and wraps around the fr ee margin of the anterior leaflet Although the width of the anterior leaflet is la ger than the posterior leaflet, both leaflets   e approximately equal in sur face area. In addition, both leaflets a e really continuous as demonstrated at the commissur es, and do not extend entir ely to the annulus. ALC, anter olateral commissur e; PMC, poster omedial commissur e; PV, pulmonar y valve.

between the mitral and aortic valve towards the peripheral and most posterior portion of the fibrous skeleton. The two trigones are connected anteriorly with a thick band of collagenous connective tissue (the mitral-aortic fibrous continuity), which lies between the aortic and mitral valve and which forms the annulus for the entire anterior mitral leaflet. The anterior leaflet occupies only 40% of the total annular perimeter, with the entire basal portion of the anterior leaflet being attached to rigid collagen tissue opposite the aortic valve, which allows commissural attachments to be very close to the trigones. These characteristics allow rigid support of the anterior leaflet. The trigones project connective tissue laterally and posteriorly, surrounding the posterior leaflet to form the remainder of the annulus. The posterior annulus is thinner and weaker than the anterior annulus – as the connective tissue progresses posteriorly it gradually tapers to leave the posterior area around the central scallop with only loose connective tissue almost completely devoid of collagen fibers. This provides less annular support for the posterior leaflet, especially near the central scallop,[10,11] allowing the annulus to stretch in this area, under the stress of ventriculoatrial dilatation.

The dimensions of the annulus are characterized by a height (anterior-posterior dimension) to width (transverse dimension) ratio of 3:4 (Figure 2.1).[7]

Chordae tendineae

The chordae tendineae are tendinous supporting structures that originate from the tips of the papillary muscles and fan out by branching before inserting into the ventricular surface of the leaflet (Figure 2.5).[3] Chordal insertion is equally spaced (0.5 mm apart) on the margin of the leaflet edge, which promotes symmetrical motion. Normal chordae tendineae are arranged in an architectural alignment and spacing allowing each chorda to remain free from touching each other. Each chorda remains free from the other chordae and from the ventricular myocardium at all phases of the cardiac cycle. Occasionally, some chordae may originate directly from the ventricular myocardium and insert into the leaflets. Small false chordae may originate from the ventricular myocardium and attach to the papillary muscles, and are thought to act as supporting apparatus for the latter. Aberrant chordae – chordae that are attached from myocardium to myocardium – have unknown significance and probably serve no real purpose. Variations in the number of chordae and in the branching or insertion patterns account for the major aberrations of the chordae tendineae.

Chordal systems differ according to whether they are attached to the anterior or posterior leaflets (see Figure 2.2).[3,12–16] Chordae to the

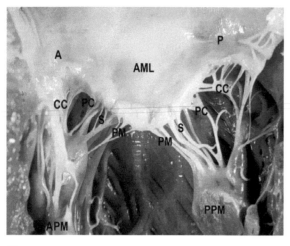

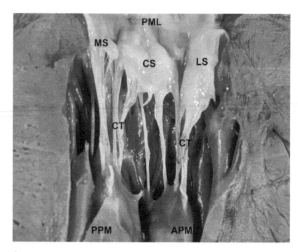

a

b

Fig. 2.2 Normal anterior and posterior leaflet anatom . (a) The anterior mitral leaflet (AML) is triangular i shape with a br oad base of attachment and a r ounded apical contour. The body of the leaflet is thin an translucent in comparison to the leaflet ma gin. Chordal inser tion to the ventricular sur face of the fr ee margin thickens the leaflet and p oduces the rough zone, which aids in pr oviding for maximum leaflet coaptation. Bot papillar y muscles supply chor dae tendineae in an oblique, symmetrical fashion to the anterior leaflet. Th oblique orientation of the chor dae allows for maximum and unr estricted movement of the anterior leaflet Anterior leaflet cho dae tendineae ar e labeled accor ding to their point of attachment to the leaflet, and t some degree, to their shape. AML, Anterior mitral leaflet; A, anterior commissu e; P, posterior commissur e; CC, commissural chor ds; APM, anterior papillar y muscle; PPM, posterior papillar y muscle; PM, paramedical chordae; S str ut chordae; PC, paracommissural chor dae. (b) The posterior mitral leaflet (PML) is ectangular in shape. It has a lar ger circumference than the anterior leaflet and attaches to a la ger por tion of the annulus. The three scallops of the posterior leaflet a e readily identifiable with the central scallop (CS) being the la gest scallop. MS, medial scallop; LS, lateral scallop. Both papillar y muscles (PPM and APM) supply evenly spaced, parallel chordae tendineae (CT) to the posterior leaflet. This parallel a rangement, a result of the shor ter distance between the papillar y muscles posteriorly in the ventricle, allows the chor dae to act as suppor ting columns for the ' passive' or 'buttressing' posterior leaflet (see text for details). The a rangement of the chordae tendineae is such that each chor d remains free of the others during all phases of the car diac cycle.

posterior leaflet project and attach to the ventricular surface of the leaflet in a parallel manner. These chordae act as supporting columns to the posterior leaflet. Branching posterior leaflet chordae insert into the central scallop at the free edge, the body (mid surface), or the basal portion near the annulus. Chordae to the lateral and medial scallops insert in a more variable arrangement. Chordae to the anterior leaflet are projected in an oblique manner, which aids in opening and closing of the leaflet. Anterior leaflet chordae insert into the ventricular surface of the leaflet at the leaflet margin (primary chordae) or slightly behind the free edge (secondary chordae).

Chordae to the anterior leaflet can be further subdivided into paramedial, central strut, or paracommissural chordae, depending on their position on the anterior leaflet's free edge.

The commissures have a unique chordal system that provides an anchor for the hinge point[3,13] (see Figure 2.3). Each papillary muscle gives rise to a single commissural chorda which fans out distally into about five small chordae inserting into the corner of both leaflets, at the free edges of the commissural tissue. Due to the slightly oblique position of the valve in the annulus fibrosus in relation to the papillary muscles, the commissural chordae to the posterior medial commissure are

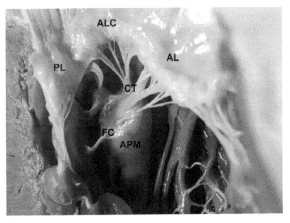
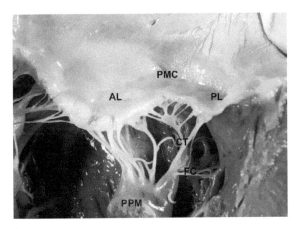

a   b

Fig. 2.3 Normal anterior and posterior commissures. Each commissure receives one chorda tendinea (CT) from its respective papillary muscle (APM and PPM). Commissural chordae are broad at their origin, project perpendicularly and fan out to intersect the commissural portion of each leaflet. In this manner, adequate support is provided to the whole commissure serving as a hinge point for leaflet motion. (a) Anterolateral commissure (ALC). (b) Posteromedial commissure (PMC). Due to the oblique orientation of the mitral valve in the fibrous skeleton in relation to the position of the papillary muscles, the commissural chordae to the posteromedial commissure are usually thicker, longer, and more widely branching than the chordae to the anterolateral commissure. This may be the reason why the leaflet tissue surrounding the anterolateral commissure is less likely to prolapse (a feature that provides a good reference point at surgery for demonstrating prolapse in other areas). AL, anterior leaflet; FC, false chords; PL, posterior leaflet

usually more widely spaced, thicker, and longer, than the chordae to the anterior lateral commissure. The proper identification of the commissures can therefore be aided by identifying the respective commissural chordal pattern.

Papillary muscles

The papillary muscles originate as muscular projections or columns from the ventricular myocardium, between the apical and middle portion of the ventricular chamber (Figure 2.6).[17,18] The exact positioning of both papillary muscles may vary considerably. The anterior papillary muscle usually arises from the lateral border of the anterior wall, and the posterior papillary muscle usually originates from the medial aspect of the posterior wall where it abuts the ventricular septum. There is usually only one anterior papillary muscle with often

two or three posterior papillary muscles. The volume or mass of the anterior and posterior muscle groups are usually equal.

When a papillary muscle group is present the individual muscles wrap around each other in a concave-convex fashion, allowing the whole group to act as a single unit during contraction. The base and body of the papillary muscles are anchored to the ventricular free wall by muscular or tendinous chordae known as false chords, which are believed also to serve as channels for Purkinje fibers. The tips or heads of the papillary muscles taper into tendinous projections to give rise to the chordae tendineae. Each papillary muscle group gives off chordae tendineae in a symmetrical fashion to their respective halves of both the anterior and posterior leaflets (see Figure 2.5). It is well established that the papillary muscles play a vital part in valve integrity and valve motion.

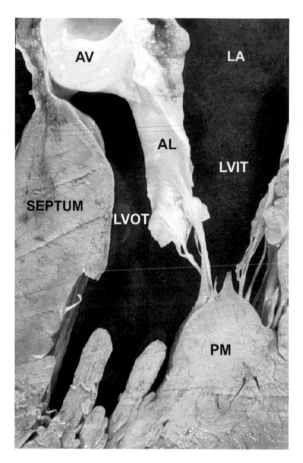

Fig. 2.4 Anatomical specimen demonstrating how the mitral valve pr oduces functional left ventricular inflow and outflow tracts. Unlike the right ventricle the left ventricle has no tr ue anatomical inflow an outflow tracts. The inflow and outflow tracts e produced by the nor mal anatomical r elationship of the mitral valvular apparatus in its posterior position and orientation in the left ventricle. LA, left atrium; LVIT, left ventricular inflow tract; VOT, left ventricular outflow tract; PM, papillar y muscle; AL, anterior mitral leaflet; V, aortic valve; SEPTUM; inter ventricular septum.

The blood supply to the papillary muscles is highly variable.[19] The anterior papillary muscle is supplied by the second septal branch of the left anterior descending artery and by a branch of the circumflex artery. The posterior papillary muscle is usually supplied from septal branches of the posterior descending artery, in addition to a small branch of the circumflex artery. The confluence of coronary artery branches for each papillary muscle joins into a single central artery or remains as a meshwork of small branches. These vessels taper and project longitudinally into the muscle. This framework of blood supply probably allows the head of the muscle to be more prone to ischemia. When the blood supply is left-dominant, the posterior papillary muscle is especially prone to ischemia. In addition to blood supply, the papillary muscles are also perfused by the diffusion of oxygen from blood in the ventricular cavity.

NORMAL MULTIPLANE TRANSESOPHAGEAL ECHOCARDIOGRAPHIC VALVE ANALYSIS

Transesophageal echocardiography (TEE) has allowed many of the intricacies of the mitral valve apparatus to be elucidated.[20–28] It is now widely recognized that function of the mitral valve depends on the normal function and integrity of the leaflets, annulus, chordae tendineae, papillary muscles, and subjacent left ventricular myocardium. Abnormalities in any of these components, either individually or in combination, produce dysfunction of the mitral valve unit. Multiplane TEE can define mitral valve structure and function. To obtain a comprehensive and accurate description of the whole mitral apparatus it is useful to have a systematic approach when performing the multiplane TEE examination. Beginning with the multiplane TEE transducer in the stomach the papillary muscle structure can be assessed along with their interaction with the left ventricle. With slow withdrawal of the probe into the esophagus the chordae tendineae, and the valve leaflets including commissural areas and annulus, can be assessed in succession (see Figures 2.8–2.11). With a careful and systematic TEE assessment, a three-dimensional picture of the whole mitral apparatus can be constructed.

With the multiplane TEE transducer at 0°, 40–45 cm from the incisors in the transgastric position, the probe is slightly anteflexed and maneuvered to obtain a short axis view of the left ventricle at the mid papillary muscle level (Figures 2.16, 2.18). Depending on the position

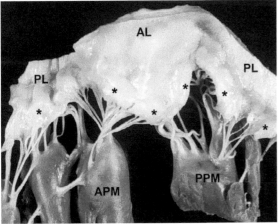

a

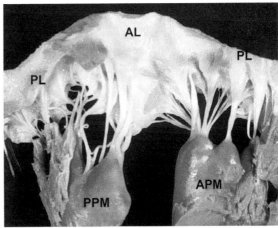

b

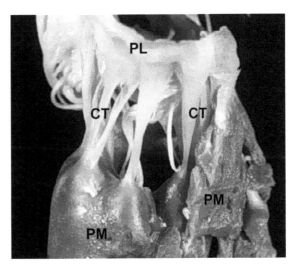

c

Fig. 2.5 Normal mitral valve anatomy. (a) Postmortem mitral valve specimen viewed from the atrial aspect of the leaflets. Chordae tendineae attach to the undersurface of the leaflet margins producing hooding of the leaflet edge for the rough zone (stars). The greater thickness of the rough zone of the leaflet margin provides greater surface area for leaflet coaptation. In addition, false chordae tendineae are demonstrated bridging one papillary muscle to another. (b) Postmortem mitral valve specimen viewed from the ventricular aspect of the leaflets. Chordae tendineae insert into the ventricular or undersurface of the leaflet margin. Chordae tendineae only insert to the peripheral margin of the anterior leaflet. (c) Postmortem mitral valve specimen viewed from a lateral ventricular aspect of the posterior leaflet surface. The parallel projection of chordal insertion to the posterior leaflet from the papillary muscles is demonstrated nicely. Chordae tendineae insert into the whole undersurface of the posterior leaflet including the leaflet margin, the body of the leaflet and the annular insertion portions. This chordal arrangement again lends credence for the pressure support function of the posterior mitral leaflet. AL, anterior leaflet; PL, posterior leaflet; AP anterior papillary muscle; PPM, posterior papillary muscle; CT, chordae tendineae.

in the chest, either vertical or horizontal, the transducer may to be rotated from 0° to about 15° to obtain a true, non-oblique short axis view of the left ventricle. With the depth of the echocardiographic image set to 12–16 cm, the normal left ventricle should fill most of the image sector and allow good visualization of the papillary muscles for examination. The papillary muscles are visualized in the short axis of the left ventricle in cross-section. The posteromedial papillary muscle is at the top of the echocardiographic display at approximately 1 o'clock, and the anterolateral papillary muscle is located between 4 and 5 o'clock.

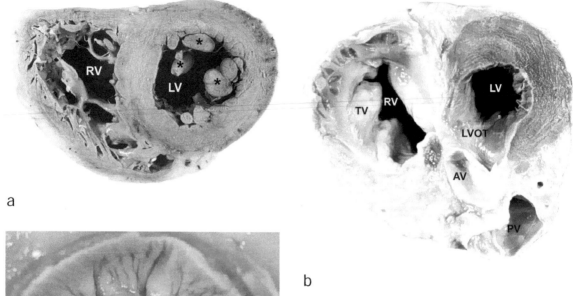

a

b

c

Fig. 2.6 Short-axis anatomical preparations corresponding to the standard echocardiographic short-axis views obtained from the gastric window at 0°. (a) Ventricular short axis at the papillary muscle level. (b) Ventricular short axis at the basal level. (c) Short-axis orientation of the mitral valve as typically projected from the transesophageal gastric window. RV, right ventricle; LV, left ventricle; TV, tricuspid valve; LVOT, left ventricular outflow tract; AV, aortic valve; PV, pulmonary valve; A1,A2,A3, anterior mitral leaflet; P1,P2,P3, posterior mitra leaflet

The exact position of the papillary muscles varies in different patients, and this is better appreciated by TEE imaging than by transthoracic echocardiography. Both papillary muscles are normally situated in the longitudinal, posterior half of the left ventricle. Therefore in the short axis view the distance between the papillary muscles in the inferior aspect of the left ventricle is less than half the distance around the anterior aspect of the left ventricle. The anterolateral papillary muscle is usually larger than the posteromedial muscle and usually comprises one muscle, in contrast to the posteromedial muscle, which is made up of a group of two or more smaller muscles. Both papillary muscles should appear in close approximation with the ventricular myocardium, and should have the same texture as the surrounding myocardium. The size or diameter of the papillary muscles should be slightly smaller than the myocardial thickness. Occasionally, both papillary muscles may exhibit isolated hypertrophy,[19] appearing thicker or slightly out of proportion to the ventricular myocardium, but are in normal positions in the ventricular cavity.

The transducer is then rotated 90° from the true cross-section to assess the papillary muscles longitudinally (Figure 2.19). In the long axis view, the papillary muscles appear in the middle of the echocardiographic image. In the apex-up orientation, with the transducer at

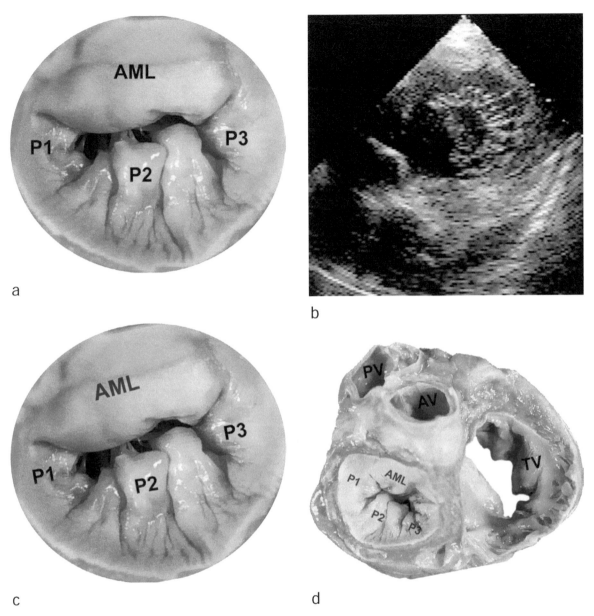

Fig. 2.7 Orientation of the mitral valve fr om different perspectives in the operating r oom. It is helpful to understand the orientation of the mitral valve fr om different perspectives so that meaningful and accurate communication can occur between the sur geon, the echocar diographer, and the anesthesiologist, especially during mitral valve r eparative procedures. (a) Sur geon's anatomical view. (b) Shor t-axis echo image. (c) Echocar diographer's orientation. (d) Anesthesiologist' s anatomical perspective fr om the head of the operating table. AML, anterior mitral leaflet; P1,P2,P3, posterior mitral leafle

the top of the screen, the posteromedial muscles with multiple heads appear directly at the top of the image and project towards the base of the heart, with the anterolateral muscle at the bottom of the image. Either papillary muscle may be better defined with minor angulations of the probe. The papillary muscles take origin from the myocardium in the mid third of the

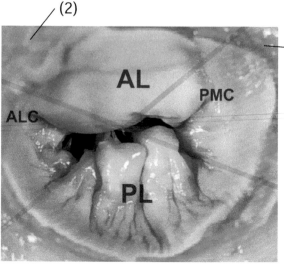

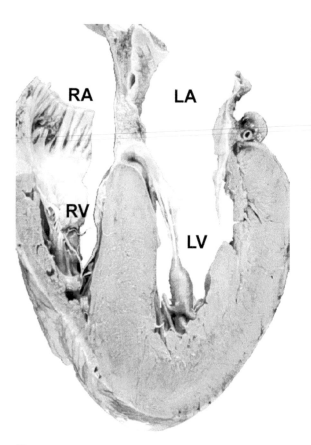

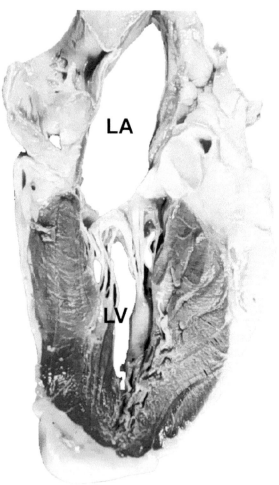

a

b

c

Fig. 2.8 Anatomical preparations demonstrating the orientation of the mitral valve depicted in the standard transesophageal echocardiography (TEE) views and short axis plane. In TEE the mitral valve plane is visualized from many different perspectives as the TEE transducer is moved through the esophagus. This often leads to confusion when attempting to accurately identify the exact leaflet area visualized. (a) The standard four-chamber, frontal plane at 0° obtained from the mid- to lower esophageal windows. (b) Typically the mitral valve is cut tangentially depending upon the position of the TEE transducer within the esophagus. Lower in the esophagus the valve leaflets are imaged nearer the posteromedial commissure, imaging more of the lateral area of the anterior leaflet and medial area of the posterior leaflet (2). As the probe is slowly withdrawn towards the mid-esophagus the leaflet are imaged nearer the anterolateral commissure; imaging more of the medial area of the anterior leaflet and lateral area of the posterior leaflet (1). (c) The standard two-chamber view at approximately 60°. The TEE imaging plane cuts the mitral valve leaflets parallel to the line of closure.

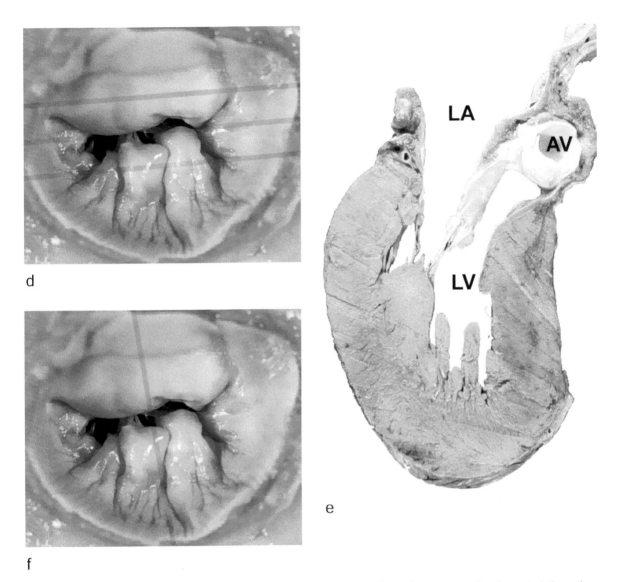

d

e

f

Fig. 2.8 (contd.) (d) With a slight r otational movement of the transducer the plane can be dir ected through the anterior leaflet and posterior leaflet line of clos e. (e) The standar d three-chamber view at 135°. (f) This view produces an imaging plane near est to tr uly cutting the mitral valve in an anterior–posterior orientation. RA, right atrium; LA, left atrium; R V, right ventricle; L V, left ventricle; A V, aortic valve; AL, anterior leaflet; PL, posterior leaflet; ALC, ante olateral commissur e; PMC, poster omedial commissur e.

ventricle, with the anterolateral muscle generally appearing longer and narrower in the longitudinal projection. In all cases, the papillary muscles should have similar size and motion. The papillary muscles are attached to the ventricle with a broad base and gradually taper to a head in a conical fashion, at the same level in the ventricular cavity. Occasionally, a small accessory papillary muscle may be seen ema-

nating from the apex. All muscles should have similar echogenicity, signifying the same muscle texture and density of the surrounding ventricular myocardium. In older patients, a small degree of increased echogenicity is frequently observed in the papillary muscle tip, signifying calcification, which probably represents the normal aging process. Normal motion of the ventricular myocardium should also be

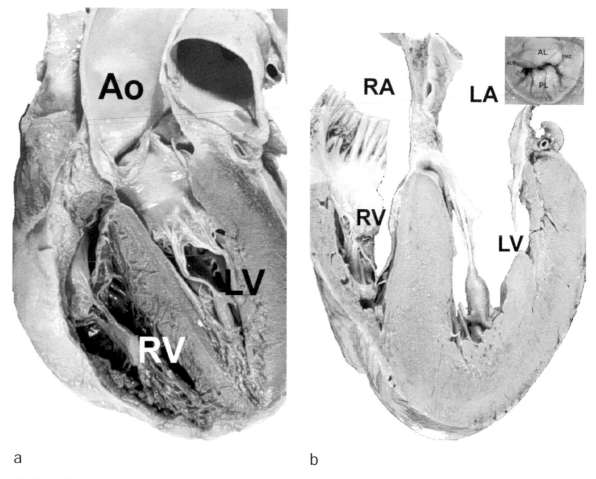

a   b

Fig. 2.9   Normal echocardiographic anatomy demonstrating mitral valve anatomy . In the lower esophageal window the mitral valve is imaged in dif ferent planes as the transducer is r otated between 0° and 180°. In examining the mitral leaflets and subvalvular apparatus it is impo   tant to have a conceptual idea of the tr ue anatomy in each plane in or der to mentally constr uct a three-dimensional perspective of the mitral anatomy . Mitral valve disease or abnor malities can mor e accurately be described and understood in this manner   . Frontal projections. (a) Anatomical pr eparation of the hear t at –10°. (b) Enlar gement of mitral apparatus –10°.

observed in relation to normal papillary muscle motion. Fractional shortening of the papillary muscle (FSPM, Figure 2.20) can be determined in this view by measuring the end-diastolic (EDL) and end-systolic longitudinal lengths (ESL), so that:

$$FSPM = [\{EDL - ESL/EDL\} \times 100].$$

Normal papillary muscle fractional shortening in is 30% ±8%.[19]

The chordae tendineae are visualized as thin horizontal, continuous structures emanating from the heads of the papillary muscles, projecting towards the annulus (base of the heart) and inserting into the ventricular surface of the leaflets (see Figure 2.17). The chordae tendineae appear as multiple, thin, linear structures that move in and out of plane between systole and diastole. Normal chordae emanate from the apex or head of the papillary muscles and

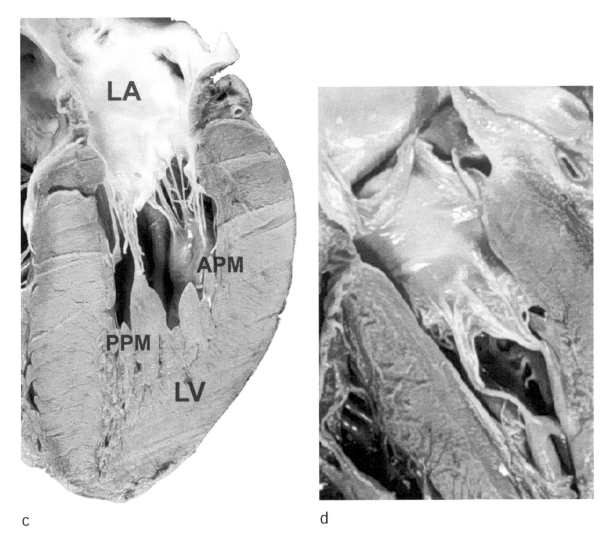

Fig. 2.9 (contd.)   (c) Anatomical preparation of the heart at 0°. (d) Enlargement of mitral apparatus 0°.

project in a straight, nearly horizontal manner as they fan out towards the leaflets. In the longitudinal projection, the chordae that insert into the posterior leaflet appear nearly horizontal, whereas the chordae to the anterior leaflet are more oblique. It should be noted that all chords, whether they insert into the anterior or posterior leaflet, should appear straight – almost under tension – in both diastole and systole. With the currently available multiplane probes,

branching of the chordae tendineae is apparent, but even in the zoom modes the image resolution does not allow for the reliable labeling of chordae as primary, secondary, or tertiary branches. Occasionally, chordae may be identified that emanate from the heads of the papillary muscles and insert into the ventricular myocardium. These chordae are frequently identified by transthoracic imaging, but are more readily apparent with transesophageal

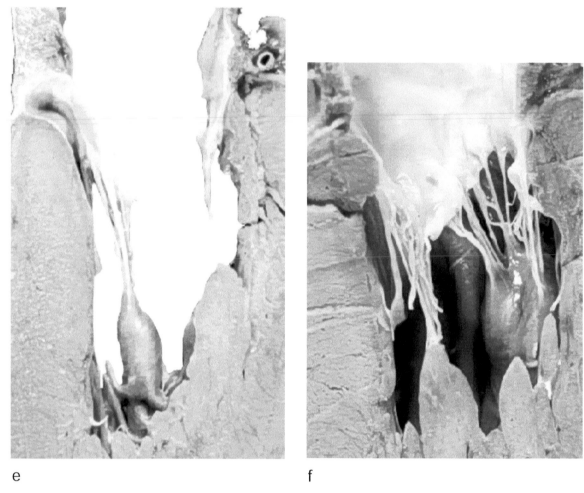

e   f

Fig. 2.9 (contd.)   (e) Anatomical pr eparation of the hear t at 30°. (f) Enlar gement of mitral apparatus 30°.

echocardiography, and are known as ventricular chordae or aberrant chordae.

The probe is slowly advanced to approximately 50 cm at 0° to the deep transgastric level, with anteflexion until the aortic root is imaged obliquely and the mitral subvalvular apparatus is well seen (see Figure 2.16). The papillary muscles are visualized obliquely with a foreshortened view of the left ventricular apex near the top of the echocardiographic screen. Usually both papillary muscles are visualized between 0° and 20°. The central portions of both

papillary muscles are easily inspected along with the chordae tendineae. The chordae tendineae appear straight, all about the same width, and lie in a vertical position in the image. The valve leaflets, however, are too foreshortened to be fully appreciated, especially when they are normal or show hooding, but it is possible to distinguish the anterior from the posterior leaflet. In our experience, this is the best view to assess the chordae tendineae. Elongation of the chordae is easily seen, as the chordae appear redundant, bowed, and curvi-

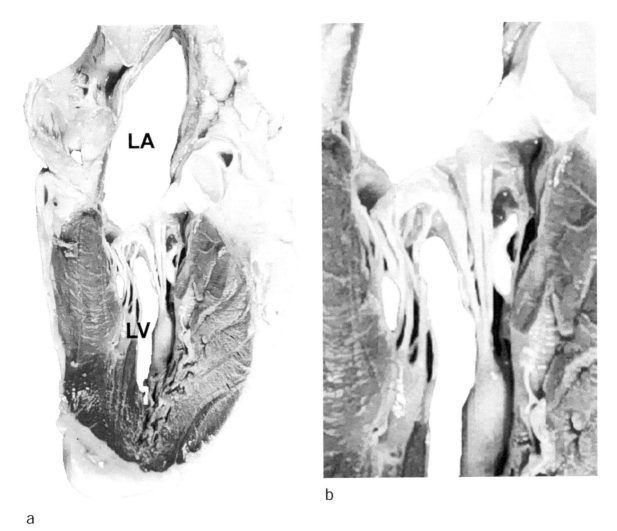

LA

LV

b

a

Fig. 2.10 Normal echocardiographic anatomy demonstrating mitral valve anatomy (continuation of Figure 2.9). Longitudinal projections. (a) Anatomical preparation of the heart at 60° with (b) enlargement of mitral apparatus.

linear, instead of straight. The chordae to the anterior leaflet appear to project at an angle away from the papillary head, and the chordae to the posterior leaflet appear to be parallel and vertical. With further rotation of the transducer from 45° to 50°, a sweep of the whole subvalvular apparatus is completed and nearly all of the chordae can be assessed.

The multiplane probe is then slightly withdrawn at 90° to center the annulus and leaflets in the echocardiographic image. With slight angulations of the probe, the full breadth of the anterior, posterior, or both leaflets are seen vertically, opening and closing with changes in the cardiac cycle. The mitral annular plane is readily apparent, separating the left ventricle (to the left of the image) and the left atrium (to the right of the image), and the normal mitral valve leaflets do not protrude significantly past this imaginary plane towards the left atrium. During diastole when the two leaflets are imaged, the posterior leaflet is seen at the top of

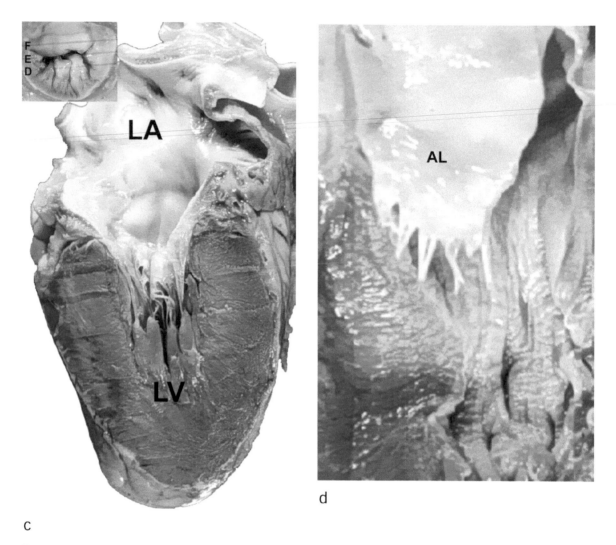

c

d

Fig. 2.10 (contd.) (c) Anatomical pr eparation of the hear t at 75° with *en face* view of the mitral leaflet illustrating rotational cuts and cor responding enlargements showing (d) pr edominately anterior leaflet

the echocardiographic image and the anterior leaflet at the bottom of the image. Rotating the transducer from 90° to 135° shifts the image towards the left ventricular outflow tract and the aortic root, displaying the anterior leaflet continuous with the aortic root at the bottom of the display. Care should be taken in assessing the thickness of the leaflets at the points of

chordal insertion so as not to overestimate leaflet thickness.

The transducer is returned to 0° and the probe is withdrawn towards the lower esophageal level (about 35 cm from the incisors) to image the base of the left ventricle and project the mitral valve leaflets and annular plane *en face* (Figures 2.12 and 2.21). The probe

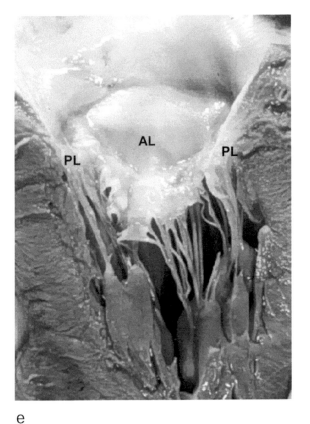

e

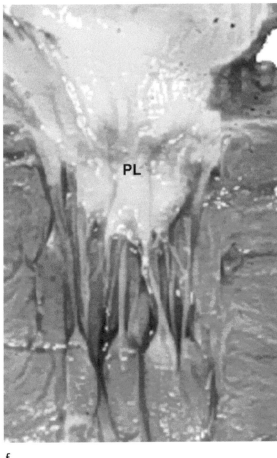

f

Fig. 2.10 (contd.) (e) Anterior and posterior leaflets near line of closu e, and (f) pr edominately posterior leaflet

is slightly angulated or the transducer is rotated to accommodate the oblique nature of the mitral annulus at this level, until the maximum opening of the valve orifice at the leaflet tips is visualized. The opening and closure of the valve leaflets may be timed with the cardiac cycle and the best appreciation of leaflet motion is obtained in this view. The anterior leaflet will be seen to the left and slightly rotated inferiorly in the image towards the ventricular septum and right ventricle. The posterior leaflet will be displayed directly opposite the anterior leaflet slightly superior and to the right, towards the

left ventricular free wall margin. The commissures are apparent as the points of continuity between the anterior and posterior leaflet. The posteromedial commissure is at the top of the image, in the same orientation as the posteromedial papillary muscle position, and the anterolateral commissure at the bottom of the image corresponds to the position of the respective papillary muscle. The leaflets appear shaggy and non-continuous during movement, due to hooding of the chordal attachments as they move in and out of the imaging plane. The leaflets on cross-section should move continu-

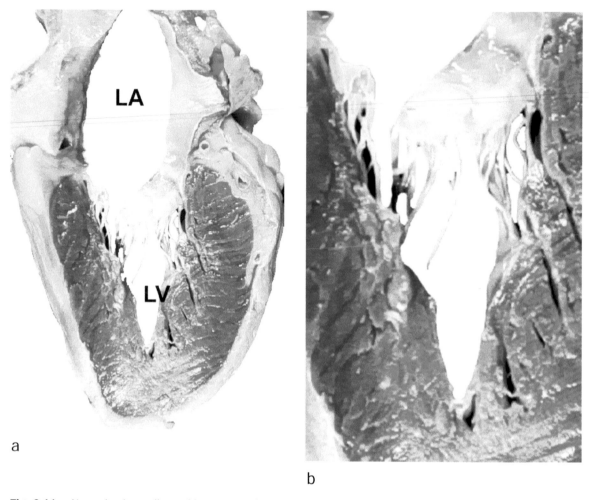

a

b

Fig. 2.11 Normal echocardiographic anatomy demonstrating mitral valve anatomy (continuation of Figur es 2.9 and 2.10). (a) Anatomical pr eparation of the hear t at 110° with (b) enlar gement showing mitral apparatus.

ously with the cardiac cycle, without areas of chaotic motion. During early diastole when the valve opens, the mitral orifice resembles the letter 'D'. When the valve leaflets are normal the leaflet margins approximate the shape and dimension of the annulus. If the whole annulus is visualized, the diameter of the annulus can be measured constructing a line between the two commissures. The anterior leaflet appears straight and the posterior leaflet concave, and both leaflets join at the commissures. During mid-diastole the leaflets slowly start to approximate in a crescentric fashion, with most motion in the anterior leaflet becoming convex to the posterior leaflet. During atrial systole, both leaflets again open abruptly to form a circular orifice. During ventricular systole both leaflets approximate, as the ventricle becomes smaller, again the anterior leaflet appearing to move more towards the posterior leaflet in a convex manner. When the leaflets are totally closed during systole the line of closure resembles a 'smile', with a symmetrical crescent-shaped configuration. During leaflet motion, the individual scallops of the posterior leaflet may be appreciated. This view represents the typical

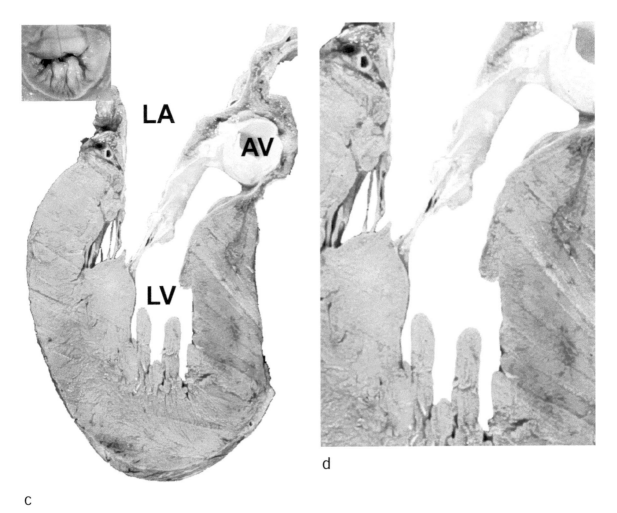

c

Fig. 2.11 (contd.)   (c) Anatomical pr eparation of the hear t at 135° with (d) enlar gement showing mitral apparatus.

exposure of the mitral valve as visualized by the cardiac surgeon, and thus is an important view for communicating leaflet abnormalities (see Figure 2.7). Both leaflets are labeled in three segments according to the normal scallops of the posterior leaflet; P1 is the anterolateral scallop, P2 is the central scallop, and P3 is the posteromedial scallop. The anterior leaflet is subdivided into A1 to A3 based on the segment of leaflet directly opposite the posterior segment.[29]

The transesophageal echocardiographic probe is then withdrawn at 0° to the mid-

esophageal level (30 cm from the incisors), with the tip of the probe in a neutral position with enough flexion to ensure contact between the transducer and the esophageal wall. During withdrawal of the probe, the heart image progresses from a short axis plane of the left ventricle to a four-chamber frontal plane of the heart, then a five-chamber frontal plane of the heart (see Figure 2.13). The right ventricle is to the left of the image and the left ventricle is to the right of the image. The atrium is displayed at the top of the echocardiography sector with the ventricular apex to the bottom of the image. The mitral

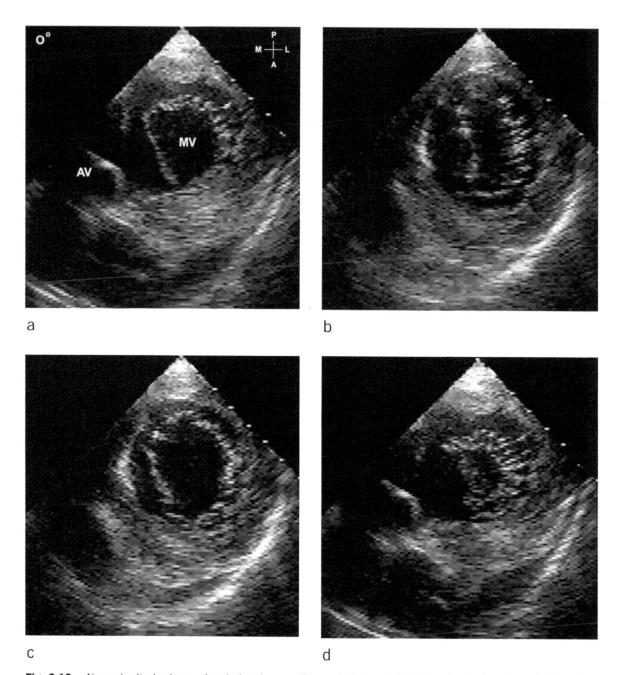

Fig. 2.12 Normal mitral valve motion during the car diac cycle in the gastric shor t axis view . In early diastole (a) the open mitral valve confor ms to a ' D' shape with the anterior leaflet to the right and the posterior leafl to the left of the echocar diographic image. In mid-diastole (b) the anterior and posterior leaflets drift close together as left ventricular filling dec eases. During atrial systole (c) the valve leaflets again separate t assume a mor e circular orifice. By late diastole (d) following atrial contraction and end systole (e) the anterio and posterior leaflets app oximate into a ' C' shape, or the typical ' smile' as described sur gically. MV, mitral valve; AV, aortic valve.

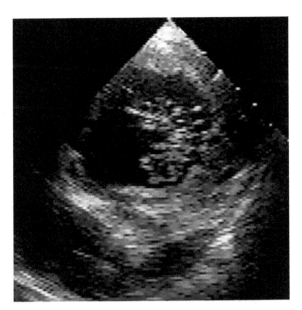

e

Fig. 2.12 (contd.)

valve should be centered in the image with slight rotation of the probe. The depth of the image sector may be decreased between 10 and 12 cm to assess the full extent of both leaflets during the cardiac cycle. Occasionally, the zoom feature may provide better delineation of the leaflet details. The two mitral leaflets open towards the left ventricular apex during diastole, producing a funnel shape to the orifice. Frequently, the subvalvular apparatus, especially the chordae tendineae, will not be visible without increasing the gain settings. The anterior leaflet will be on the left of the echocardiographic image, appear longer, and show the most motion during opening and closure. The posterior leaflet will appear to the right of the echocardiographic image towards the lateral left ventricular wall. The posterior leaflet will appear shorter and move less, with slight but noticeable billowing of the leaflets compared with the anterior leaflet during closure. The rate of movement of the anterior leaflet appears greater than that of the posterior

leaflet, with the anterior leaflet opening parallel to the ventricular septum and the posterior leaflet nearly parallel to the posterolateral ventricular wall.

Due to the oblique position of the mitral valve annulus in relation to the transesophageal echocardiographic probe, the valve appears tilted, so that the imaging plane through the valve leaflets cuts the valve tangentially, often producing confusion in accurately identifying the exact area of the leaflet (see Figure 2.8). When imaging the valve at 0° in the frontal plane, the valve leaflets are imaged nearer the posteromedial commissure at the lower esophageal position, imaging more of the lateral area of the anterior leaflet and medial area of the posterior leaflet (A3, P1). As the probe is slowly withdrawn, the leaflets are transected in a successive manner more towards the middle of the leaflets (A2, P2). With further withdrawal of the probe, the anterolateral commissure portion of the leaflet is reached at the mid-esophageal level, and the medial portion of the anterior leaflet and the lateral region of the posterior leaflet are visualized (A1, P3). With this maneuver, the complete free margins of both leaflets may be inspected. This is most helpful in evaluating the point of closure of the leaflets during systole. The frontal plane provides an excellent view to visualize the annular plane and excessive motion of the valve leaflets. An imaginary line can be drawn from the points of attachment of both leaflets to the annulus. With normal mitral valve closure the points of approximation of the free edge of both leaflets should not extend past the annular plane or protrude into the left atrium. Due to the saddle shape of the normal mitral valve leaflets during closure, the body of the leaflets may billow or extend minimally past this plane, but the exact point of closure or approximation normally will not. Normal billowing of the body of the leaflet should not protrude more than 1 cm past the annular plane. When evaluating the line of closure in all of these views, the rough zone of the free margins of both leaflets should give the impression that both leaflets coapt, so that the leaflet surface area of contact is at least 1–2 mm. Evaluation the line

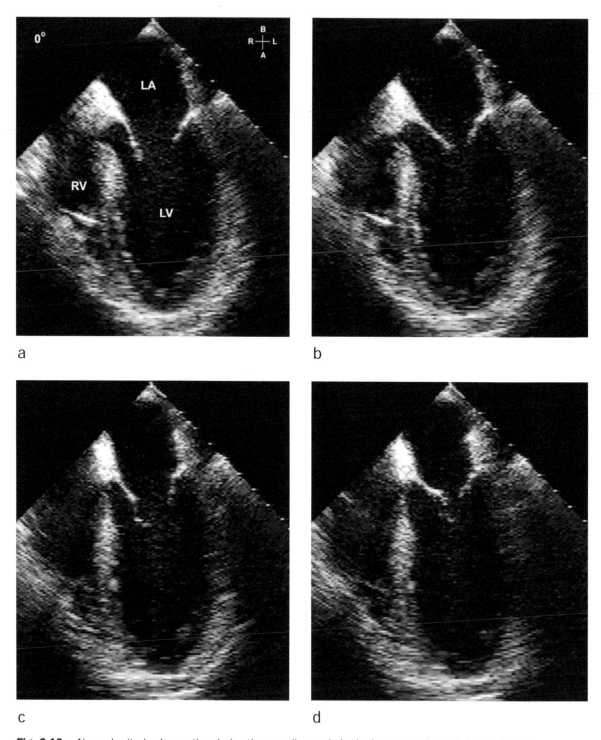

Fig. 2.13 Normal mitral valve motion during the car diac cycle in the lower esophageal view at 0°. The anterior leaflet is in the left of the image sector and the posterior leaflet is on the right. The anterior leaf appears longer and exhibits gr eater motion than the posterior leaflet. Both leaflets open and close in trapdoor fashion. (a) Early diastole. (b) Mid-diastole. (c) Atrial systole. (d) Late diastole.

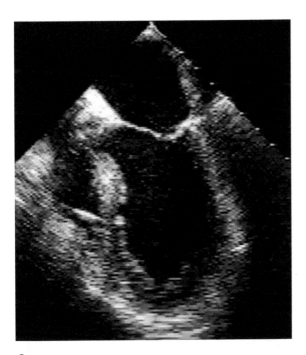

e

Fig. 2.13 (contd.) (e) End systole. LA, left atrium; LV, left ventricle; R V, right ventricle.

of closure in all of these views, the rough zone of the free margins of both leaflets should give the impression that both leaflets coapt sufficiently. With normal closure the point of contact of both leaflets should be at least 1–2 mm. Normal valve leaflets should not appear to be barely reaching one another. When the mitral valve is viewed sagittally, the leaflets appear to open into the left ventricle like a trapdoor, with the anterior leaflet moving predominately. During closure of the valve, the anterior leaflet swings up to meet the posterior leaflet in the plane of the annulus. Thus the anterior leaflet has been referred to as the velocity or active leaflet and the posterior leaflet as the passive leaflet.

In the five-chamber frontal plane, with the transesophageal echocardiographic probe in the mid-esophagus, measurements can be made of the mitral valve unit (Figure 2.22). When there is subtle dilatation of the annulus, the length of the anterior leaflet may be com-

pared with the length of the annulus, providing an important ratio to assess normal annulus dimensions.[30] This measurement can be readily made in this view by multiplane transesophageal echocardiography, and the ratio of the anterior leaflet/annulus length should be about 0.9. A ratio less than 0.9 suggests that the annulus is so dilated that the anterior leaflet cannot reach the posterior leaflet for adequate approximation and the leaflet will appear to be barely reaching the other during closure.

Another important assessment, easily made with TEE, is the aorto-mitral annulus angle or angle of closure (Figure 2.23).[31] In the normal mitral valve, there is an obtuse angle between the anterior mitral leaflet and the aortic root to signify normal annulus size as well as lack of excessive leaflet tissue and redundancy. This allows forward blood flow during diastole to be oriented toward the ventricular apex, and pushes the line of leaflet closure far from the left ventricular outflow tract, preventing impingement or obstruction by the mitral apparatus.

From 0° the transducer can be rotated slowly to 180° to obtain the full circumference of the mitral annulus and leaflets, exemplifying the true utility of multiplane transesophageal echocardiography (see Figures 2.13–2.15). With some currently available probes the transducer can be rotated past 0° to –10°, which opens into the left ventricular outflow tract or five-chamber view (see Figure 2.9). Rotating the transducer from 0° to 60° or 75° images the mitral plane in a two-chamber view, with the left atrium in the top of the image sector and the left ventricle to the bottom of the image (see Figure 2.14). The anterior and posterior mitral leaflets will be imaged parallel to the line of closure and, with slight manipulation of the probe shaft, either the anterior or posterior leaflet will be imaged in its full breadth from commissure to commissure. Either leaflet will appear as a continuous line traversing the annular plane. As the transducer is further rotated through 110°–135°, the mitral leaflets will be imaged in a three-chamber view, with the posterior leaflet now towards the left of the

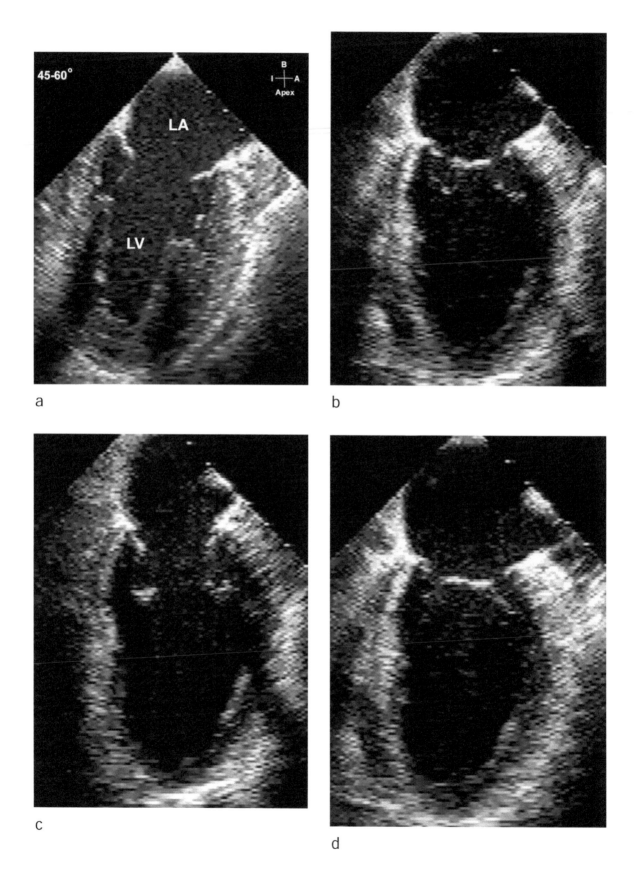

a

b

c

d

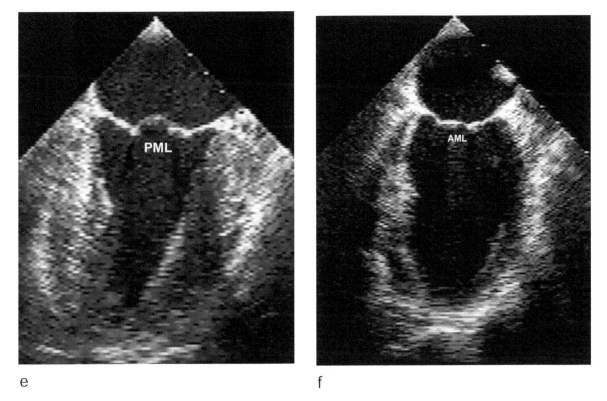

e   f

Fig. 2.14 Normal mitral valve motion during the car diac cycle in the lower esophageal view at 45–60°. The anterior leaflet appears in the middle of the annular plane bo dered by the posterior leaflet on both sides. Th anterior leaflet moves in and out of the mitral plane during the ca diac cycle, while the posterior leaflet swing back and for th. The pr obe can be slightly r otated to focus the examination on the anterior or posterior leafle during closure. (a) Early diastole. (b) Mid-diastole. (c) Atrial systole. (d) Late diastole. (e) Pr edominately posterior leaflet during end systole – note scalloping of the leaflet. (f) edominately anterior leaflet during en systole. LA, left atrium; L V, left ventricle; PML, posterior mitral leaflet; AML, anterior mitral leafle

image sector, and the anterior leaflet to the right and continuous with the aortic root to form the left ventricular outflow tract (see Figure 2.11).

MULTIPLANE DOPPLER EXAMINA TION OF THE NORMAL MITRAL V ALVE

The mitral valve directs the flow of blood from the left atrium to the left ventricle. During diastole the open mitral valve is funnel shaped, and gives rise anatomically and physiologically to the left ventricular inflow tract. During systole the mitral valve maintains the forward flow of blood by closing, thereby preventing significant regurgitation of blood into the left atrium. The closed mitral valve leaflets, along with the supporting subvalvular apparatus, protect the left atrium and contiguous pulmonary structures from the high pressures generated in the left ventricle, but do not interfere with the outflow tract during left ventricular contraction. The architecture of the mitral valve is finely adapted to fulfil these functions and when disease affects the mitral apparatus, abnormal hemodynamics are produced that may be identified by Doppler techniques.

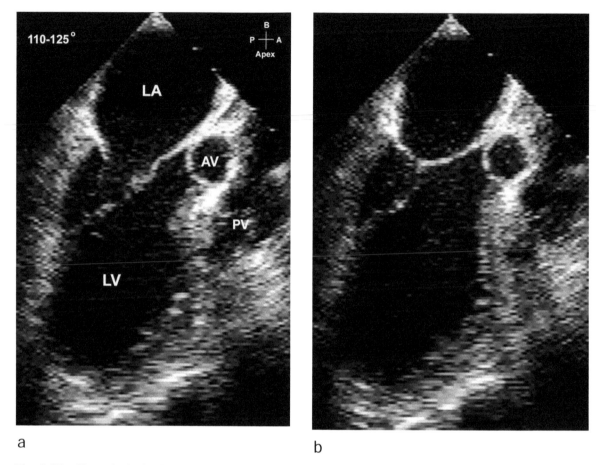

Fig. 2.15 Normal mitral valve motion during the car diac cycle in the lower esophageal view at 110–125°. The anterior leaflet is on the right of the echo image with the posterior leaflet on the left. As in the orientation the anterior leaflet appears la ger and exhibits gr eater excision. This view however , represents the tr uest anterior–posterior cut to the mitral valve plane. (a) Early diastole. (b) Mid-diastole.

The principles for transesophageal echocardiographic Doppler assessment of mitral valvular hemodynamics are identical to those for transthoracic measurements and calculations. Routinely, there is no clear advantage in Doppler echocardiography obtained from the transesophageal exam over the transthoracic exam, and one would rarely expect to obtain different information from the transesophageal echocardiogram. One exception to this rule might be the recording of pulmonary venous flow for assessment of mitral insufficiency, which is usually easier with transesophageal windows.

Although Doppler recordings may be made in any of the mitral valve views described in this chapter, the most important views are those that present the left ventricular inflow tract parallel to the transducer beam. Views obtained from the mid- and lower esophagus allow good windows for directing the Doppler beam through the left atrium and the left ventricular inflow tract (Figure 2.24).

Usually, pulsed Doppler is used to measure the low flow velocities of blood generated from diastole and atrial systole through the left ventricular inflow tract, producing the e- and a-wave morphology without a detectable gradi-

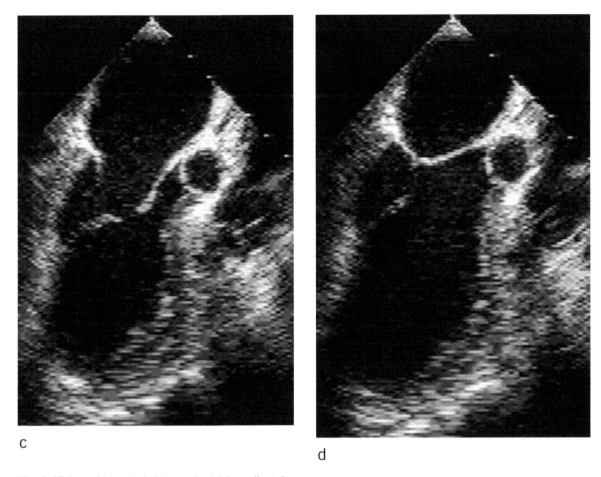

c

d

Fig. 2.15 (contd.)   (c) Atrial systole. (d) Late diastole.

ent. Continuous wave Doppler is usually necessary to measure mitral inflow when increased and disturbed flow is produced, promoting aliasing due to a transmitral gradient. As with transthoracic measurements, color Doppler may help to direct the Doppler beam in a parallel direction toward the inflow tract. By contrast, with the transthoracic echocardiogram, in which the atrium is usually black during this part of the cycle, blood flow can be mapped easily with transesophageal echocardiography as it fills the left atrium. Jets of orange-red flow empty from the pulmonary veins, collecting and mixing in the body of the left atrium. Diastolic forward flow increases as it enters the funnel-shaped mitral inflow orifice, and the converging flow is shown as patterns of hemispherical aliasing recorded near the open leaflets. As blood flows through the valve and fills the left ventricular cavity undisturbed, red-orange laminar flow is recorded at alternating velocities as the leaflets open with early diastolic filling, and slowly approximate before re-opening with atrial systole. Diastolic filling flow is detected as it swirls and turns through 180 degrees at the ventricular apex, before blue laminar flow is again recorded in the left ventricular outflow area. A small area of increased velocity and aliasing is usually detected in the outflow tract, hugging the proximal ventricular septal wall below the aortic valve. During early systole, especially

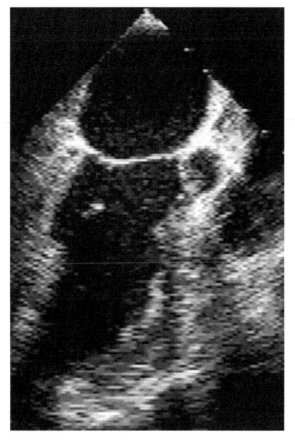

e

Fig. 2.15 (contd.)   (e) End systole. PV , pulmonary valve.

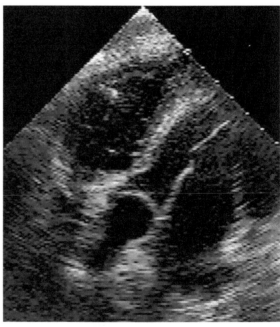

a

Fig. 2.16   Deep transgastric view of the mitral valve. The mitral valve apparatus is nicely demonstrated in the deep transgastric view . The chordae tendineae and papillar y muscles ar e not overshadowed or hidden by coexistent leafle abnormalities due to the close appr oximation of the mitral apparatus to the TEE pr obe. Pathology, including abnormalities in motion of the chor dae tendineae and papillar y muscles, is r eadily demonstrated during diastole and systole. (a) Diastolic frame at 0°. (b) Systolic frame at 0°.

b

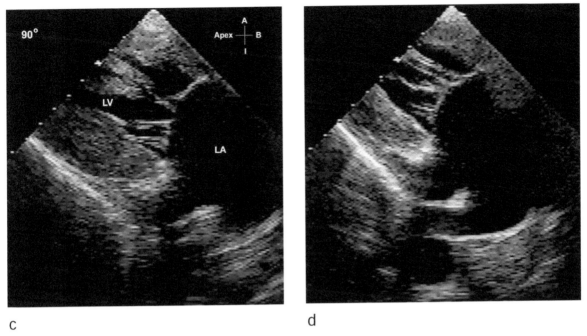

c

d

Fig. 2.16 (contd.) (c) Diastolic frame at 90°. (d) Systolic frame at 90°. The chor dae tendineae should appear straight during both diastole and systole. Redundancy or excessive motion of the chor dae is easily demonstrated especially during systole suggesting chor dal elongation and occasionally systolic anterior motion (SAM). LA, left atrium; L V, left ventricle; R V, right ventricle; A V, aortic valve; LVOT, left ventricular outflow tract

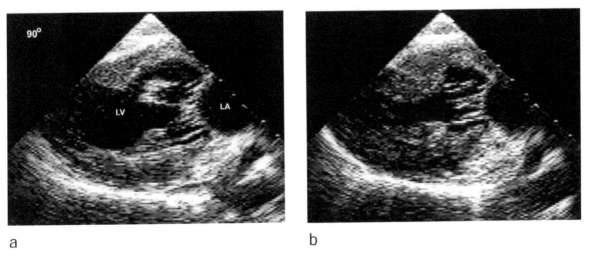

a

b

Fig. 2.17 Gastric views of the mitral subvalvular apparatus. In the gastric view at 90° the chordae tendineae and papillary muscles ar e easily demonstrated during diastole and systole. The chor dae to the posterior leafle appear parallel in orientation during diastole (a) and systole (b).

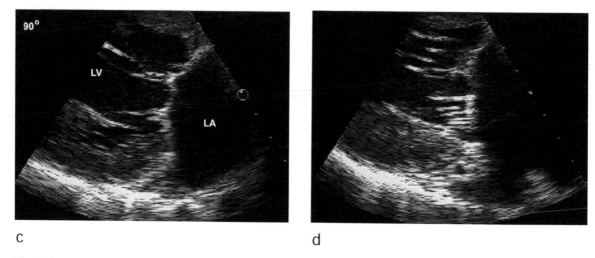

c

d

Fig. 2.17 (contd.) With slight rotation of the probe the chordae to the anterior leaflet are demonstrated with their oblique orientation during diastole (c) and systole (d). With annular dilatation chordae assume an oblique orientation to the posterior leaflet, similar to the anterior leaflet chordae. LA, left atrium; LV, left ventricle.

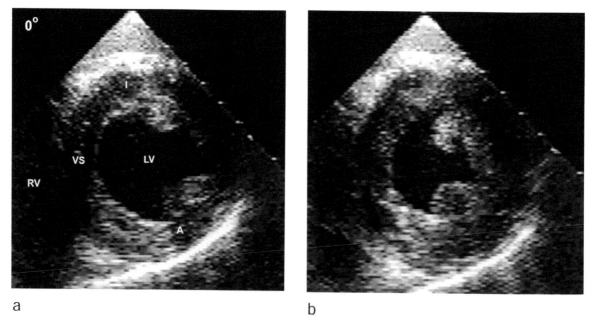

a

b

Fig. 2.18 Gastric views of the papillary muscle. In the gastric view at 0° at the mid-ventricular level the papillary muscles are seen in short axis. The posterior papillary muscle is seen at the top of the image and the anterior papillary muscle is seen at the bottom of the image. Both papillary muscles are seated in the posterior third of the ventricle during (a) diastole and (b) systole, which promotes a smaller posterior circumferential dimension than anterior dimension. This dimension is important in that it ensures blood flow in a posterior direction from the left ventricular inflow and also promotes a parallel chordal arrangement to the posterior mitral leaflet. LV, left ventricle; RV, right ventricle; VS, ventricular septum.

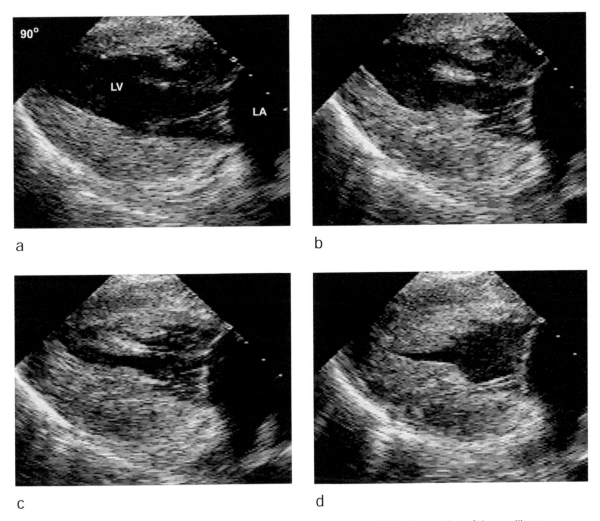

Fig. 2.19 Gastric views of the papillar y muscle. In the gastric view at 90° the motion of the papillar y muscles may be assessed thr oughout the car diac cycle. Fractional shor tening of the papillar y muscle can be measured. (a) Early diastole. (b) Mid-diastole. (c) Atrial contraction. (d) Systole. L V, left ventricle; LA, left atrium.

with lower aliasing velocity settings, low velocity backward flow may be recorded initially as the leaflets push blood flow back into the left atrium during closure, to approximately 1 cm from the annulus. At completion of leaflet apposition, blood flow stops completely. Physiological or normal regurgitation is defined by small jets of flow reversal detected close to the mitral annular plane. Single or multiple color flow jets with small jet areas and low flow velocities are imaged without significant turbulence or variance.

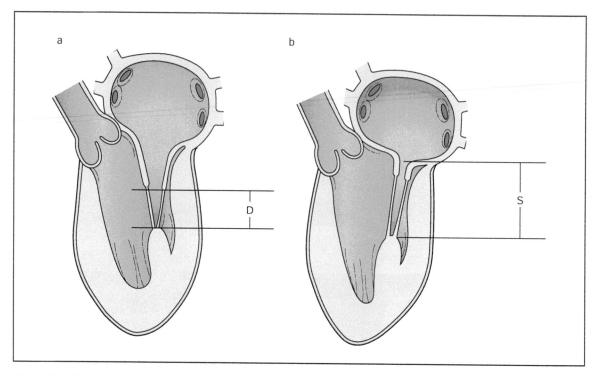

Fig. 2.20 Diagram demonstrating measur ements of the mitral subvalvular apparatus. Fractional shor tening of the papillar y muscle can be easily deter mined by measuring the end-diastolic (a) and end-systolic (b) longitudinal lengths as r epresented in the diagram. Nor mal motion of the ventricular myocar dium should also be obser ved in relationship to nor mal papillar y muscle motion.

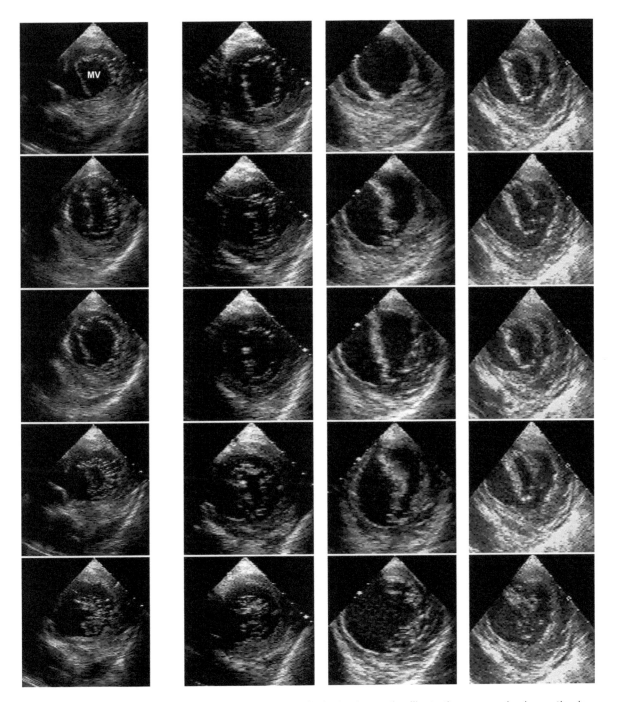

Fig. 2.21 Short-axis echocardiographic visualization of mitral valve motion illustrating normal valve motion in comparison to types I, II and III mitral motion according to the Carpentier classification scheme. M, mitral valve.

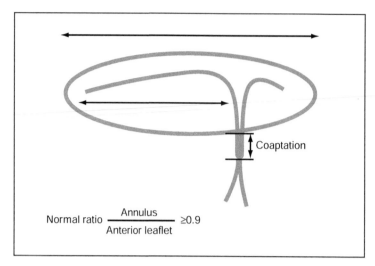

Normal ratio $\dfrac{\text{Annulus}}{\text{Anterior leaflet}} \geq 0.9$

Fig. 2.22 Diagram demonstrating measurements with TEE for mitral annular dilatation. When ther e is dilatation of the annulus, the length of the anterior leaflet may be compa ed to the length of the annulus and pr ovides an important ratio for evaluating annular dimensions. A ratio less than 0.9 suggests that the annulus is so sufficiently dilated that the anterior leaflet cannot r each the posterior leaflet for adequate closur e.

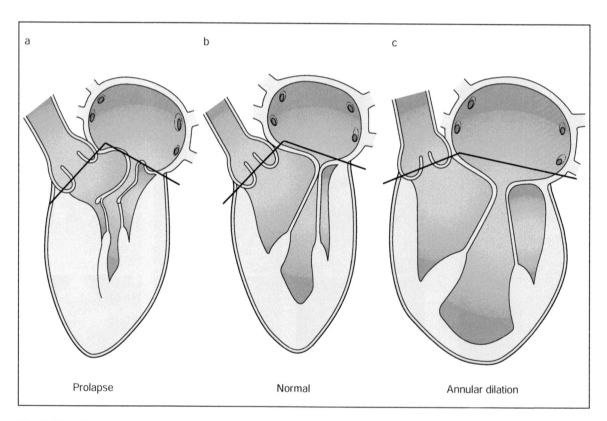

Prolapse Normal Annular dilation

Fig. 2.23 Diagram demonstrating the aor to-mitral angle. The aor to-mitral angle may be easily visualized for semi-quantitative or dir ect measur ement with multiple TEE. (a) In mitral valve pr olapse excess tissue, predominantly of the posterior leaflet, pushes the valvular apparatus towa ds the left ventricular outflow trac causing the aor to-mitral angle to become mor e acute. (b) The nor mal aor to-mitral angle appr oximately 90°–110°,allows for the functional delineation of the left ventricular inflow and outflow tracts. (c) Annul dilatation of the mitral valve pr oduces an obtuse angle with the posterior leaflet being pulled away f om the anterior leaflet educing the leaflet su face area available for coaption.

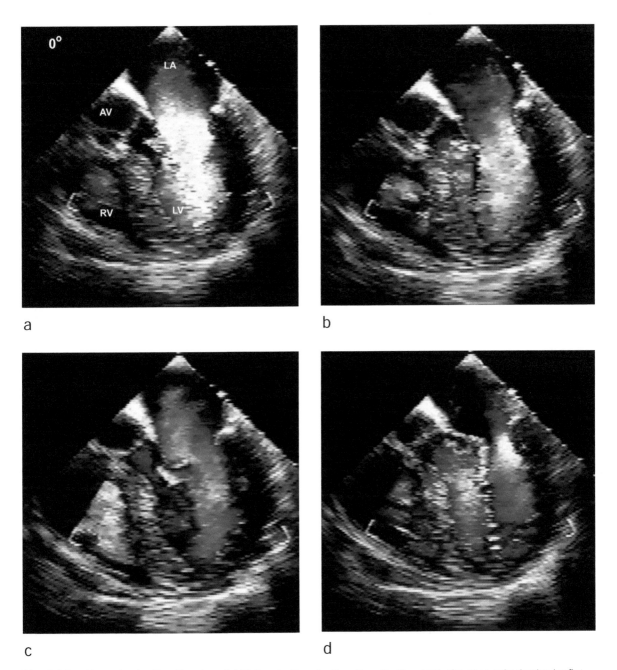

Fig. 2.24 Normal color flow Dopple . (a) High velocity color flow Doppler th ough the open mitral valve leaflet in early diastole r ecorded in the low esophageal window at 0°. (b) As diastole pr ogresses the velocity of the color flow signal sta ts to decr ease and flow cu ves around the ventricular apex towar ds the left ventricular outflow tract. (c) Mid-diastole blood flow velocities dec ease substantially as the valve leaflets begin to clos further. (d) With atrial systole higher velocity flow is again ecorded in the left ventricular inflow tract.

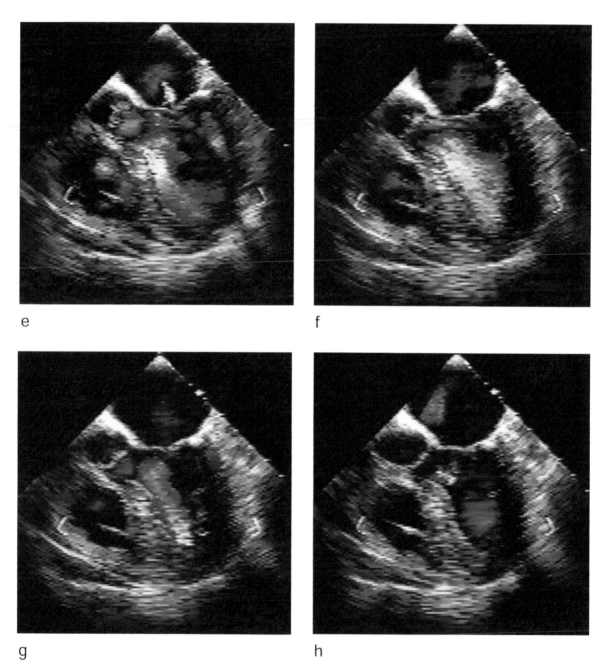

Fig. 2.24 (contd.) (e) With further closure of the mitral leaflets, eversal of blood flow is noted backwa d towards the left atrium. (f, g) With complete mitral valve closur e and the star t of systole, higher velocity blood flow is noted in the left ventricular outflow tract towa ds the aor tic valve. (h) At end systole only low velocity flow is detected in the left atrium or left ventricle.

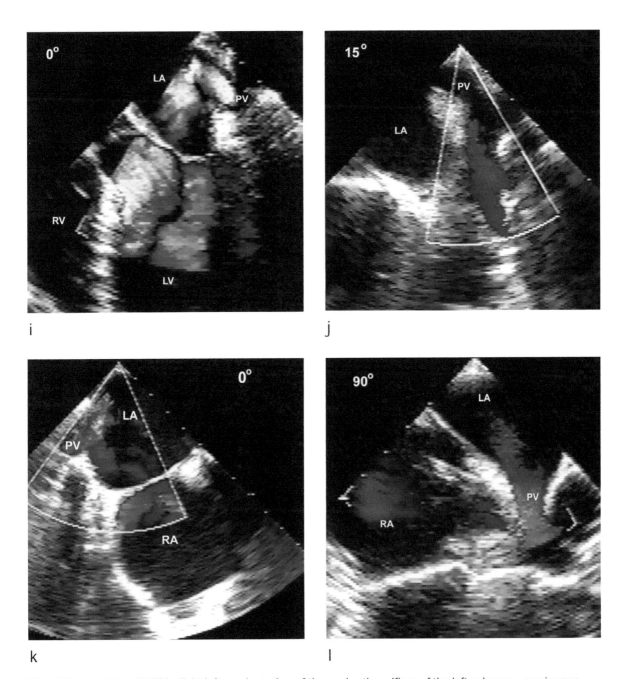

Fig. 2.24 (contd.) (i) With slight leftwar d rotation of the pr obe the orifices of the left pulmona y veins ar e visualized with low velocity pulmonar y venous flow seen entering the left atrium in early diastole. (j) Rotatin the transducer to appr oximately 15° the left pulmonar y veins ar e visualized. Pulsed Doppler can be easily performed in this view to inter rogate and r ecord the pulmonar y venous flo . (k) Retur ning the pr obe to 0°, with mild withdrawal and rightwar d rotation of the pr obe the origin of the right pulmonar y veins is visualized entering the left atrium. (l) At the same level and r otation of the transducer to 90° the full extent of the right pulmonar y vein and low velocity color flow is ecorded.

REFERENCES

1. Ranganathan N, Lam JHC, Wigle ED, Silver MD. Morphology of the human mitral valve. II. The valve leaflets. Circulation 1970;41:459–467.
2. Edwards JE, Burchell HB. Pathologic anatomy of mitral insufficiency. Proc Staff Meet Mayo Clin 1958;33:497.
3. Lam JHC, Ranganathan N, Wigle ED, Silver MD. Morphology of the human mitral valve. II. Chordae tendineae: a new classification. Circulation 1970;41:449–458.
4. Olson LJ, Subramanian R, Ackermann DM, et al. Surgical pathology of the mitral valve: a study of 712 cases spanning 21 years. Mayo Clin Proc 1987;62:22–34.
5. Dean AI Jr. The movements of the mitral cusps in relation to the cardiac cycle. Am J Physiol 1916;40:206.
6. Rushmer RF, Finlayson BL, Nash AA. Movements of the mitral valve. Circ Res 1956;4:337.
7. Carpentier A, Deloche A, Dauptain J, et al. A new reconstructive operation for correction of mitral and tricuspid insufficiency. J Thorac Cardiovasc Surg 1971;61:1–13.
8. Zimmerman J, Bailey CP. The surgical significance of the fibrous skeleton of the heart. J Thorac Cardiovasc Surg 1962;44:701.
9. Komeda M, Glasson JR, Bolger AF, et al. Three-dimensional dynamic geometry of the normal canine mitral annulus and papillary muscles. Circulation 1996;49:II159–63.
10. Titus JL. Anatomy and pathology of the mitral valve. In: Surgery for acquired mitral valve disease. Ellis FH Jr. (ed). Philadelphia: Saunders, 1967.
11. Little RC. Effect of atrial systole on ventricular pressure and closure of the A-V valves. Am J Physiol 1951;166:289.
12. Brock RC. The surgical and pathological anatomy of the mitral valve. Br Heart J 1952;14:489.
13. Rusted IE, Scheifley CH, Edwards JE. Studies of the mitral valve. I. Anatomic features of the normal mitral valve and associated structures. Circulation 1952;6:825.
14. Chiechi MA, Lees WM, Thompson R. Functional anatomy of the normal mitral valve. J Thorac Surg 1956;32:378.
15. Van der Spuy JC. The functional and clinical anatomy of the mitral valve. Br Heart J 1958;20:471.
16. Silverman ME, Hurst JW. The mitral complex. Interaction of the anatomy, physiology and pathology of the mitral annulus, mitral valve leaflets, chordae tendineae and papillary muscles. Am Heart J 1968;76:399–418.
17. Sarris GE, Miller DC. Role of the mitral sub-valvular apparatus in left ventricular systolic mechanics. Sem Thorac Cardiovasc Surg 1989;1:133–143.
18. Roberts WC, Cohen LS. Left ventricular papillary muscles. Circulation 1972;46:138–153.
19. Madu EC, D'Cruz IA. The vital role of papillary muscles in mitral and ventricular function: Echocardiographic insights. Clin Cardiol 1997;20:93–98.
20. Pandian NG, Hsu TL, Schwartz SL, et al. Multiplane transesophageal echocardiography. Imaging planes, echocardiographic anatomy, and clinical experience with a prototype phased array OmniPlane probe. Echocardiography 1992;9:649–666.
21. Bansal RC, Shakudo M, Shah PM, Shah PM. Biplane transesophageal echocardiography: Technique, image orientation, and preliminary experience in 131 patients. J Am Soc Echocardiography 1990;3:348–366.
22. Pai RG, Tanimoto M, Jintapakorn W, et al. Volume rendered three-dimensional anatomy of the mitral annulus using transesophageal echocardiography. Circulation 1993;88:341–349.
23. Stumper O, Fraser AG, Ho SY, et al. Transesophageal echocardiography in the longitudinal axis: correlation between anatomy and images and its clinical implications. Br Heart J 1990;64:282–288.
24. Schneider A, Schwartz S, Pandian N, et al. Multiplane transesophageal echocardiography provides more precise echocardiography-anatomic definition and functional assessment of the normal and pathologic mitral valve and its apparatus. J Am Coll Cardiol 1993;21:83A.
25. Salutri A, Becker AE, Van Herwerden L, et al. Three-dimensional echocardiography of normal and pathologic mitral valve: a comparison with two-dimensional transesophageal echocardiography. J Am Coll Cardiol 1996;27:1502–1510.

26. Chandraratna PAN, Aronow WS. Mitral valve ring in normal versus dilated left ventricle. Cross-sectional echocardiographic study. Chest 1981;79:151–154.

27. Come PC, Riley MF. M-mode and cross-sectional echocardiographic recognition of fibrosis and calcification of the mitral valve chordae and left ventricular papillary muscles. Am J Cardiol 1982;49:461–466.

28. Glasson JR, Komeda M, Daughters GT, et al. Loss of three-dimensional canine mitral annular systolic contraction with reduced left ventricular volumes. Circulation 1996;94:II152–158.

29. Deloche A, Jebara VA, Relland JYM, et al. Valve repair with Carpentier techniques. The second decade. J Thorac Cardiovasc Surg 1990;99:990–1001.

30. Assoun B, Diebold B, Abergel E, et al. Morphology-function relationship after mitral valve repair (abstr). Circulation 1992;86(suppl I):I–724.

31. Mihaileanu S, Marino JP, Chauvaud S, et al. Left ventricular outflow obstruction after mitral valve repair (Carpentier's Technique): Proposed mechanisms of disease. Circulation 1988; 78(suppl I):I–78–84.

3

Mitral Stenosis

Transesophageal echocardiographic assessment of mitral stenosis • Doppler evaluation of mitral stenosis • Percutaneous balloon mitral valvuloplasty

Mitral stenosis is the most common cause of left ventricular inflow obstruction. The most common cause of mitral stenosis is rheumatic carditis, despite its decline in developing countries since the introduction of penicillin. Transesophageal echocardiography offers no real advantage over transthoracic techniques in rheumatic mitral stenosis, unless the patient does not have a suitable transthoracic acoustic window. The real advantage of transesophageal echocardiography in mitral stenosis is in diagnosing associated cardiac pathology such as mitral insufficiency, thrombi in the left atrial cavity and appendage, and assessing the integrity of the atrial septum. Transesophageal echocardiography is particularly helpful in assessing the suitability for, and predicting the results of, percutaneous balloon mitral valvuloplasty, surgical repair and/or commissurotomy. In diagnosing the other causes of mitral or left ventricular inflow obstruction – congenital mitral stenosis, parachute mitral valve, mitral arcade, supravalvular mitral ring, cor triatriatum, left heart or mitral apparatus tumors or thrombi, bacterial or non-bacterial endocarditis, and severe mitral annular calcification – transesophageal echocardiogra-

phy has a distinct advantage over transthoracic echocardiography.

Rheumatic mitral stenosis in the adult may be categorized by: leaflet thickening occurring from fibrosis or calcification; commissural fusion; and stenosis produced in conjunction with fusion, shortening, and calcification of the subvalvular apparatus. These three processes may occur independently but usually occur in combination and with various degrees of severity. Commissural fusion is produced from localized inflammation in areas of reduced motion occurring as a result of annular dilatation during the acute process. The fusion may be isolated, with the other portions of the leaflet remaining totally pliable and free of disease. Leaflet fibrosis, thickening, and calcification frequently occur with commissural fusion. Over time, progressive fibrosis occurs leading to restriction, contracture and immobility of the leaflets, starting at the edges and extending to the body of the leaflet. Thickening and fusion of the chordae tendineae follows, producing narrowing and stenosis of the subvalvular area. In many cases this is the predominant pathology of obstruction to inflow. [1,2]

TRANSESOPHAGEAL ECHOCARDIOGRAPHIC ASSESSMENT OF MITRAL STENOSIS

The transesophageal echocardiographic assessment of mitral stenosis includes (1) an anatomic description of the morphology and mobility of the mitral valve and the subvalvular apparatus, (2) an evaluation of the severity of stenosis by estimating the valve orifice area using planimetry and Doppler methods, (3) an evaluation of the effects produced by the hemodynamics of obstruction (left atrial enlargement, pulmonary hypertension, right heart enlargement, and biventricular function), (4) the identification of associated abnormalities (left atrial thrombus, patent foramen ovale or atrial septal defect), and (5) a thorough evaluation of the other valves including the assessment of associated mitral regurgitation.

Assessment of the mitral valve and subvalvular apparatus

The best views for assessment of the mitral subvalvular apparatus in mitral stenosis are the deep transgastric frontal view (50–55 cm from the incisors, 0°) and the transgastric longitudinal view (40 cm from the incisors, 90–120°). In both views the papillary muscles and chordae tendineae are not affected by acoustic shadowing or ghosting from calcified and thickened mitral leaflets. The papillary muscles will appear hypertrophied, and the chordae tendineae should be evaluated for shortening or retraction, fusion or thickening, and calcification. In mild cases of mitral stenosis the only recognizable differences in the subvalvular apparatus will be slight increases in chordal thickening and minor increase in echogenicity of these structures. Calcification of the subvalvular area may present as small, discrete areas of increased echogenicity. In more severe cases of mitral stenosis the papillary muscles, chordae tendineae and points of chordal insertion to the leaflets can appear as one continuous thick structure without identifiable points of demarcation between them. The chordae tendineae in severe calcific mitral stenosis may be very thick, shortened and fused, and appear to cause retraction or eversion of the leaflets.

Estimating the area of the mitral valve orific

The transesophageal echocardiographic probe is withdrawn to the proximal transgastric position, and the transducer can be rotated between 0° and 20° to image the mitral valve *en face*. This can be difficult, since the valve is frequently oblique to the probe and the imaging plane from this position in the esophagus. The mitral commissures will be visible and will appear to be thickened and fused, especially near the outer margins. Depending on the degree of fusion and scarring of each individual commissure, the usually central mitral orifice may be displaced or distorted, in addition to being narrowed, producing the classic fish-mouth appearance of the leaflets during diastole. The extent of commissural fusion will determine the severity of mitral stenosis, and in mild and moderate stenosis will cause an abrupt opening movement of the leaflets. With small adjustments in the probe in anteflexion, an assessment of the mitral orifice can be made by planimetry. Accurate planimetry of the valve orifice depends on obtaining a true short-axis view of the leaflet tips, viewing the valve as far as possible enface, and locating the smallest orifice area between the valve leaflets and subvalvular apparatus. Care must be taken to image the valve at the level of the tips of the mitral valve leaflets and not at the base of the mitral valve funnel, to avoid overestimation of the valve area. Ignoring significant narrowing of the subvalvular area will result in underestimation of the valve area. In heavily calcified valves, adjustment of the echocardiographic equipment must be set appropriately to avoid blooming of the thickened leaflets and overestimation of the degree of stenosis, with measurements made from the inside edge of the valve leaflets. Stoddard and colleagues[3] have shown an excellent correlation betwen mitral valve areas obtained by planimetry from both the transesophageal and transthoracic echocardiographic approaches. Mitral valvotomy or commissurotomy usually produces distortion of the mitral orifice, so that measurements of the orifice area by planimetry may be less accurate than measurements made using other techniques. After valvotomy the valve shows expansion in the orifice dimension along its horizontal axis from commissure to commissure, usually without an obvious change in leaflet opening. In any event, the hallmark of mitral stenosis after valvotomy is that the commissures freely move and are not fused, without significant change in the remainder of the valvular apparatus. Reports have varied about the accuracy of planimetry measurements in mitral stenosis,[3] but in our experience valves can easily and accurately be categorized as mild, moderate, or severe, using the transesophageal echocardiographic probes currently available.

Assessment of other effects and abnormalities

With further withdrawal of the probe to the lower and mid-esophageal positions, and with the scope in the neutral or slightly anteflexed position, the mitral valve is imaged in profile in the four-chamber horizontal view at 0°. Thickening and diastolic doming of the anterior and posterior leaflets is readily apparent. Frequently, the subvalvular apparatus will not be visible due to acoustic shadowing from the thickened and calcified leaflets. In mild mitral stenosis, only the distal leaflet tips will appear thickened and immobile. The body of the leaflets present visually with the "hockey stick" or "bent-knee deformity", indicating diastolic doming. As the disease progresses, the body of the leaflets thickens and becomes visibly less mobile, until the diastolic doming disappears and the valve leaflets show either minimal excursion or appear immobile from diastole to systole. Rotating the transducer from 0° to 135° may adequately assess the anterior and posterior leaflets, along with the commissures.

With the transesophageal echocardiographic probe in the upper esophageal position and continued slight anteflexion at 0°, the basal short-axis plane of the heart visualizes the left atrium, atrial septum, and the left atrial appendage. The left atrium enlarges sequentially with worsening degrees of stenosis, often reaching 6–7 cm in severe mitral stenosis. Frequently, spontaneous contrast [4–6] or "echo smoke" is visualized in the left atrium and left atrial appendage, characterized by an echocardiographic appearance of swirling and sludging of slowly moving blood cells secondary to rouleaux formation. The left atrium should be carefully inspected for the presence of thrombus. The most frequent site of thrombus[7] is the left atrial appendage, followed by the superior aspect (roof) of the left atrium, the area around the pulmonary vein orifices, and the secundum atrial septum. The left atrium must be fully examined by scanning from 0° to 90° and moving the probe from a somewhat neutral position to full anteflexion, in the upper esophageal position.

It may be helpful to examine the left atrium in stages, starting with the left atrial appendage. The left atrial appendage at 0° has a narrow orifice and projects longitudinally in a twisting, tapering fashion, frequently out of plane. It is necessary to rotate the transducer slowly to 90° to image the full extent of the appendage. When there are prominent pectinate muscles, the appendage may appear cystic and it may be difficult to distinguish the pectinate muscles from thrombi. In this circumstance, it may be helpful to use the zoom feature, with or without color Doppler, to observe blood flow in the area. Color flow Doppler usually surrounds and enhances a thrombus. It is also occasionally helpful to place the M-mode cursor through the area in question to look for chaotic motion, as seen with some thrombi. With slow withdrawal of the transesophageal echocardiographic probe and rotation of the transducer from 0° to 90°, the body of the left atrium is visible with the areas around the pulmonary veins, atrial septum and foramen ovale, followed by visualization of the roof of the atrium around the level of the aorta and pulmonary artery.

Thrombi vary in size and may appear either well laminated to the atrial wall or freely mobile. It is not uncommon to visualize spontaneous contrast associated with the thrombi, especially in the presence of atrial fibrillation. It is therefore extremely important to carefully observe areas near spontaneous contrast to fully exclude the presence of thrombi.

To complete the examination in mitral stenosis, pulmonary venous flows[8] are evaluated, especially when there is significant mitral insufficiency, the right heart is assessed for chamber enlargement, right ventricular function, and tricuspid and pulmonic flows are assessed to estimate pulmonary artery pressures and to rule out pulmonary hypertension.

DOPPLER EVALUATION OF MITRAL STENOSIS

Accurate estimates of the transmitral gradient and mitral valve orifice area may be made with conventional and color Doppler in the four-chamber esophageal views, using the same techniques as those of transthoracic echocardiography.[9–12] High pulsed repetition frequency or continuous wave Doppler can be used to measure the transmitral gradient. The mitral inflow jet can be easily interrogated and positioned directly parallel to the transducer imaging plane, with the aid of color Doppler and minor adjustments of the transesophageal echocardiographic transducer. The characteristic Doppler features of mitral stenosis are increased peak velocity, reduced rate of decrease in velocity with time and, in patients in sinus rhythm, augmentation of the velocity signal due to atrial contraction. The increased transmitral blood flow velocity profile and its slow decline indicate a pressure gradient across the valve continuing throughout diastole. The pressure gradients across the mitral valve at any time are estimated with the modified Bernoulli equation ($P1 - P2 = 4[V_{max}]^2$). Peak and mean transvalvular gradients obtained with the modified Bernoulli formula correlate closely with those calculated at cardiac catheterization using the Gorlin formula, and can be measured online with most currently available echocardiographic equipment.[10] Although pressure gradients provide an indication of the presence of obstruction, they are dependent upon the transvalvular volumetric flow and driving pressures through the orifice, which are dictated by the patient's hemodynamic status, therefore they may not accurately reflect the severity of obstruction.[13]

The mitral valve orifice area can be measured with Doppler by estimating the transmitral pressure half-time (PHT) during diastole.[14–29] In mitral stenosis, the measured transmitral gradi-

ent is maximal near the onset of diastole and declines in a linear fashion. The transmitral pressure half-time is calculated as the time required for the initial maximum gradient to fall by 50%. The more severe the degree of obstruction of the mitral orifice, the longer the time of pressure fall off. The mitral pressure half-time can be calculated from the velocity signal as the time interval over which the velocity falls from its maximum to minimum value divided by the square root of 2. The normal pressure half-time is less than 100 msec. Since the transmitral pressure gradient and blood flow velocity are related by a square power function, mitral valve orifice area is calculated as MVA = 220/pressure half-time.[15] Mild mitral stenosis has a pressure half-time of 160 msec or less with a valve area greater than 2 cm². In severe mitral stenosis the pressure half-time is greater than 220 msec with a valve area less than 1 cm². There has been concern that the angle of incidence produced by the Doppler interrogation of the mitral valve inflow with transesophageal echocardiography might negatively influence the mitral valve area and maximal gradient. Stoddard and colleagues[16] have shown that Doppler transesophageal echocardiography compares favorably to the transthoracic approach.

Atrioventricular compliance[17,18] and other hemodynamic variables[19] that influence the transmitral gradient may cause inaccurate measurement of the mitral valve area by the pressure half-time method. The pressure half-time method for calculating the mitral valve area results in significant overestimation of the true valve area in situations such as aortic regurgitation,[20–22] mitral regurgitation,[23–24] exercise,[13] pregnancy, decreased diastolic performance of the left ventricle, and immediately after balloon valvuloplasty.[30]

Mitral valve area may also be calculated using the law of continuity.[28] The continuity principle states that volume flow per unit of time through a stenosis is equal to the volume flow either proximal or distal to the stenosis, provided the cardiac output remains constant during both measurements. Volume flow is assessed as the product of the flow velocity integral (FVI) and the cross-sectional area (CSA) of the flow stream. $FVI_1 \times CSA_1$ (normal zone) = $FVI_2 \times CSA_2$ (stenotic zone). In patients with mitral stenosis, the normal zone blood flow velocity and vessel diameter is measured either in the proximal aorta or the proximal pulmonary artery. The blood flow velocity integral across the stenotic mitral valve is obtained with continuous wave Doppler, and the cross-sectional area of the stenosis is calculated. Mitral valve areas calculated from Doppler measurements using the continuity equation correlate closely with those areas calculated during cardiac catheterization, irrespective of varying hemodynamic conditions or in conditions (as described above) that may affect the pressure half-time. In cases of aortic insufficiency, the normal zone volume flow measurements should be made in the pulmonary artery instead of the aorta to avoid overestimation of the mitral valve area. In patients with significant mitral regurgitation, the increased velocity related to the regurgitant volume tends to underestimate the mitral valve area, limiting the use of the continuity equation in cases of mixed mitral stenosis and regurgitation.

Color Doppler provides other methods for estimating mitral stenosis. It identifies flow convergence surrounding the opening of the mitral orifice on the atrial side, and a characteristic "flame" jet of increased velocity and disturbed forward flow through the stenotic mitral orifice in diastole. The mitral valve orifice may be measured by color Doppler mapping of the proximal isovelocity surface area (PISA) combined with the continuous wave Doppler interrogation of the flow jet through the mitral inflow.[16–20] As flow enters a narrowed orifice from a larger chamber, the convergence of flow is depicted by color flow Doppler as a series of radial, uniform layers or isovelocity surface areas proximal to the stenosis. By identifying PISA and quantifying the volume flow rate, the stenotic area can be calculated using the continuity equation. Initial studies have identified these isovelocity layers as hemispheric, and allow the calculation of flow as the product of the surface area and its aliasing velocity.

The flow convergence region proximal to the stenotic mitral orifice during diastole is easily recorded in the lower esophageal position with the transducer at 0°–90°, to give the best representation of the anterior and posterior leaflets as they form a funnel opening. Flow is recorded at a low aliasing velocity (V_n) by adjusting the color flow baseline to obtain the largest isovelocity from the area, and the radius (r) at peak diastole is measured. Flow rate is corrected by adjusting for the inflow angle formed by the mitral valve leaflets (measured angle α divided by 180°). The peak flow velocity through the mitral valve is recorded with continuous wave Doppler (V_{peak}). Mitral valve area is then calculated as:

$$MVA = 2\pi r^2 \times \alpha/180° \times V_n/V_{peak}.$$

The width of the mitral valve orifice can be measured with biplane or multiplane transesophageal echocardiography in two orthogonal planes, with color Doppler visualization of the flow jet through the mitral inflow. The minor axis of the flow jet can be measured at 0° in the four-chamber view, and the major axis of the flow jet can be measured at 90° in the two-chamber view. The mitral valve area (MVA) can be measured simply by calculating the shape of the mitral valve orifice as an ellipse, using the major (M1) and minor axis (M2) of the flow jet:

$$MVA = \pi \times (M1)/2 \times (M2)/2.$$

Chen and colleagues[31] reported that, in patients with mitral stenosis, there was a very strong correlation between mitral valve areas calculated using transesophageal echocardiographic data, and those derived by the Gorlin formula using cardiac catheterization data (r = 0.94; standard error of estimate = 0.13 cm^2).

PERCUTANEOUS BALLOON MITRAL VALVULOPLASTY

Although mitral stenosis is usually adequately defined by transthoracic echocardiography, transesophageal echocardiography is usually necessary for patients undergoing percutaneous mitral valvotomy.[32–40] Transesophageal echocardiography may be helpful to identify an occasional case of congenital mitral stenosis that has emerged in adulthood and might not be ideal for valvuloplasty. Transesophageal echocardiography is also extremely helpful in ruling out left atrial thrombi, which are the main contraindication to balloon valvuloplasty.[41,42] Atrial thrombi are not routinely visualized by transthoracic echocardiographic imaging. These thrombi may be dislodged during the manipulation of the catheter hardware during the procedure, and are a source of cerebral or systemic embolization and untoward complications.[43]

Transesophageal echocardiography is also necessary to adequately evaluate mitral insufficiency that may not be fully appreciated on transthoracic imaging.[44–46] Moderate to severe mitral regurgitation is considered a contraindication since this can be made worse with balloon dilatation. As a rule of thumb, mitral regurgitation increases by at least one degree of severity with balloon dilatation. The acoustic shadowing that is usually present on transthoracic imaging due to a calcified mitral valve or the eccentricity of a regurgitant jet means that mitral regurgitation can easily be overlooked. Mitral regurgitant jets may be difficult to detect by transthoracic echocardiography, especially in cases of previous commissurotomy.

Although transesophageal echocardiographic imaging is well suited to describe these contraindications, transthoracic echocardiography is adequate for most patients in determining the echocardiographic score index for mitral stenosis. In a few patients with poor transthoracic windows, transesophageal echocardiography may be helpful in predicting the anticipated success of the balloon valvuloplasty by accurately defining the extent of the stenotic pathology.[47–49] Wilkins and colleagues[32] have described an echocardiographic scoring system in an attempt to predict which patients would benefit from this procedure (Table 3.1). The score index grades stenotic pathology on a scale of 0–4, higher scores representing more

Table 3.1   Anatomic classification of the mitral valve (ilkins' score, Massachusetts General Hospital)

Leaflet mobility
Highly mobile valve with only leaflet tips   estricted
Leaflet mid and base por tions have nor mal mobility
Valve continues to move for ward in diastole, mainly fr om the base. No or minimal for ward movement of the leaflets in diastol

Subvalvar thickening
Minimal thickening just below the mitral leaflet
Thickening of chor dal structures extending up to one thir d of the chor dal length
Thickening extending to the distal thir d of the chor ds
Extensive thickening and shor tening of all chor dal structures extending down to the papillar y muscles

Valvar thickness
Leaflets near nor mal in thickness (4–5 mm)
Mid-leaflets normal, considerable thickening of mar gins (5–8 mm)
Thickening extending thr ough the entir e leaflet (5–8 mm)
Considerable thickening of all leaflet tissue (>8–10 mm)

Valvar calcificatio
A single ar ea of incr eased echo brightness
Scatter ed areas of brightness confined to leaflet m   gins
Brightness extending into the mid-por tion of the leaflet
Extensive brightness thr oughout much of the leaflet tissu

abnormal valve structures. Valve mobility, thickness, and calcification, and subvalvular thickening, are all graded echocardiographically, and the individual scores are added together to give a score index between 1 and 16. Patients with a score of 8 or less have a greater than 90% likelihood of a satisfactory result with balloon dilatation. The predictors that correlate best with mitral valve splitability or subsequent area improvement are the severity of leaflet thickness, pliability, and degree of valve calcification. Cannan and colleagues[50] have shown that the echocardiographic assessment of commissural calcium is a simple predictor of outcome after percutaneous mitral valvotomy. Patients with calcium in either the medial or lateral commissures have a significantly lower rate of survival, and significantly higher incidences of repeat balloon valvotomy and mitral valve replacement, compared to patients without commissural calcium. Cannan's study also showed by Cox regression that commissural calcium together with the mitral echo score was the only significant variable for predicting outcome. Although the individual decision to proceed to valvotomy must be based on clinical considerations, the echocardiographic characteristics of the mitral apparatus may be a useful guide for deciding further treatment.

Transesophageal echocardiographic imaging may be used during the balloon valvuloplasty procedure for the positioning of catheters, puncturing the atrial septum, determining balloon sizing, and evaluating the worsening of any regurgitation after the procedure. In many interventional cardiac laboratories, transesophageal echocardiography is done routinely during the procedure in conjunction with fluoroscopy. It is also possible to undertake balloon valvuloplasty with transesophageal echocardiography alone, especially for laboratories familiar with the procedure.[43]

Transesophageal echocardiography is surprisingly well tolerated by patients during balloon valvuloplasty. In most laboratories, intravenous sedation is given during the procedure, which also allows the patient to tolerate the transesophageal echocardiographic procedure. The transesophageal echocardiographic

probe should be left in place only for as long as is necessary to allow visualization of the procedure. It is helpful to support the scope in the mouth, not allowing the scope to slacken or move frequently, which prevents gagging and minimizes aspiration. A clear advantage of multiplane transesophageal echocardiographic imaging is that it allows for less probe manipulation, which may be better tolerated by the patient. It is also important to monitor the patient's airway, making sure it is clear at all times, suctioning frequently, and ensuring that oral and topical anesthesia does not wear off during an occasionally long procedure. The transesophageal echocardiographic procedure allows a physician to be at the head of the examination table, much like an anesthesiologist during surgery, and this is often appreciated by the patient.

To aid in puncturing and crossing the atrial septum with the catheter hardware, the foramen ovale area is visualized in the lower esophageal position between 0° and 45° or the mid-esophageal position at 90°–130°. In both views, a large portion of the bodies of both the left and right atrium are visualized with the foramen ovale area positioned in the middle of the echocardiographic display. Using this approach, the atrial septum is nearly perpendicular to the imaging plane and allows the visualization of typical catheter artifact as the hardware is introduced into the appropriate position. With minor angulations, the orifice of the inferior vena cava, superior vena cava, tricuspid valve, or coronary sinus should be easily visualized to allow direction of the catheter in the appropriate position.

To visualize the catheter and the balloon as it crosses the mitral valve, standard four or two chamber views concentrating on imaging the left atrium and ventricle are obtained from the mid- to lower esophageal positions. The catheter hardware is readily identified by transesophageal echocardiography in both the left atrium and left ventricle. The size of the mitral annulus may be estimated by measuring the diameter or the length of the annulus between the posterior wall of the aortic root and the junction of the left atrium and ventricle.

Imaging during the seating of the balloon with inflation gives confidence during the procedure that the balloon is in the best position. Success is shown by increased leaflet motion after balloon deflation. Doppler interrogation of the mitral inflow to assess valve orifice area immediately following the procedure is unrewarding.

After balloon deflation the mitral valve is carefully assessed for the development or worsening of mitral regurgitation.[44-46] With balloon dilatation, the valve should split and open along both commissures, in a similar fashion to surgical commissurotomy. The mitral valve area can be calculated from measurement of the major and minor axis of the flow jet through the mitral orifice in two orthogonal views, or by planimetry of the mitral orifice in the short axis views.

Mitral regurgitation is readily apparent by color Doppler after the procedure, and a structural defect may be attributed to the cause of the regurgitation with the careful interrogation of valve anatomy. Mitral regurgitation can be measured quickly by the modified flow convergence or the vena contracta method, as long as significant distortion of the valve orifice has not been produced during the procedure.

The pulmonary venous flow pattern may be assessed by pulsed Doppler methods.[51] In mitral stenosis, the pulmonary venous systolic flow is decreased and the pulmonary diastolic flow is prolonged. After mitral valvuloplasty there is an immediate increase in pulmonary venous systolic forward flow in patients with sinus rhythm.

Echocardiographically, the procedure is successful if the mitral valve area is 1.5 cm^2 or more and mitral regurgitation is 2+ or less. Lung and colleagues[38,39] reported that the independent predictors of good functional results five years after mitral valvuloplasty were the mitral echo score, functional class and cardiothoracic index before the procedure, and the resultant valve area after balloon dilatation. Although most patients benefit from this procedure, the inherent nature of the disease process expressed by the echocardiography score index means that results in individual patients are variable. In selected patients with pliable valves, non-calcified leaflets with minimal subvalvular involvement, and little or no mitral regurgitation, the results of balloon valvotomy are similar to the surgical commissurotomy.[52,53] After the procedure, imaging of the atrial septum and Doppler techniques may be used to determine the persistence and size of a residual atrial septal defect, which usually disappears over time.[54-56] In our experience, the information obtained during the balloon procedure with transesophageal echocardiography may be used to interpret subsequent transthoracic echocardiograms done in the follow-up period, as long as acceptable transthoracic images are obtained.[57]

Case Studies

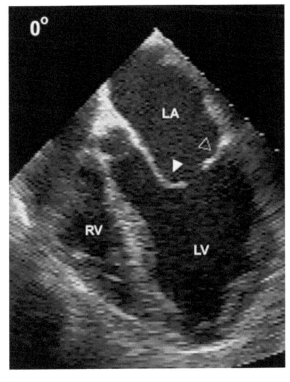

a

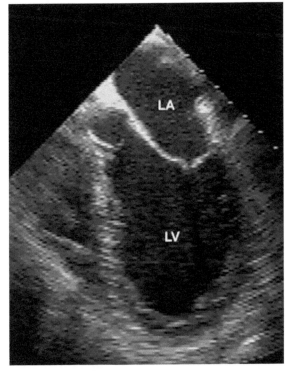

b

Case 3.1 Mild mitral stenosis. The str uctural and functional abnormalities of mitral stenosis, including fib osis, calcification and estriction of motion (diastolic doming), can be easily demonstrated with multiplane TEE in the lower esophageal window . Conventional and color Doppler evaluation of the left ventricular inflow tract is easily pe formed with a parallel plane to mitral flo . (a) Diastolic frame obtained at 0° illustrating mildly thickened mitral leaflets and diastolic doming (ar row). The anterior leaflet is towar ds the septum and the left of the image with the posterior leaflet to the right of th image. Valve opening can also be visually assessed during diastole as well as valve closur e during (b) systole. (c) Color flow Doppler in diastol demonstrating a stenotic jet (ar row) through the mitral valve.

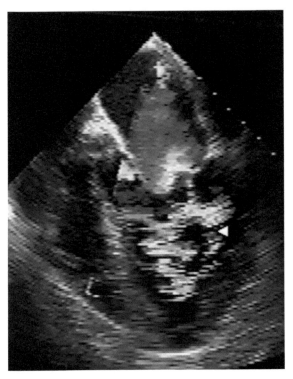

c

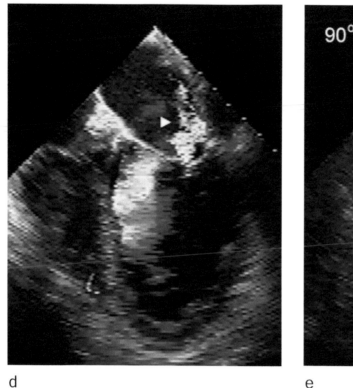

d

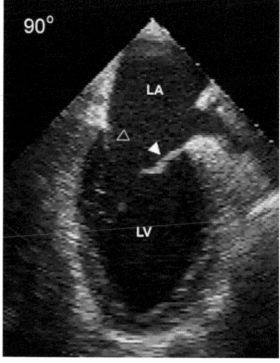

e

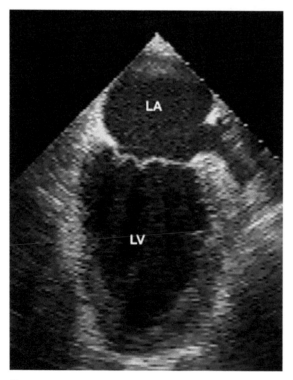

f

Case 3.1 (contd.)   (d) Color flow Doppler durin systole demonstrates a small r egurgitant jet (ar row). Rheumatic disease often pr esents as a mixed lesion with both stenosis and r egurgitation. Rotating the transducer to 90° demonstrates (e) diastolic doming (arrows) and (f) valve closur e during systole.

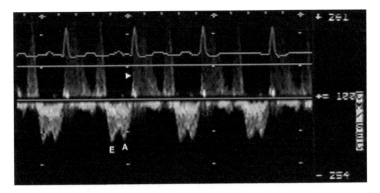

g

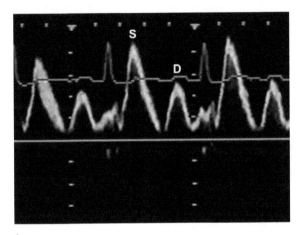

h

Case 3.1 (contd.) (g) Continuous wave Doppler thr ough a mildly stenotic mitral valve orifice demonstrate increased E and A wave velocities, with a nor mal pressur e half-time. (h) At 90° left pulmonar y venous Doppler is per formed demonstrating nor mal systolic (S) and diastolic (D) flow p ofiles. LA, left atrium; L V, left ventricle; RV, right ventricle.

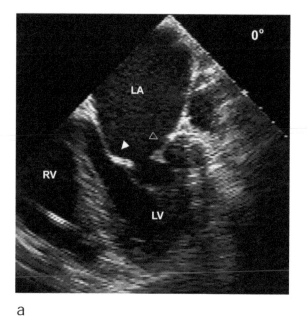

a

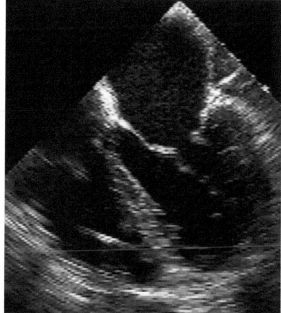

b

c

Case 3.2 Mild mitral stenosis and r egurgitation. Thickening and diastolic doming of the mitral valve leaflets with mild r estriction of opening during early diastole (a) and end diastole (b) at 0° in the lower esophageal window. (c) Systolic frame demonstrating leaflet closure.

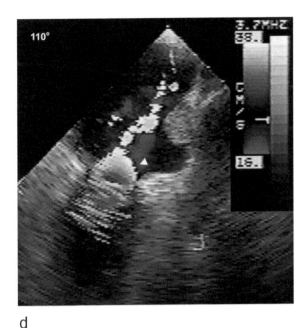

d

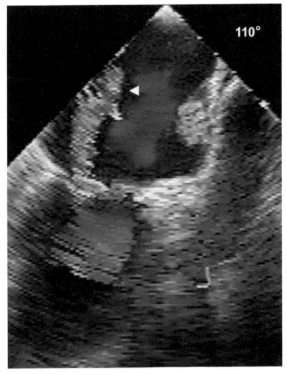

e

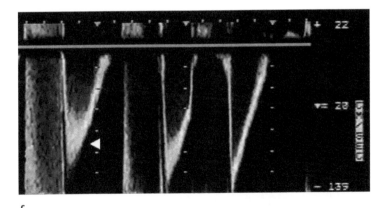

f

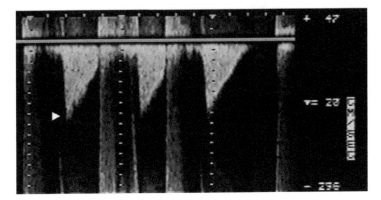

g

Case 3.2 (contd.) (d) Color flo Doppler performed with the transducer rotated to 110° demonstrating flo convergence through the stenotic mitral orifice. Flow conve gence can be best visualized by adjusting the aliasing velocity. (e) Systolic frame demonstrating a mild mitral r egurgitant jet. Color flow Doppler can also b useful for directing conventional Doppler (f) pulsed wave or (g) continuous wave thr ough the stenotic valve orifice. Conventiona Doppler demonstrates incr eased velocity of the *e* wave (arrows) and lack of an *a* wave during atrial fibrillation. Pressur e half-time can be estimated with continuous wave Doppler. LA, left atrium; L V, left ventricle; RV, right ventricle.

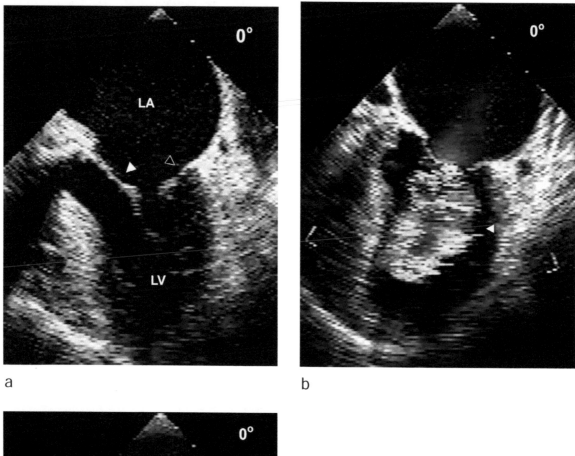

a

b

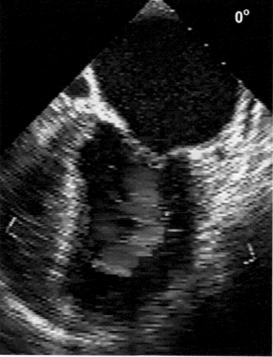

c

Case 3.3 Moderate mitral stenosis and mild regurgitation. The mitral leaflets are thickened and restricted with decreased amplitude of opening during diastole (a) and with color flow Doppler stenotic jet (b) is demonstrated. Note diastolic doming is often less noticeable as the severity of mitral stenosis increases. In systole (c) the mitral regurgitant jet is not identified until the transducer is rotated to 110° (d).

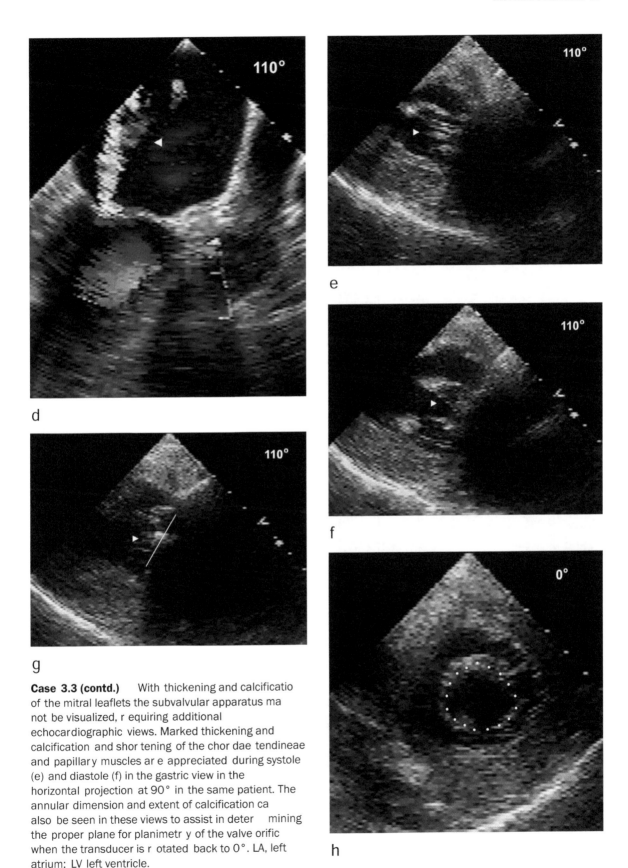

d

e

f

g

h

Case 3.3 (contd.) With thickening and calcificatio of the mitral leaflets the subvalvular apparatus ma not be visualized, r equiring additional echocardiographic views. Marked thickening and calcification and shor tening of the chor dae tendineae and papillar y muscles ar e appreciated during systole (e) and diastole (f) in the gastric view in the horizontal projection at 90° in the same patient. The annular dimension and extent of calcification ca also be seen in these views to assist in deter mining the proper plane for planimetr y of the valve orific when the transducer is r otated back to 0°. LA, left atrium; LV left ventricle.

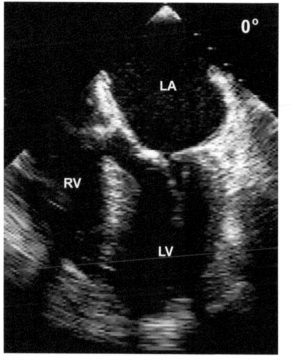

a

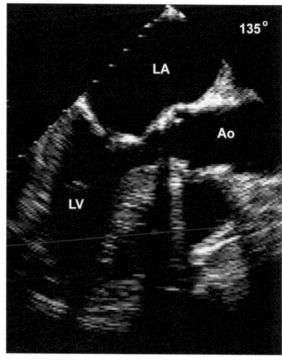

b

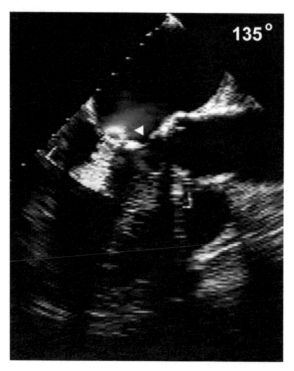

c

Case 3.4 Severe mitral stenosis. Marked thickening and calcification of the mitral valve leafle with significantly estricted opening in diastole (a) at 0° in the lower esophageal views. Rotating the transducer to 135° (b) allows fur ther interrogation of the mitral valve and in addition illustrates a stenotic aortic valve. Color flow Doppler at 135 demonstrates flow conve gence of the mitral stenotic jet during diastole (c)

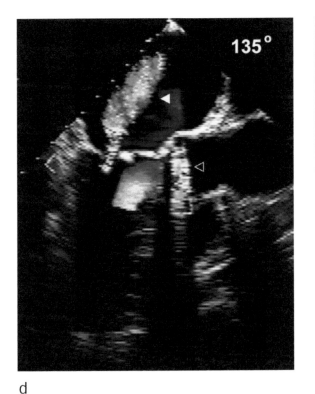

d

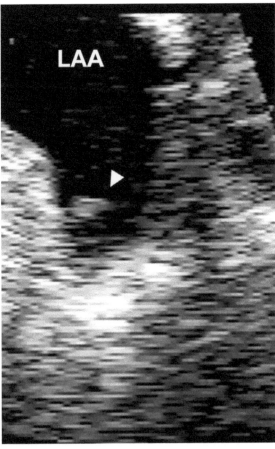

e

Case 3.4 (contd.)   and a mitral r egurgitant jet (d) with turbulent and stenotic flow ac   oss the aor tic valve during systole. (e) Visualizing the left atrial appendage demonstrates a thr   ombus at 10° in the upper esophageal view. LA, left atrium; L V, left ventricle; R V, right ventricle; LAA, left atrial appendage.

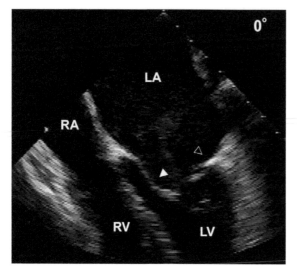

a

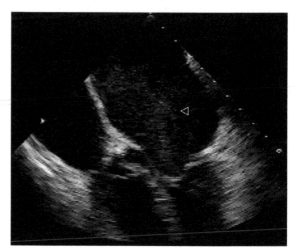

b

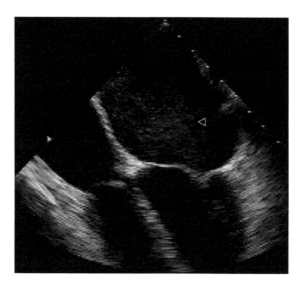

c

Case 3.5 Moderate mitral stenosis. (a) Marked left atrial enlargement with diastolic doming of the restricted and thickened leaflets. The posterior leafl is heavily calcified and exhibits seve ely restricted motion. (b) Echocar diographic smoke (ar row) identified in the body of the left atrium denoting sluggish blood flow due to the estricted mitral valve opening. (c) Closur e of the mitral valve leaflets Echocardiographic smoke (ar row). LA, left atrium; LV, left ventricle; RA, right atrium; R V right ventricle.

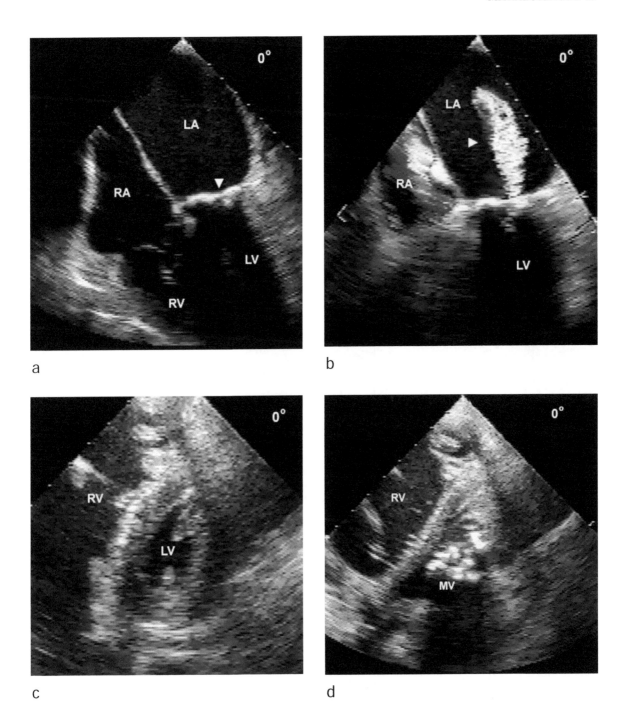

Case 3.6 Severe mitral stenosis. (a) Marked annular calcification and calcified mitral leaflets. (b) Dur
systole a mitral r egurgitant jet (ar row) is demonstrated. (c) Gastric transducer position at 0°   at the ventricular
basal level demonstrates the typical small left ventricle (L   V) of sever e mitral stenosis with a flattened septu
and a dilated right ventricle (R V) consistent with right ventricular pr essure overload. (d) With slight withdrawal
of the transducer to the esophagus the mitral valve (MV) orifice may be visualized for estimation of orifi
area.

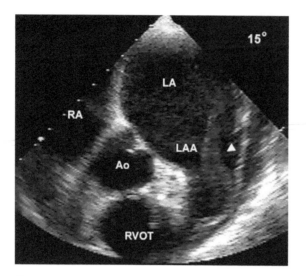

e

Case 3.6 (contd.) (e) Views of the left atrial appendage (LAA) demonstrate a thrombus and echocardiographic smoke. Pulsed wave Doppler interrogation of the left atrial appendage (f) demonstrates fibrillatory waves (arrows) with atrial fibrillation and diminished flow velocity in the appendage as a precursor for smoke and thrombus formation. LA, left atrium; RA, right atrium, RVOT, right ventricular outflow tract; AV, aortic valve.

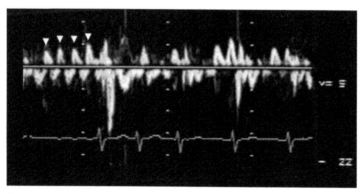

f

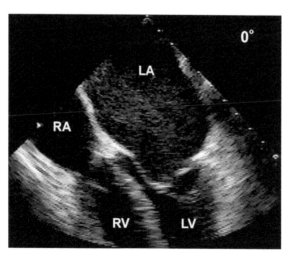

a

Case 3.7 Severe mitral stenosis. (a) Left atrial enlargement with diastolic doming of the mitral leaflets with restricted opening.

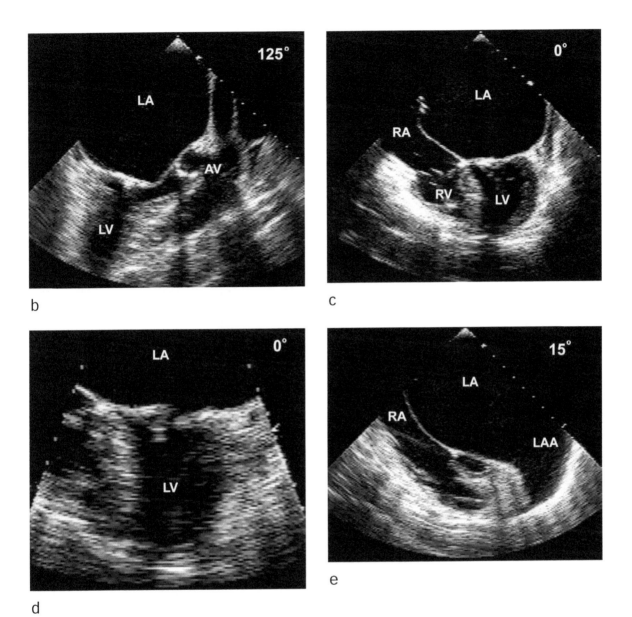

Case 3.7 (contd.) (b) Markedly enlarged left atrium in comparison to a small left ventricle with rotation of the transducer to 125°. (c) Bi-atrial enlargement with small ventricular cavities in a patient with rheumatic disease illustrating a restrictive component from associated pericardial involvement. (d) Annular plane exhibiting marked calcification. (e) Marked left atrial enlargement including the left atrial appendage (LAA). LA, left atrium; LV, left ventricle; RA, right atrium; RV, right ventricle; AV, aortic valve.

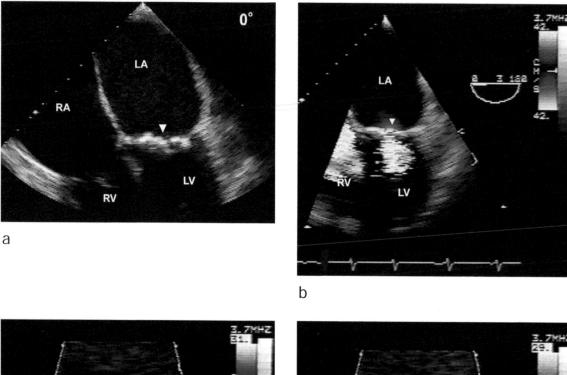

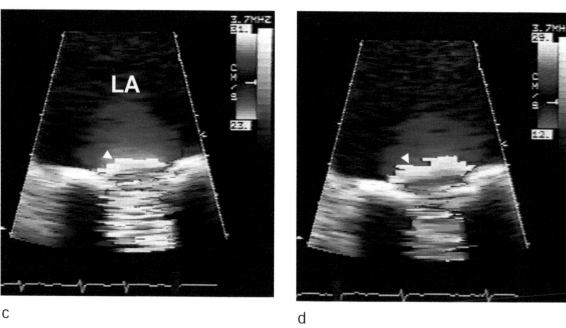

Case 3.8 Calculation of the mitral valve orifice in mitral stenosis. The PISA method can be utilized t measure the stenotic valve orifice a ea. (a) Stenotic mitral valve obtained in the lower esophageal view at 0°. The leaflets a e thickened and calcified and mitral valve opening is not eadily identified. (b) Color flow Doppl demonstrating the mitral stenotic jet during diastole. With nor mal aliasing velocity and standar d echocardiographic depth settings the pr oximal flow conve gence is not well visualized. Utilizing the zoom or RES feature of the echocar diographic equipment this ar ea can be magnified for measu ement. Decreasing the color flow aliasing velocity and shifting the baseline allows for better visualization (c,d,e) of the a ea of firs alias (arrow) allowing mor e accurate measur ement of the radius and deter mining the angle of the mitral leaflets.

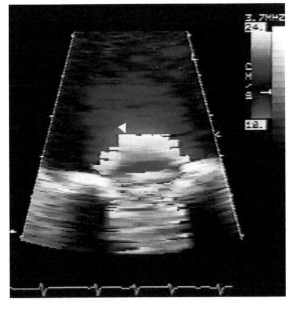

e

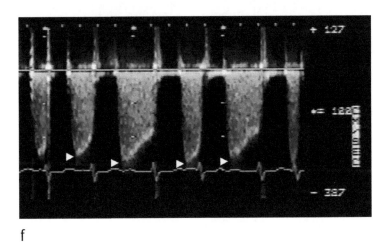

f

Case 3.8 (contd.)   (f) Continuous wave Doppler r ecording of mitral stenosis, demonstrating an averaged maximum velocity (ar rows) of 2.9 m/sec. Mitral r egurgitation is also demonstrated above the baseline during systole.   LA, left atrium; RA, right atrium; L V, left ventricle; R V, right ventricle.

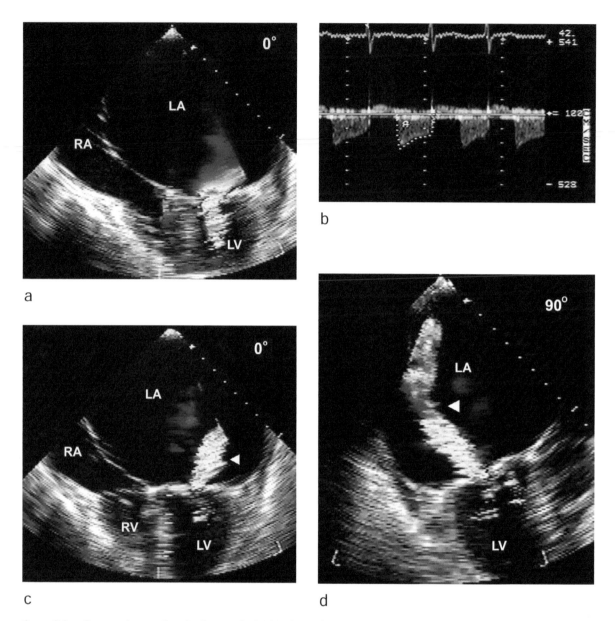

Case 3.9 Severe rheumatic mitral stenosis. (a) Marked left atrial enlar gement, with color flow Dopple demonstrating a mitral stenotic jet. (b) Continuous wave Doppler dir ected by the color flow stenotic jet in (a), exhibits incr eased maximal gradient and a pr olonged pressure half-time. (c) Color flow Dopple demonstrating an associated mitral r egurgitant jet (ar row). (d) The same color flow Doppler egurgitant jet visualized in (c) as visualized at 90°.

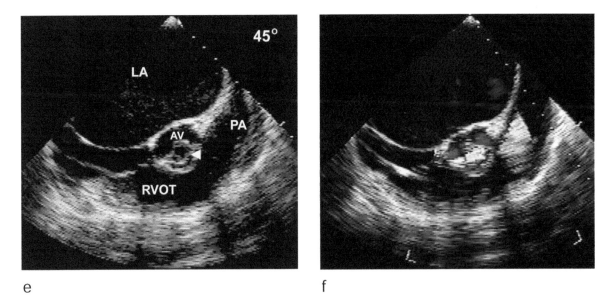

e   f

Case 3.9 (contd.)   (e) Visualization of the aor tic valve in the upper esophageal view at 45°. The aor tic valve is stenotic with r eduction of valve ar ea during systole. Multiple valvular lesions fr equently occur in r heumatic disease. (f) The aor tic valve during diastole exhibits marked calcification during closu e. LA, left atrium; PA, pulmonary arter y.

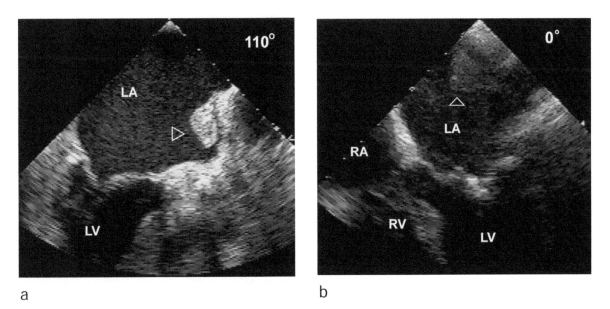

a   b

Case 3.10   Left atrial thr ombi are frequently associated with mitral stenosis. (a) Left atrial thr ombus at the origin or left atrial appendage (ar row). (b) Left atrial thr ombus (arrow) attached to the superior , posterior wall of the left atrium.

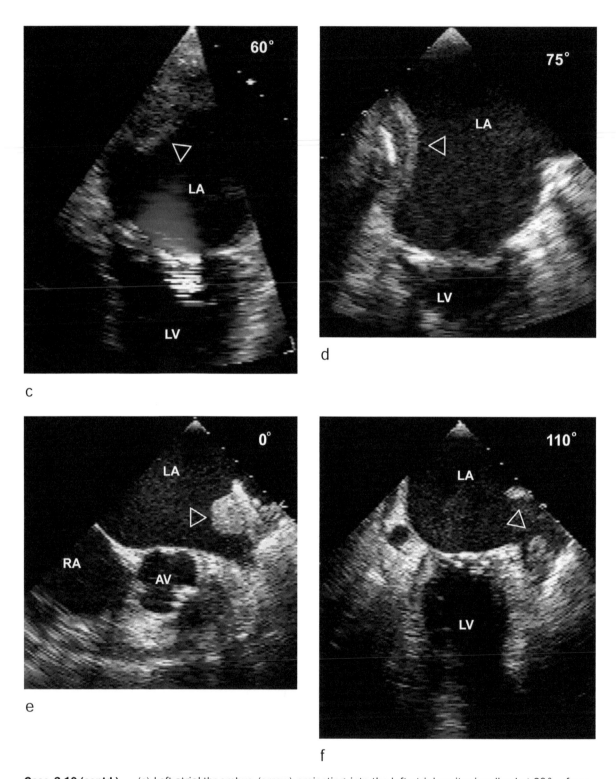

Case 3.10 (contd.) (c) Left atrial thr ombus (arrow) projecting into the left atrial cavity visualized at 60° from the lower esophageal window . (d) A laminated left atrial thr ombus (arrow) attached to the posterior wall of the left atrium visualized at 75°. (e) A left atrial appendage thr ombus (arrow) protruding into the body of the left atrium. (f) Left atrial thr ombus buried in the apex of the left atrial appendage. LA, left atrium; L V, left ventricle; LAA, left atrial appendage.

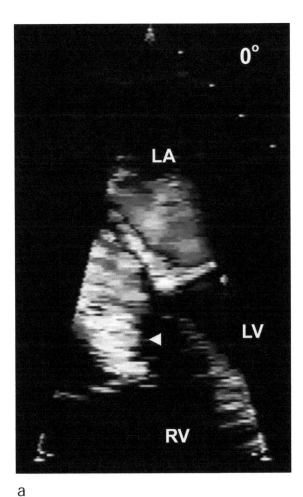

a

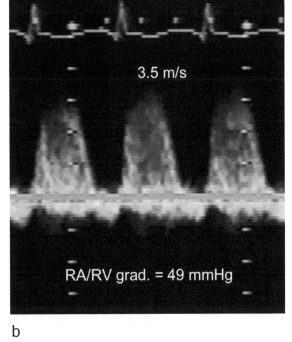

b

Case 3.11 Coexistent abnormalities associated with mitral stenosis. (a) T ricuspid regurgitation demonstrated by color flow Dopple . (b) Continuous wave Doppler guided by the color flow egurgitant jet in (a). The maximum velocity r ecorded is gr eater than 3 m/sec, consistent with pulmonar y hypertension. (c) Atrial septal aneur ysm (arrow).

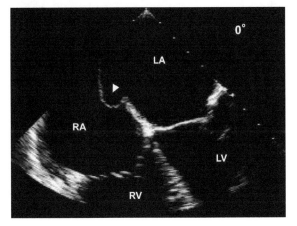

c

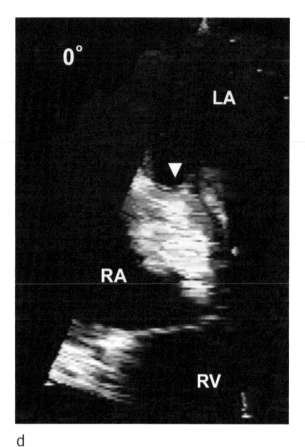

d

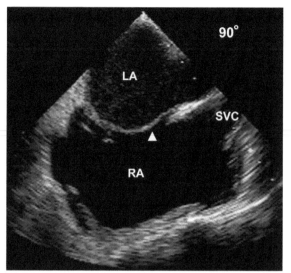

e

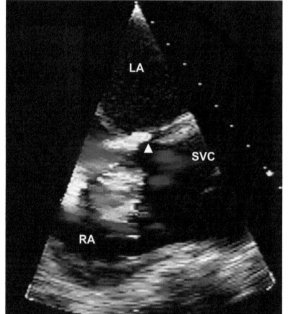

f

Case 3.11 (contd.) (d) Tricuspid regurgitation jet in the same patient wraps ar ound and outlines the atrial septal aneur ysm. (e) The bicaval view obtained at 90° in the upper esophageal position, visualizing the atrial septum. Thinning of the atrial septum is noted in the r egion of the foramen ovale. (f) Color flow Doppler in the same patient demonstrating a left to right shunt (ar row) in the r egion of the atrial septum. LA, left atrium; RA, right atrium; SVC, superior vena cava.

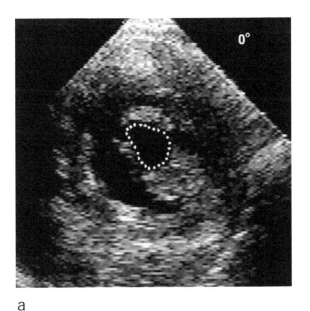

a

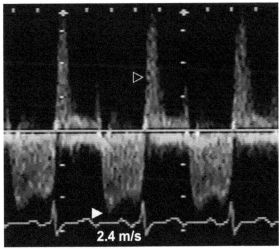

b

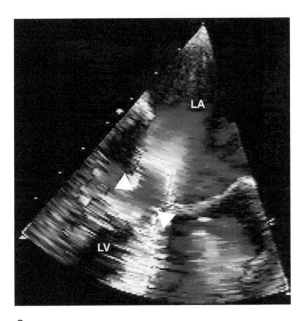

c

Case 3.12   Measurement of mitral valve ar ea in mitral stenosis. (a) Planimetr y of the valve orific (dotted circle) can be per formed in the shor t-axis views. Care must be taken in or der to measur e the valve area in the appr opriate plane. In addition, heavily calcified valves may p oduce blooming of the echo interface and obscur e the tr ue valve opening, overestimating the severity of stenosis.
(b) Continuous wave Doppler thr ough the mitral valve orifice. The maximum and mean gradients, as well as the pressur e half-time, may be measur ed with continuous wave Doppler. A newer method for calculating mitral valve ar eas utilizes the vena contracta of the stenotic color flow jet. With the ven contracta method, the mitral valve ar ea is calculated by measuring the width of the color flow jet at th level of the stenotic valve orifice (vena contracta) i one (c) or two perpendicular planes (d).

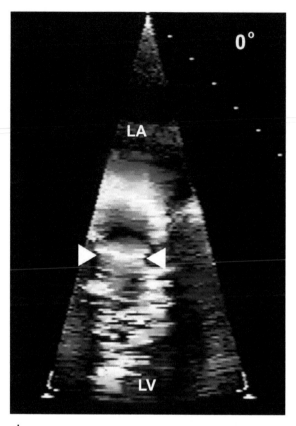

d

Case 3.12 (contd.)   (d). LA, left atrium; L V, left ventricle.

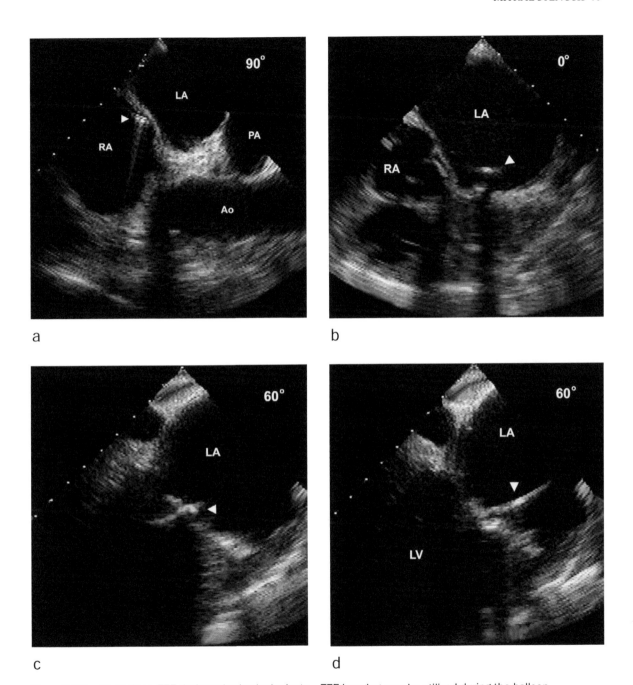

a

b

c

d

Case 3.13 Multiplane TEE during mitral valvuloplasty . TEE imaging may be utilized during the balloon valvuloplasty procedure for the positioning of catheters, puncturing the atrial septum, deter mining balloon sizing and evaluating valve opening and mitral r egurgitation after balloon dilatation. A clear advantage of multiplane TEE imaging is that it rapidly obtains multiple views with minimal pr obe manipulation. (a) View of the atrial septum and ideal catheter position (ar row) for crossing the atrial septum. The balloon catheter (arrow) is advanced into the left atrium (b), and acr oss the mitral valve (c) and (d). LA, left atrium; RA, right atrium; Ao, aor ta; LV, left ventricle; LAA, left atrial appendage.

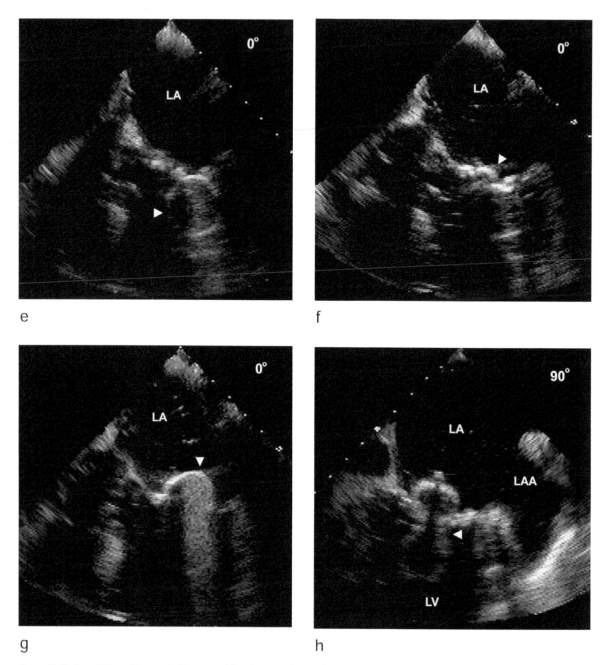

Case 3.13 (contd.) Proper balloon position (ar row) is confi med in the stenotic orifice (e) and (f). P ogressive inflation of the balloon at 0° and 90° (g–l).

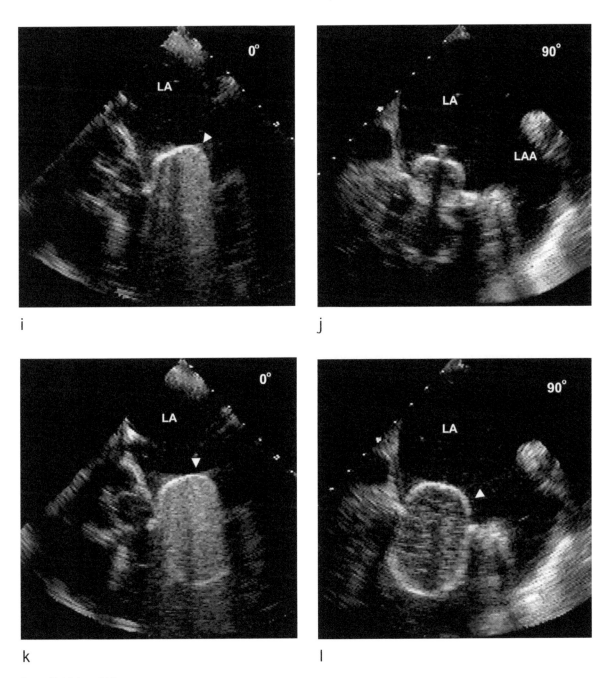

i

j

k

l

Case 3.13 (contd.)

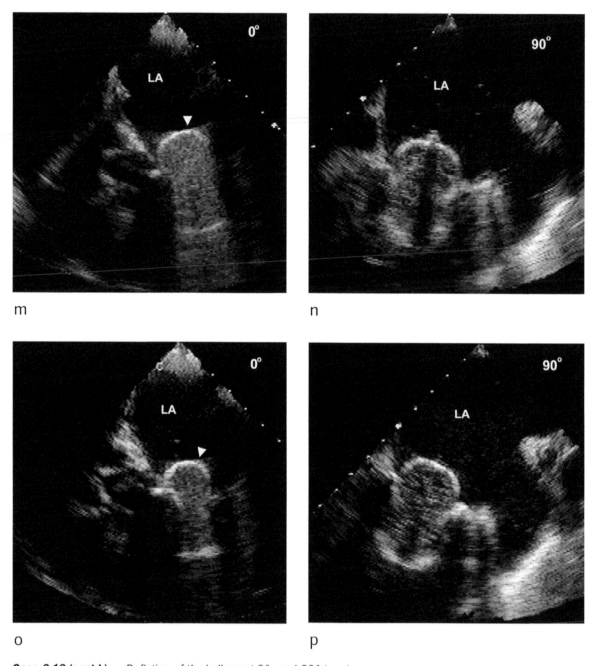

m

n

o

p

Case 3.13 (contd.)   Deflation of the balloon at 0° and 90° (m–r).

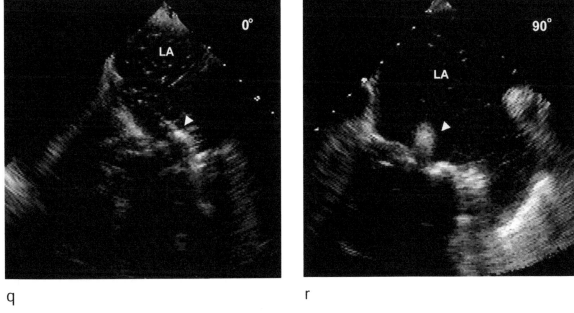

q   r

Case 3.13 (contd.)

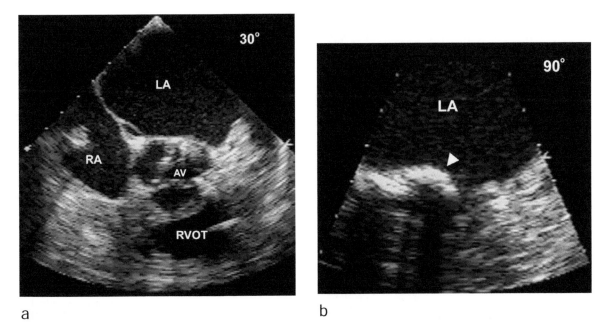

a   b

Case 3.14   Following the procedure, a TEE examination is per formed to deter mine the development of new mitral regurgitation and residual shunting acr oss the atrial septum. (a) Small defect in the atrial septum following the removal of the balloon catheter . (b) Mitral valve closur e, with point of leaflet coaption (a row). Heavy calcification is noted in the annular plane.

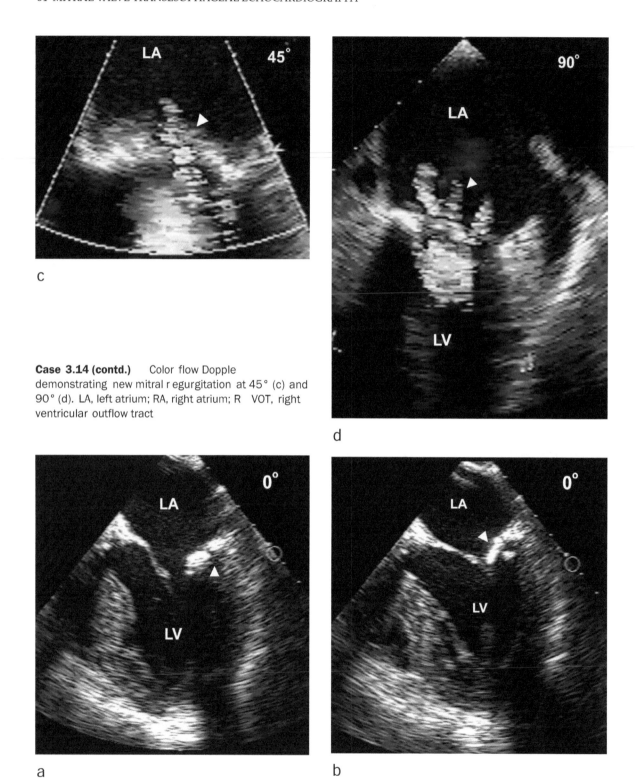

Case 3.14 (contd.) Color flow Dopple demonstrating new mitral r egurgitation at 45° (c) and 90° (d). LA, left atrium; RA, right atrium; R VOT, right ventricular outflow tract

Case 3.15 Mitral annular calcification. Calcification of the posterior mitral annulus (row) during diastole at 0° (a) and 90° (c), and during systole at 0° (b) and 90° (d).

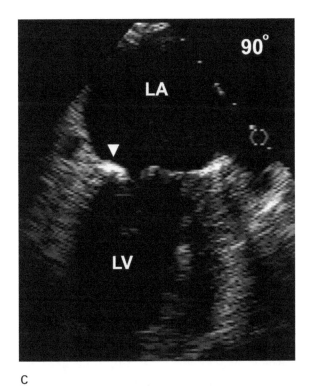

c

d

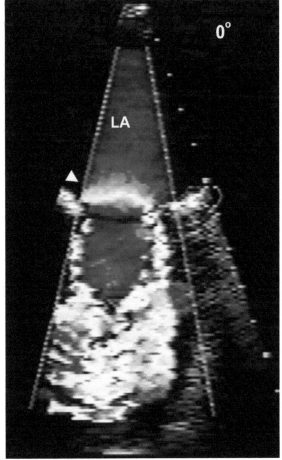

e

Case 3.15 (contd.) (e) Color flow Doppler th ough the mitral valve orifice during diastole demonstratin turbulence (arrow).

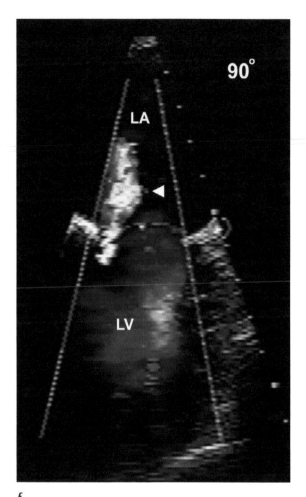

f

Case 3.15 (contd.) Mild mitral regurgitation (arrow) during systole (f). LA, left atrium; L V, left ventricle.

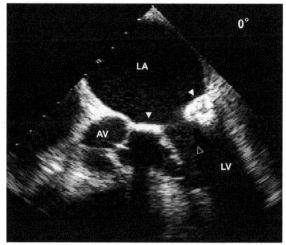

a

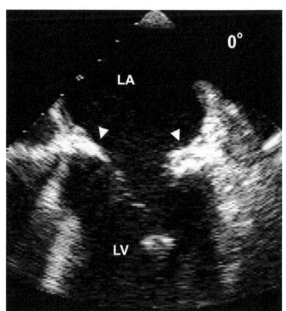

b

Case 3.16 Severe mitral annular calcification. (a) Severe calcification of the anterior and posterio annulus of the mitral valve (ar rows). Calcificatio extends in the posterior leaflet. (b) Adequate motio is exhibited by the anterior leaflet during diastole however, the posterior leaflet appears seve ely restricted.

c

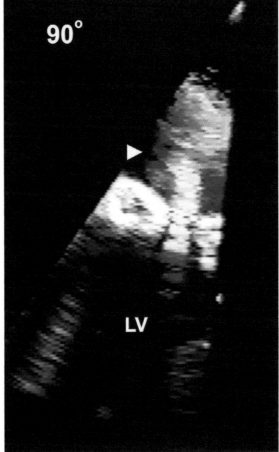

e

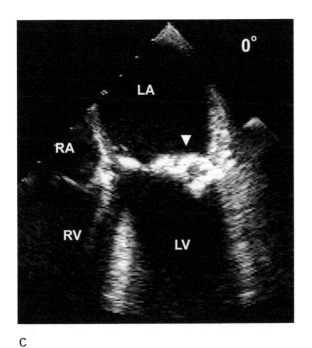

d

Case 3.16 (contd.)   (c) During systole only the annulus is visualized during valve closur e. (d) Color flow Doppler r ecorded during diastole demonstrates a high velocity turbulent jet (ar row), resembling the flow jet of mitral stenosis. (e) Color flow Dopple demonstrating a mitral r egurgitant jet (ar row) during systole. LA, left atrium.

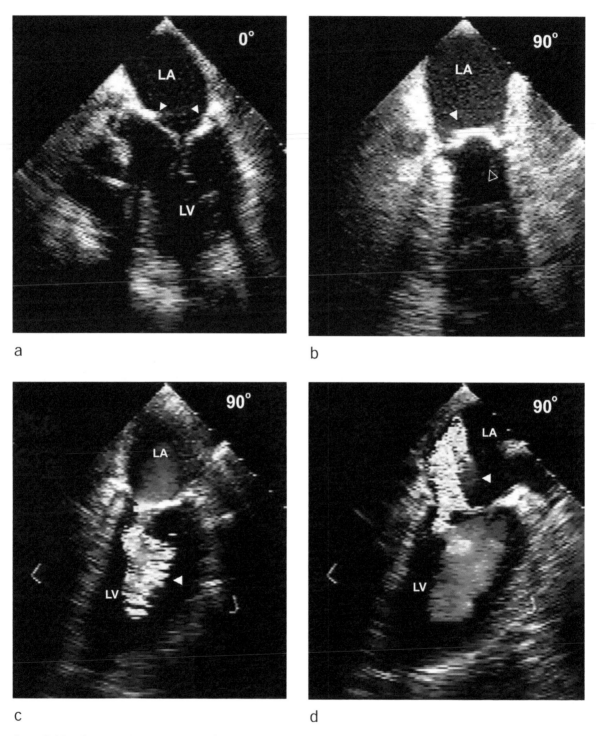

Case 3.17 Severe mitral annular calcification. (a) Seve e calcification of the anterior and posterior annulus o the mitral valve (ar rows). (b) During systole only the annulus is visualized during valve closur e. (c) Color flo Doppler recorded during diastole demonstrates a high velocity turbulent jet (ar row). (d) Color flow Dopple demonstrating mitral regurgitant jet (arrow) during systole.

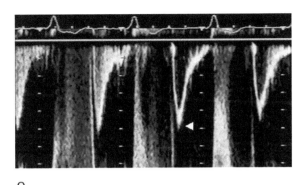

e

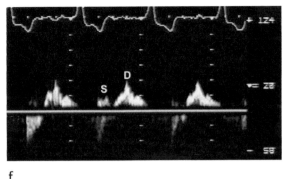

f

Case 3.17 (contd.) (e) Pulsed wave Doppler dir ected by the color flow jet demonstrating inc eased *e* wave velocity and mitral r egurgitation. (f) Pulsed wave Doppler of pulmonar y venous flow demonstrating flow eversal during systole suggesting significant mitral egurgitation. S, systolic flow; D, diastolic fl .

REFERENCES

1. Gordon SPF, Douglas PS, Come PC, Manning WJ. Two-dimensional and Doppler echocardiographic determinants of the natural history of mitral valve narrowing in patients with rheumatic mitral stenosis: implications for follow-up. J Am Coll Cardiol 1992;19:968–973.
2. Sagie A, Freitas N, Padial LR, et al. Doppler echocardiographic assessment of long-term progression of mitral stenosis in 103 patients: valve area and right heart disease. J Am Coll Cardiol 1996;28:472–479.
3. Stoddard MF, Prince CR, Ammash NM, Goad JL. Two-dimensional transesophageal echocardiographic determination of mitral valve area in adults with mitral stenosis. Am Heart J 1994;127:1348–1353.
4. Chen Y-T, Kan M-N, Chen J-S, et al. Contributing factors to formation of left atrial spontaneous echo contrast in mitral valvular disease. J Ultrasound Med 1990;91:51–55.
5. Daniel WG, Nellessen U, Shroder E, et al. Left atrial spontaneous echo contrast in mitral valve disease: an indicator for an increased thromboembolic risk. J Am Coll Cardiol 1988;11:1204–1211.
6. Yamamoto K, Ikeda U, Seino Y, et al. Coagulation activity is increased in the left atrium of patients with mitral stenosis. J Am Coll Cardiol 1995;25:107–112.
7. Roberts WC. Morphologic features of the normal and abnormal mitral valve. Am J Cardiol 1983;51:1005–1028.
8. Klein AL, Bailey AS, Cohen GI, et al. Effects of mitral stenosis on pulmonary venous flow as measured by Doppler transesophageal echocardiography. Am J Cardiol 1993;72:66–72.
9. Currie PJ, Hagle DJ, Seward JB, et al. Instantaneous pressure gradient: a simultaneous Doppler and dual catheter correlative study. J Am Coll Cardiol 1986;7:800–806.
10. Nishimura RA, Rihal CS, Tajik AJ, Holmes DR. Accurate measurement of the transmitral gradient in patients with mitral stenosis: a simultaneous catheterization and Doppler echocardiographic study. J Am Coll Cardiol 1994;24:152–158.
11. Kim WY, Bisgaard T, Nielsen SL, et al. Two-dimensional mitral flow velocity profiles in pig models using epicardial Doppler echocardiography. J Am Coll Cardiol 1994;24:532–545.
12. Pu M, Griffin BP, Vandervoort PM, et al. Intraoperative validation of mitral inflow determination by transesophageal echocardiography: comparison of single-plane, biplane and thermodilution techniques. J Am Coll Cardiol 1995;26:1047–1053.
13. Dahan M, Paillole C, Martin D, Gourgon R. Determinants of stroke volume response to exercise in patients with mitral stenosis: a Doppler echocardiographic study. J Am Coll Cardiol 1993;21:384–389.

14. Libanoff AJ, Rodbard S. Atrioventricular pressure half-time: measure of mitral valve orifice area. Circulation 1968;38:144–150.

15. Hatle L, Angelsen B, Tromsdal A. Noninvasive assessment of atrioventricular pressure half-time by Doppler ultrasound. Circulation 1979; 60:1096–1104.

16. Stoddard MF, Prince CR, Tuman WL, Wagner SG. Angle of incidence does not affect accuracy of mitral stenosis area calculation by pressure half-time: application to Doppler transesophageal echocardiography. Am Heart J 1994;127:1562–1572.

17. Triposkiadis F, Wooley CF, Boudoulas H. Mitral stenosis: left atrial dynamics reflect altered passive and active emptying. Am Heart J 1990;120:124–132.

18. Karp K, Teien D, Bjerle P, Eriksson P. Reassessment of valve area determinations in mitral stenosis by the pressure half-time method: impact of left ventricular stiffness and peak diastolic pressure difference. J Am Coll Cardiol 1989;13:594–899.

19. Braverman AC, Thomas JD, Lee RT. Doppler echocardiographic estimation of mitral valve area during changing hemodynamic conditions. Am J Cardiol 1991;68:1485–1490.

20. Moro E, Nicolosi GL, Zanuttini D, et al. Influence of aortic regurgitation on the assessment of the pressure half-time and derived mitral-valve area in patients with mitral stenosis. Eur Heart J 1988;9:1010–1017.

21. Flachskampf FA, Weyman AE, Gillam L, et al. Aortic regurgitation shortens Doppler pressure half-time in mitral stenosis: clinical evidence, in vitro simulation and theoretic analysis. J Am Coll Cardiol 1990;16:396–404.

22. Grayburn PA, Smith MD, Gurley J, et al. Effect of aortic regurgitation on the assessment of mitral valve orifice area by Doppler pressure half-time in mitral stenosis. Am J Cardiol 1987;60:322–326.

23. Bryg RJ, Williams GA, Labovitz AJ, et al. Effect of atrial fibrillation and mitral regurgitation on calculated mitral valve area in mitral stenosis. Am J Cardiol 1986;57:634–638.

24. Fredman CS, Pearson AC, Labovitz AJ, Kern MJ. Comparison of hemodynamic pressure half-time method and Gorlin formula with Doppler and echocardiographic determinations of mitral valve area in patients with combined mitral stenosis and regurgitation. Am Heart J 1990;119:121–129.

25. Wranne B, Ask P, Loyd D, Eng D. Analysis of different methods of assessing the stenotic mitral valve area with emphasis on the pressure gradient half-time concept. Am J Cardiol 1990; 66:614–620.

26. Knutsen KM, Bae EA, Sivertssen E, Grendahl H. Doppler ultrasound in mitral stenosis. Assessment of pressure gradient and atrioventricular pressure half-time. Acta Med Scand 1982;211:433–436.

27. Lloyd D, End D, Ask P, Wranne B. Pressure half-time does not always predict mitral valve area correctly. J Am Soc Echocardiogr 1988;1:313–321.

28. Nakatani S, Masuyama T, Kodama K, et al. Value and limitations of Doppler echocardiography in the quantification of stenotic mitral valve area: comparison of the pressure half-time and the continuity equation methods. Circulation 1988;77:78–85.

29. Faletra F, Pezzano A, Rossana F, et al. Measurement of mitral valve area in mitral stenosis: Four echocardiographic methods compared with direct measurement of anatomic orifices. J Am Coll Cardiol 1996;28:1190–1197.

30. Thomas JD, Wilkins GT, Choong CY, et al. Inaccuracy of mitral pressure half-time immediately after percutaneous mitral valvotomy. Dependence on transmitral gradient and left atrial and ventricular compliance. Circulation 1988;78:980–993.

31. Chen C, Schneider B, Koschyk D, et al. Biplane transesophageal color Doppler echocardiography for assessment of mitral valve area with mitral inflow jet widths. J Am Soc Echocardiogr 1995;8:121–131.

32. Wilkins GT, Weyman AE, Abascal VM, et al. Percutaneous balloon dilatation of the mitral valve: an analysis of echocardiographic variables related to outcome and the mechanism of dilatation. Br Heart J 1988;60:299–308.

33. Condit JR, Benoit SB, Gottdiener JS. Transesophageal echocardiography is of no additional diagnostic value to transthoracic echocardiography in the evaluation of mitral stenosis for balloon mitral valvuloplasty. Circulation 1993;88:I–351.

34. Jaarsma W, Visser CA, Suttorp MJ, et al. Transesophageal echocardiography during percutaneous balloon mitral valvuloplasty. J Am Soc Echocardiogr 1989;2:380–385.

35. Cormier B, Vahanian A, Michel P-L, et al. The contribution of transesophageal echocardiography in the ultrasound assessment of percutaneous mitral valvuloplasty (abstr). J Am Coll Cardiol 1989;13:51–A.

36. Otto CM, Davis KB, Holmes DR, et al. Methodologic issues in clinical evaluation of stenosis severity in adults undergoing aortic or mitral balloon valvuloplasty. Am J Cardiol 1992;69:1607–1616.

37. Casale PN, Whitlow P, Currie PJ, Stewart WJ. Transesophageal echocardiography in percutaneous balloon valvuloplasty for mitral stenosis. Cleve Clin J Med 1989;56:597–600.

38. Lung B, Cormier B, Ducimetiere P, et al. Immediate results of percutaneous mitral commissurotomy. A predictive model on a series of 1514 patients. Circulation 1996;94:2124–2130.

39. Lung B, Cormier B, Ducimetiere P, et al. Functional results 5 years after successful percutaneous mitral commissurotomy in a series of 528 patients and analysis of predictive factors. J Am Coll Cardiol 1996;27:407–414.

40. Orange SE, Kawanishi DT, Lopez BM, et al. Actuarial outcome after catheter balloon commissurotomy in patients with mitral stenosis. Circulation 1997;95:382–389.

41. Manning WJ, Reis GJ, Douglas PS. Use of transesophageal echocardiography to detect left atrial thrombi before percutaneous balloon dilatation of the mitral valve: a prospective study. Br Heart J 1992;67:170–173.

42. Kronzon I, Tunick PA, Glassman E, et al. Transesophageal echocardiography to detect atrial clots in candidates for percutaneous transseptal mitral balloon valvuloplasty. J Am Coll Cardiol 1990;16:1320–1322.

43. Orme EC, Wray RB, Mason JW. Balloon mitral valvuloplasty via retrograde left atrial catheterization. Am Heart J 1989;117:680–683.

44. Abascal VM, Wilkins GT, Choong CY, et al. Mitral regurgitation after percutaneous balloon mitral valvuloplasty in adults: evaluation by pulsed Doppler echocardiography. J Am Coll Cardiol 1988;11:257–263.

45. Mahan EF III, Ballal RS, Nanda NC. Mitral valve tear complicating percutaneous valvuloplasty: diagnosis by transesophageal Doppler color flow mapping. Am Heart J 1991;122:238–241.

46. O'Shea JP, Abascal VM, Wilkins GT, et al. Unusual sequelae after percutaneous mitral valvuloplasty: a Doppler echocardiographic study. J Am Coll Cardiol 1992;19:186–191.

47. Reid CL, McKay CR, Chandraratna PAN, et al. Mechanisms of increase in mitral valve area and influence of anatomic features in double-balloon, catheter balloon valvuloplasty in adults with rheumatic mitral stenosis: a Doppler and two-dimensional echocardiographic study. Circulation 1987;76:628–636.

48. Marwick TH, Torelli J, Obarski T, et al. Assessment of the mitral valve splitability score by transthoracic and transesophageal echocardiography. Am J Cardiol 1994;22:194A.

49. Levin TN, Feldman T, Balasia B, et al. Commissural morphology to predict outcome after balloon mitral valvotomy. Circulation 1993;88:I–35.

50. Cannan CR, Nishimura RA, Reeder GS, et al. Echocardiographic assessment of commissural calcium: a simple predictor of outcome after percutaneous mitral balloon valvotomy. J Am Coll Cardiol 1997;29:175–180.

51. Jolly N, Arora R, Mohan J, Khalilullah M. Pulmonary venous flow dynamics before and after balloon mitral valvuloplasty as determined by transesophageal Doppler echocardiography. Am J Cardiol 1992;70:780–784.

52. Farhat MB, Boussadia H, Gandjbakhch I, et al. Closed versus open mitral commissurotomy in pure noncalcific mitral stenosis: Hemodynamic studies before and after operation. J Thorac Cardiovasc Surg 1990;99:639–644.

53. Lau K-W, Ding Z-P, Hung J-S. Percutaneous transvenous mitral commissurotomy versus surgical commissurotomy in the treatment of mitral stenosis. Clin Cardiol 1997;20:99–106.

54. Vasan RS, Shrivastava S, Kumar MV. Value and limitations of Doppler echocardiographic determination of mitral valve area in Lutembacher syndrome. J Am Coll Cardiol 1992;20:1362–1370.

55. Yoshida K, Yoshikawa J, Akasaka T, et al. Assessment of left-to-right atrial shunting after

percutaneous mitral valvuloplasty by transesophageal color Doppler flow-mapping. Circulation 1989;80:1521–1526.

56. Kronzon I, Tunick PA, Goldfarb A, et al. Echocardiographic and hemodynamic characteristics of atrial septal defects created by percutaneous valvuloplasty. J Am Soc Echocardiogr 1990;3:64–71.

57. Palacios IF, Tuzcu ME, Weyman AE, Newell JB, Block PC. Clinical follow-up of patients undergoing percutaneous mitral balloon valvotomy. Circulation 1995;91:671–676.

4

Mitral Regurgitation

Classification of mitral r egurgitation • Quantification of mitral r egurgitation • Echocardiographic diagnosis of mitral r egurgitation • Diastolic mitral regurgitation • Estimation of the severity of mitral regurgitation • Prediction of ventricular function after sur gical correction • Papillary muscle dysfunction • Mitral annular calcificatio

Mitral regurgitation is a very complex disease and has been poorly understood in the past. Unlike mitral stenosis, for which the cause is almost always rheumatic disease resulting in predictable mitral valve lesions, there are many disease processes that may render a mitral valve incompetent (Table 4.1).[1] With the eradication of rheumatic disease in most parts of the world, degenerative valve disease, bacterial and non-bacterial endocarditis, congenital heart disease, and diseases of the left ventricle including ischemia and cardiomyopathy, are increasingly implicated as the cause of mitral regurgitation. In addition, each disease process may cause a variety of mitral lesions that can singly or in combination adversely affect the structural integrity of the mitral valve apparatus.

Table 4.1 Etiology of mitral r egurgitation	
n = 520	%
Degenerative	63
Ischemic	14
Rheumatic	13
Endocarditis	6
Congenital	4

Acute or chronic mitral regurgitation is common in cardiac patients. The natural history of mitral insufficiency is highly variable and depends on the etiology and the rate of progression of mitral lesions in the individual patient. Survival is largely dependent on the rate of deterioration of left ventricular function and the development of other co-morbid factors.[2] Recently, Ling and colleagues[3,4] have described the natural history of mitral regurgitation due to flail mitral leaflets. Patients with flail mitral leaflets that are managed medically have a 6.3% yearly mortality, and early surgical correction reduces mortality by almost 70%.

In the past, mitral valve replacement was the only option for treating patients with severe symptoms who failed medical therapy. Irrespective of the cause, mitral valve replacement has not been a panacea for the treatment of mitral regurgitation, because of high morbidity and mortality.[5] Despite the progress made in other open-heart procedures, significant improvement in survival for patients with mitral regurgitation and mitral valve replacement has not occurred. Valvular reconstructive techniques have been developed to treat mitral regurgitation, stemming from the need to avoid anticoagulation and the relatively high cost of mitral valve replacement.[6–9]

Enthusiasm for mitral valve repair has quickly grown because of a low operative risk and excellent short-term and long-term results, without the need for anticoagulation. With the introduction and success of mitral valve reconstructive techniques, patients with severe mitral regurgitation are now being considered as surgical candidates at a younger age, before they develop symptoms and have irreversible cardiac dysfunction. It is not a coincidence that many of the strides made in better appreciating and treating mitral disease, particularly regurgitation, have paralleled developments and improvements in echocardiographic technology. As image resolution and Doppler techniques have improved, especially with the introduction of transesophageal echocardiography, mitral valve anatomy and function can be visualized in detail.

Mitral regurgitation can result from primary disease in any one of the component parts of the mitral valve leaflets or subvalvular apparatus.[1] Rheumatic disease, bacterial endocarditis, non-bacterial endocarditis (lupus erythematosus), myxomatous degeneration, fibroelastic deficiency, or trauma, may all damage the mitral leaflets, elongate or rupture the chordae tendineae. The papillary muscles may malfunction transiently or permanently secondary to ischemia, infarction, or infiltrative disease. The mitral valve annulus may dilate secondary to ventricular enlargement, or calcify secondary to degenerative disease, preventing normal annular motion. Mitral regurgitation may also result from the disruption of the valvular structures, which may occur with increased muscle mass or hypertrophy commonly associated with increased ventricular pressures during systole, such as in aortic stenosis and obstructive hypertrophic cardiomyopathy. In dilated cardiomyopathy, mitral regurgitation may result from changes in left ventricular cavity shape, with the ventricle becoming more spherical than ellipsoid. Distorted ventricular geometry produces multiple abnormalities in mitral architecture. The papillary muscles are displaced along the long axis of the heart so they are further apart than normal. Since there is no change in chordae tendineae length, leaflet motion is altered and the leaflets are unable to coapt normally.

Transesophageal echocardiography has enabled us to:

- Establish the presence of mitral regurgitation
- Determine the patho-etiology of mitral regurgitation
- Quantify the severity of mitral regurgitation
- Determine the severity of left ventricular dysfunction and pulmonary hypertension
- Make preoperative and postoperative evaluations of mitral valve surgery.

To provide a consistent and logical framework for defining the pathology of mitral regurgitation, it is helpful to describe mitral valve lesions with echocardiography on the basis of a functional approach rather than specifically describing each particular abnormality.

CLASSIFICATION OF MITRAL REGURGITATION

Abnormal structural integrity of the mitral valve can easily be categorized according to the classification described by Carpentier,[6] defining the leaflet motion responsible for the lack of leaflet approximation during systole. Mitral valve motion in mitral regurgitation may be simply and logically described as: type I, normal valve mobility; type II, increased leaflet mobility; and type III, restricted valve mobility (Figure 4.1). In conjunction with this classification, specifics of mitral anatomy can be defined echocardiographically or visually at the time of surgery to elucidate further the cause of mitral insufficiency (Table 4.2). Adopting this classification of mitral regurgitation helps establish effective communication between the echocardiographer and the surgeon, helping to define the surgical methods necessary for a successful repair.

Many studies comparing the results of transesophageal echocardiography, transthoracic echocardiography, and epicardial echocardiography with surgical valve analysis have used this functional classification of mitral valve disease. The ESMIR group[10] recently reported that the correct prediction of surgical strategy in mitral regurgitation was 86% with transthoracic

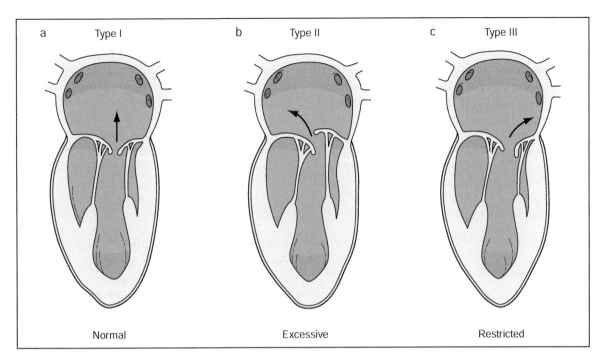

Fig. 4.1 Mitral valve motion in mitral r egurgitation has been classified by Carpentier and colleagues int three groups. This is a useful method for describing the abnor mality responsible for mitral r egurgitation, often alluding to the pathology , as well as in communicating mitral valve str uctural abnormalities to the sur geon in the operating r oom. Mitral valve motion is described accor ding to the principal abnor mality noted, since mitral dysfunction is often caused by coexisting abnor malities. (a) Type I mitral r egurgitation results from annular dilatation. (b) Type II mitral r egurgitation results from excessive leaflet motion during closu e producing prolapse during diastole. (c) Type III mitral r egurgitation is pr oduced by r estrictive motion of one or both leaflets

Table 4.2	Carpentier's functional classification of mitral valve diseas
Type	*Description*
Type I **Normal leaflet motio**	Annular dilatation Leaflet perforation Cleft leafle
Type II **Leaflet prolapse**	Chordal rupture Chordal elongation Papillary muscle r upture Papillary muscle elongation
Type III **Restricted leaflet motio**	Commissur e fusion or thickening Chordal fusion or thickening RWMA/LV aneur ysm

echocardiography, and 89% with monoplane transesophageal echocardiography. These findings are similar to those reported by Stewart and colleagues,[11] who accurately defined mitral regurgitation by epicardial and transesophageal echocardiography. Two-dimensional imaging and Doppler accurately diagnosed 93% of surgical patients with posterior leaflet prolapse or flail, 94% of anterior leaflet prolapse or flail, 44% of bileaflet prolapse or flail, 75% of papillary muscle elongation or rupture, 91% of restricted leaflet motion or rheumatic thickening, 72% of ventricular-annular dilation, and 62% of leaflet perforation or cleft.

Type I valve motion

In type I mitral regurgitation, the valve motion is normal, and most of the regurgitation is produced by annular dilatation. Although the valve leaflets are normal they are not long enough to adequately produce the required surface area for approximation of the rough edges of both leaflets. Therefore regurgitation is produced from inadequate sealing of the leaflets during systole. Other causes of type I mitral regurgitation include discrete leaflet perforation and cleft mitral valve.

Annular dilatation usually occurs as a result of an enlarging left ventricle (ventriculo-annular dilatation).[12–15] Studies of the mitral annulus have shown it to be dynamic rather than a fixed structure, normally changing its orifice shape and chamber dimensions during systole and diastole. Most of the motion in the annulus occurs in its posterior circumference situated in the atrioventricular groove. Histologically, the posterior aspect of the annulus is composed of loose connective tissue, devoid of collagen, since the collagen fibers that project posteriorly from the trigones taper and thin out before reaching the entire circumference of the annulus. Therefore the posterior region is the weakest and most vulnerable aspect of the annulus when stretching under tension. With excessive dilatation of the ventricle, the mitral annulus enlarges or 'gives' in the posterior aspect, allowing the annulus to assume a more geometrically circular shape,

rather than the normal D shape during systole. This dilatation means that the anterior leaflet does not approximate to the posterior leaflet on the basis of a fixed leaflet length. The chordae tendineae to the posterior leaflet may be slightly elongated and assume a more oblique angle, rather than having their normal parallel orientation, thus tethering the posterior leaflet and not allowing the necessary motion for both leaflets to coapt properly. With transesophageal echocardiography, the annulus appears enlarged with normal leaflet motion. The loss of surface area for coaptation of the leaflets is readily appreciated in the lower esophageal position, when imaging the mitral level from the four-chamber and two-chamber views obtained from 0° to 135°. In addition to evaluating leaflet approximation with these views, a ratio of the length of the annular ring diameter can be compared with the height of the anterior leaflet – annular dilatation exists with ratios less than 0.9. Imaging from the transgastric position with the transducer at 0°, the mitral annulus has a D shape in normal patients and a circular shape when dilated (see Figure 2.21). The posteromedial commissure is directly at the top of the image sector, and the anterolateral commissure is at the bottom of the screen. The anterior leaflet appears to the left, next to the septum, and is geometrically convex. The posterior leaflet appears to the right and is geometrically concave. The pattern of leaflet opening and closing when annular dilatation occurs is readily distinguishable from normal when visualizing the valve *en face* by transesophageal echocardiography in the horizontal transgastric view. Normally during systole, the line of leaflet approximation or closure illustrates a "smile" shape which is distorted when dilatation occurs. Opening is more circular in shape, as described above. The posterior position of the line of closure should be easily appreciated relative to the center of the valve plane, which shifts centrally with dilatation. Color flow Doppler imaging from the lower esophageal position, in the horizontal or longitudinal views of the left heart, usually helps to show any centrally projected regurgitant jet(s) into the left atrium.

Papillary muscle dysfunction has been noted in patients with dilated and poorly contracting left ventricles.[16] Papillary-muscle abnormalities have also been described in cardiomyopathic diseases involving the left ventricle. There is significant elongation and thinning of papillary muscle in idiopathic dilated cardiomyopathy. Left ventricular enlargement tends to alter the spatial relation between the papillary muscles rather than affecting their motion. With significant dilatation, the papillary muscles are pulled further into the left ventricular cavity, producing incompetence of the mitral valve by affecting the apposition of the leaflets during systolic closure.

In cases of cleft mitral valve or leaflet perforation, mitral valve leaflet opening and closing are normal and the specific defect may not be readily apparent. Cleft mitral valves are occasionally observed in the adult as an isolated finding not associated with atrioventricular canal defects.[17–20] The clefts may be partial or complete, and when complete, may be confused with an accessory leaflet or an anatomic tricuspid leaflet. Associated with the cleft deformity in the leaflet are accessory chordae, which insert into the margins of the cleft and originate from the ventricular septum. The cleft is usually found in the anterior leaflet and, viewing the valve *en face* in short axis, appears as a line of opening perpendicular to the usual line of leaflet closure during diastole. This finding may be confused with scalloping of the leaflet. In transverse or longitudinal long axis views, the cleft in the leaflet can be confused with the normal orifice opening during diastole or mild prolapse with billowing during systole, if careful scanning is not performed. Another characteristic of a cleft leaflet that distinguishes it from a prolapsed leaflet, is that there is minor leaflet thickening in comparison to that seen in mitral valve prolapse from myxomatous degeneration. When scanning between 0° and 135°, the cleft should be distinguishable from the normal orifice by demonstrating both openings and by the fact that the cleft is usually eccentric to the normal location of the orifice in respective views. Color Doppler is usually very helpful in demonstrating systolic and diastolic turbulent high-velocity flow through the cleft orifice, which is readily distinguishable from normal.

Leaflet perforations usually occur as a result of trauma (wrongly placed catheters) or as a common consequence of bacterial endocarditis. The cause is usually apparent from the patient's clinical history and not readily distinguishable on echocardiography, unless obvious vegetation is present. Leaflet perforations may occur on either leaflet, and may or may not be involved with the line of leaflet closure. Leaflet perforations are visualized echocardiographically in long-axis views as small areas of leaflet prolapse, or with color Doppler as high velocity jets in non-suspect areas of the mitral valve plane with no obvious defect.

Type II valve motion

Type II motion is due to leaflet prolapse and is present when the free edge of either leaflet overrides the annular plane and orifice during systole, preventing coaptation of the leaflets.[21–28] This is different from billowing or floppy mitral leaflets, in which excessive leaflet tissue protrudes or prolapses beyond the annular plane into the left atrium, with the point of leaflet coaptation below the plane of annulus (Figure 4.2). It is not unusual, however, to observe billowing valve leaflets associated with prolapse, causing lack of apposition of the leaflets. This type of valve motion is frequently produced by degeneration of the valve structures from chronic rheumatic disease; myxomatous degeneration; fibroelastic deficiency; or a combination of any of these. The hallmark of degenerative valve disease is excessive leaflet tissue, shown echocardiographically by altered leaflet thickening and increased length, resulting in redundant leaflet motion.[27] With the progression of degenerative disease, isolated annular dilatation[22] without ventricular enlargement can result with subsequent mitral annular calcification. Type II motion may also be caused by isolated chordal or papillary muscle elongation and/or rupture.[29–34]

Mitral valve prolapse is now a well-recognized cause of mitral regurgitation, largely due

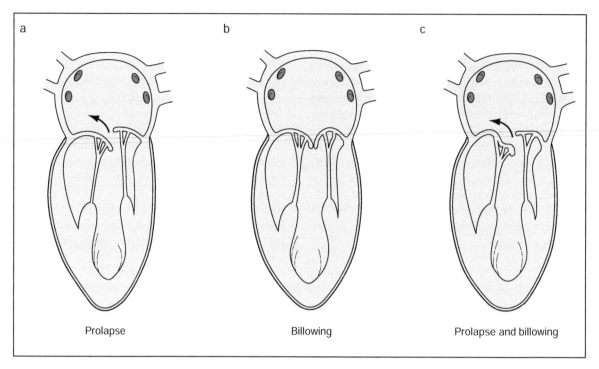

Fig. 4.2 Diagram demonstrating mitral valve motion with pr olapse. Mitral valve pr olapse is pr oduced when the mitral valve apparatus allows for excessive leaflet motion during diastole p omoting the lack of leafle coaptation during closur e. Billowing of the leaflet due to excessive tissue p oduces protrusion of the body of the leaflet into the left atrium during diastole without a fecting leaflet closu e. Mitral valve pr olapse of myxomatous origin often pr oduces prolapse and billowing of the mitral apparatus. It is impor tant to distinguish true prolapse from billowing in the diagnosis of mitral r egurgitation, especially when defining valvula abnormalities prior to mitral valve r epair.

to improvements in echocardiography. In the early history of mitral valve prolapse, diagnosis was difficult because of the relatively poor imaging resolution of available echocardiographic equipment. With transthoracic echocardiography, the mitral valve depth is usually out of the range for good visualization of the leaflets. Pronounced billowing of the leaflets is commonly misdiagnosed as prolapse with transthoracic imaging, even under multiple views. Excellent images are necessary to be sure which leaflet is prolapsing. Coexisting abnormalities, such as elongated chordae and ruptured small chords, can be very difficult to detect if examination is not thorough and meticulous. A definitive diagnosis can usually be made with transesophageal echocardiographic imaging from the esophagus under

higher imaging frequencies. It is paramount, however, even with transesophageal echocardiographic imaging, that a systematic approach be followed in analyzing the full mitral valve unit in patients with prolapse, to follow the progression of disease, or to give the cardiac surgeon the necessary information for a successful repair when the disease has reached that stage.

The transgastric and deep transgastric views are ideal for assessing the subvalvular apparatus in mitral valve prolapse, and for establishing continuity for the papillary muscles, chordae tendineae, and valve leaflets (see Figures 2.16–2.19, 2.21). The papillary muscles and chordae tendineae should be scanned from 0° to 135° in both views to identify focal areas of echogenicity, indicating fibrosis or calcific lesions, representing friction-type lesions when either are elongated, redundant, or displaced. Areas with high frequency or vibratory movement in the chordae or papillary muscles during the cardiac cycle suggest rupture of the supporting apparatus. In the deep transgastric views, sweeping from 0° to 45°, the papillary muscles are imaged obliquely, but the chordal apparatus is well visualized. Elongation and redundancy of the chordae may be noted by comparing chordal length among the chordal groups – in many cases significant bowing of the chordae can be seen during the cardiac cycle.

The four-chamber and two-chamber left ventricular views from the lower and mid-esophageal positions from 0° to 110° enable the best evaluation of the valve leaflets. The leaflets are easily identified as anterior and posterior in relation to the commissures. In the four-chamber, view slowly withdrawing the scope, the posterior commissural area is shown from the lower esophageal position; the mid-portion of the leaflets is seen in the mid-esophagus position, and the anterior commissural area in the upper esophageal position. Rotating the transducer from 0° to 90° allows the leaflets to be imaged together, or in full-length individual cuts. The mitral annular plane should be constructed mentally, and leaflet motion for each segment of the anterior and posterior leaflets in relation to the ventricular side of the annulus should be labeled as excessive, normal, or restricted. By contrast with transthoracic echocardiography, billowing or prolapse of the leaflet margins is distinguishable using the many views obtained with multiplane transesophageal echocardiography. At about 45° to 90°, the mitral leaflets are imaged parallel to the line of closure. Each leaflet will appear as a continuous echocardiographic line traversing the annular plane. With subtle medial or lateral rotation of the probe, either the anterior or posterior leaflet will be visualized. The posterior leaflet will be essentially linear with minor bulging illustrating the three scallops. The anterior leaflet will appear more curvilinear in the center of the valve plane, with the lateral and medial scallops of the posterior leaflet on either side of the anterior leaflet – this will be especially apparent when the leaflets are open during diastole. In this view, prolapse or flail of the opposite leaflet will usually appear as a smaller, free linear or curvilinear echo, superior to the annulus and the other leaflet on the atrial side. Flail segments are easily noted and are represented by the leaflet overriding the other leaflet in the frontal planes, generally with short segments of the ruptured chorda attached, showing either high-frequency movement or actual prolapse back and forth between the atrial and ventricular cavities during the cardiac cycle. Leaflet thickness[35] may also be assessed in this view. In degenerative mitral-valve prolapse the leaflets may thicken in diastole when they are slack and unstressed as the result of leaflet redundancy, overlap, prominent interchordal hooding, and the presence of excessive tissue. In systole, when the leaflets are under tension from ventricular forces, the leaflets appear thinner. Leaflet thickness can be assessed by measuring the percentage change in leaflet width from diastole to systole, which is normally 22–34%. In patients with mitral valve prolapse, the percentage change in leaflet thickness from diastole to systole averages 54–62%.

In all these views, the direction of the regurgitant jet(s) is illustrated using color Doppler. The long-axis planes are ideal for determining which leaflet is involved, although the short axis planes are better for determining the specific segment of the abnormal leaflet.[11] The number of jets and their origin should be noted. Careful scanning will prevent the improper labeling of a single jet as multiple when tangentially cut out of plane. In large jets that fill the left atrium, it may be necessary to decrease the color and image gain so as to correctly identify the origin of the jet. The origin should be described as anterior/posterior (i.e. towards one of the two commissures), or central (i.e. having a central location along the line of leaflet coaptation during closure), or emanating from outside of the plane. Color Doppler flow mapping may also be helpful to define prolapsing leaflet tissue, showing an eccentric regurgitant flow jet in the opposite direction of the leaflet that is prolapsing.[36] With degenerative prolapse of the anterior leaflet, the regurgitant jet is directed posteriorly, and with posterior leaflet prolapse the regurgitant jet is directed anteriorly. By contrast, rheumatic prolapse results in the predominant fibrosis of one leaflet – the normal leaflet protrudes above the abnormal one, and the regurgitant jet is directed toward it. When there is bi-leaflet rheumatic or degenerative disease involvement producing prolapse of both leaflets, the jet is directed centrally into the left atrium, or is slightly eccentric if one leaflet prolapses more than the other. There may be many jets, showing that there are multiple discrete areas that do not approximate properly. It is important to identify the presence of multiple jets in more than one view.

It is also possible to derive the pathological cause of prolapse echocardiographically by noting mitral lesion patterns common to specific disease states. In rheumatic prolapse, the predominant lesion in most cases is isolated prolapse of the anterior leaflet secondary to elongated or ruptured chordae tendineae or papillary muscles. Both leaflets may be slightly thickened or retracted with shortening and fusion of the chords, and only a few show annular dilatation.[37–39] Myxomatous degeneration is characterized by excessive tissue on all the scallops of the posterior leaflet.[40,41] When there is associated anterior leaflet prolapse, it is most prominent in the posteromedial half of the leaflet (A2, A3). Myxomatous degeneration is frequently observed in younger patients, and as the disease progresses both leaflets appear thickened, with extensive hooding of the rough zone. Chordae to both leaflets elongate and appear thickened and redundant. Excessive tissue of the posterior leaflet tends to push the anterior leaflet and line of closure forward, which in small ventricles narrows the aorto-mitral angle, to produce systolic anterior motion (SAM) of the valve leaflets and chordal apparatus. Patients with fibroelastic deficiency and prolapse have thinner leaflets and lack of billowing. Prolapse is usually limited to the central scallop (P2) of the posterior leaflet with some degree of annular dilatation. The chordae appear thinner but redundant, with or without

minor ruptures, and the left ventricle is commonly hypertrophic. Prolapse of ischemic origin usually results in thickening and increased echogenicity of the chordae tendineae and papillary muscles. Normal-appearing leaflets are occasionally seen, with ruptured chordae near the leaflet edge insertion points.

Papillary muscle rupture, either partial or complete, is an uncommon complication of acute myocardial infarction, and is associated with high mortality.[42–46] There is a significant increase in the incidence of posteromedial papillary muscle rupture compared with anterolateral muscle rupture in myocardial infarction. Rupture may occur near the head of the papillary muscle partially involving the chordal attachments. Rupture of the whole muscle results in complete detachment of the papillary muscle from the ventricular myocardium, producing a flail mitral leaflet. Regional wall motion abnormalities are usually detected in the myocardium subjacent to the papillary muscle, and are hypokinetic, rather than akinetic or dyskinetic as might be expected. Transthoracic echocardiography imaging is usually adequate for the diagnosis of papillary muscle rupture, but transesophageal echocardiography may be required in patients with poor acoustic windows in cases of partial rupture, or when the ruptured papillary muscle head does not prolapse into the left atrium. Transesophageal echocardiography will also reveal papillary muscle hemorrhage[47,48] in acute mitral regurgitation, showing a markedly irregular echolucency in a papillary muscle with ventricular systolic thinning of the myocardium, preventing coaptation of the mitral leaflets.

Transesophageal echocardiography illustrates the anatomical abnormalities of papillary muscle rupture with more certainty than transthoracic echocardiography, but both techniques adequately define abnormal regional wall motion involvement, and the use of Doppler with either technique defines the severity of the resultant mitral regurgitation. Moursi and colleagues[46] have shown that an accurate diagnosis of ruptured papillary muscle can be made with biplane or multiplane transesophageal echocardiography. In 90% of their patients, the ruptured papillary muscle head showed relatively large-amplitude erratic motion in the left ventricular cavity even when the ruptured muscle did not prolapse into the left atrium. In 70% of the patients the residual papillary muscle still attached to the ventricular wall also showed a prominent but less erratic motion than the free papillary muscle head portion. From these findings, transesophageal echocardiography reliably detected all patients with papillary muscle rupture in a retrospective analysis.

When there is partial rupture of the papillary muscle, the involved leaflet still appears flail, but the muscle does not prolapse into the left atrium. Careful inspection of the papillary muscle in multiple planes usually shows partial attachment of the papillary muscle to the ventricular myocardium. Prominent mitral leaflet prolapse occurs in all patients with papillary muscle rupture. Even though each leaflet receives support from both papillary muscles, one leaflet is usually observed to prolapse more than the other. When the pulmonary veins are interrogated with Doppler, systolic flow reversal is recorded. With color Doppler, the mitral regurgitant jet usually fills the entire atrium.

Type III valve motion

Type III motion is shown by restricted leaflet motion in which a leaflet does not open normally during diastole. Echocardiographically, it appears that only one leaflet is moving while the other leaflet is fixed in a diastolic position, producing lack of coaptation (see Figure 2.21). This type of leaflet motion may result from commissural fusion or thickening, from chordal fusion or thickening, or, more commonly, from left ventricular infarction with or without aneurysm formation. As with type II motion, annular dilatation may be present, since one leaflet may be restricted and the other leaflet prolapsing.

Even though mitral regurgitation has been readily attributed to ischemic papillary muscle dysfunction, the functional consequence of mitral regurgitation secondary to isolated ischemic papillary muscle dysfunction is unclear.[49–51] Regional wall motion abnormalities of the left ventricle are frequently observed in patients with papillary muscle dysfunction. It has been suggested that papillary muscle motion or function should be assessed together with the motion of the left ventricular wall subjacent to the particular papillary muscle. In patients with prior myocardial infarctions[52] a reduction in percentage of papillary muscle fractional shortening to 15±14% has been observed, compared with normal patients (30±8%). In patients with posterior myocardial infarction, the posteromedial papillary muscle motion was reduced, and appeared more echodense than the anterolateral muscle. Mintz and colleagues[42] reported that the posterior leaflet was retracted, rigid, and non-mobile in patients with a prior infarct and severe mitral regurgitation. The severity of associated mitral regurgitation is related to the degree of contractility and dilation of the left ventricle. Significant mitral regurgitation is rare with normal left ventricular systolic function. Kaul and colleagues[51] showed that ischemic mitral regurgitation is not related to acute papillary muscle dysfunction or to regional wall motion abnormality produced experimentally in the laboratory, but rather to global left ventricular dysfunction. The prevalence of severe mitral regurgitation is greater when there is both anterior and posterior papillary muscle dysfunction.

Sporadic or diffuse mitral annular calcification (MAC) may coexist with all three types of valve motion.[53] MAC occurs in degenerative disease irrespective of annular dilatation. MAC probably represents the breakdown and degeneration of the annulus followed by calcification, especially in the posterior segment which is composed of loose connective tissue. Sporadic or extensive annular calcification may occur, may distort the orifice, and can influence results unfavorably.

QUANTIFICATION OF MITRAL REGURGITATION

It has become increasingly important to define accurately the severity of mitral regurgitation. Even though there are methods to describe the quantity of mitral insufficiency, none is totally acceptable. The difficulty in evaluating mitral regurgitation stems mostly from its variable presentations attributable to different mitral lesions; the inability to detect accurately and assign a meaningful value to the true quantity of regurgitant flow, and the inability to define precisely the hemodynamic significance imposed by regurgitation in different disease states. Echocardiography provides an easy, accurate, and non-invasive method to identify and serially quantify mitral regurgitation. Either method, transthoracic or transesophageal, may be used to quantify mitral regurgitation, since the same technical and physiological factors limit both echocardiographic and Doppler techniques (Table 4.3). In individual patients, however, transesophageal echocardiography may provide additional information via better imaging from the esophageal window. The excellent quality of the images obtained of the valve apparatus and the color flow jets with transesophageal echocardiography provide much more accurate information than obtained from other methods. Information from transesophageal echocardiography may also aid in the recognition and interpretation of subsequent transthoracic studies.

Patients often develop severe mitral regurgitation and left ventricular dysfunction before the onset of symptoms, highlighting the importance of assessing the degree of regurgitation by an accurate and reproducible method.

Table 4.3   Echocardiographic quantification of mitral egurgitation

	Sellers grade			
I	Mild 1+	Moderate 2+	Mod/Sev 3+	Severe 4+
Max regurg jet area[73]	1.5–4 cm^2 (130,139)	4–7 cm^2 (139,143)		>7 cm^2 (131,143)
Mosaic jet [74]	<3 cm^2 (140, 142, 143)			>6 cm^2 (135,142,143)
Jet area/left atrial area ratio[71]	<20% (135,138,140)		>35% (129,132,137)	
Pulmonary venous flo [78]	Normal	Blunted systolic flow (128,141)		Systolic flow reversal (137,143)
PISA (ROA)$^{TTE\ (100)}$	<0.1 cm^2		0.3–4.9 cm^2	≥0.5 cm^2
Vena contracta $^{mono\ (85)}$ ROA	2.6±1.0 mm	4.2±1.2 mm	6.3±1.2mm	8.6±2.2 mm >5.5cm^2 (134,136)
RSV				>60 cc (137,137,138)
Vena contracta $^{multi\ (90)}$				>6 mm (139,142)
RSV				>80 cc (133,136,139)

ROA = regurgitant orifice a ea; RSV = r egurgitant stroke volume; PISA = pr oximal isovelocity sur face area; mono = monoplane transesophageal echocar diography; multi = multiplane transesophageal echocar diography; TTE = transthoracic echocardiography; numbers in par entheses (sensitivity, specificit , positive pr edictive value).

Currently, we can at best semiquantify the hemodynamic significance of mitral regurgitation, which has serious prognostic implications for patients with mitral regurgitation. In patients with suspected mitral regurgitation, echocardiography is primarily used to identify regurgitant jets by color flow or conventional Doppler techniques (see Table 4.3). Once the presence of mitral regurgitation is documented, its severity is estimated by correlating the total quantity of regurgitant flow to an assessment of ventricular output and reserve (Table 4.4). In this way, patients with mitral regurgitation can be successfully managed with surgery, which presently offers the best outcome for patient management.

In valvular stenosis, it is widely accepted that the reduction of valve opening or the size of the hole as described by the stenotic orifice area determines the severity of valve disease. The stenotic orifice area is conceptually easier to understand and is accepted by clinicians, since it may be directly measured or calculated. Unlike stenotic valve disease, the effective

---

Table 4.4   Echocardiographic finding suggesting severe mitral regurgitation

1. Progressive end-systolic ventricular enlargement > 4 cm

2. Left ventricular end-diastole dimension ≥ 7 cm

3. Ejection fraction < 60%

4. ROA > 0.5 cm^2

5. Regurgitant volume ≥ 60 cc

6. Regurgitant fraction > 55%

7. Flail leafle

8. Color flow max egurgitant jet area > 7 cm^2

9. Regurgitant jet area/left atrial area > 35%

10. Pulmonary venous systolic flow eversal

11. Left atrial diameter > 30 mm per squar e meter of BSA

---

regurgitant orifice, or the hole in the valve produced by valve lesions, especially atrioventricular valves, is difficult to conceptualize since it is not readily appreciated by any method. In mitral regurgitation, the hole produced during systole by the lack of approximation during closure of the valve leaflets can be better appreciated, especially when using the functional classification. It is easy to deduce – the larger the regurgitant hole, the greater the regurgitant volume. Recently, echocardiographic and Doppler methods have been developed to measure and calculate the regurgitant orifice area. In addition to these methods, the better image resolution and multiple views of multiplane transesophageal echocardiography lead to a better appreciation of the regurgitant orifice area concept.

It is well accepted that the degree of severity of mitral regurgitation is associated with the regurgitant volume. A regurgitant volume less than 35% of the total left ventricular stroke volume can be well tolerated for long periods and does not result in significant progression of left ventricular dysfunction. Rather, regurgitant volumes greater than 50% seem to lead almost invariably to quicker clinical deterioration. Mitral regurgitation with volumes of 35–50% presents a clinical dilemma, and may or may not cause a problem depending on other coexistent conditions. In most cases, ejection fraction and the serial measurements of end-systolic and end-diastolic ventricular volumes can be used to assess ventricular performance. However, because of its high dependence on loading conditions, the ejection fraction may not reflect intrinsic left ventricular performance. End-systolic and end-diastolic volumes are markers that predict a clinical outcome after surgery in terms of perioperative mortality and morbidity, but they lack adequate sensitivity and specificity. The risk of early and late postoperative morbidity and mortality is increased in patients with impaired left ventricular performance. The potential for postoperative improvement is limited as ventricular reserve diminishes. Therefore, the ideal timing for surgical intervention probably occurs at the onset of left ventricular impairment to circumvent the small risk of perioperative events associated with current surgical techniques.

ECHOCARDIOGRAPHIC DIAGNOSIS OF MITRAL REGURGITATION

Conventional and color Doppler methods allow the detection of mitral regurgitation with a high degree of accuracy (see Table 4.3). Positioning the pulsed Doppler sample volume on the left atrial side of the mitral annulus, below the leaflet tips during systole, permits sensitive identification of backward systolic flow, which is diagnostic of mitral regurgitation. Pulsed wave Doppler mapping of the left atrium to determine the extent of the regurgitant jet is not routinely performed and is superfluous with transesophageal echocardiography. The color Doppler flow method is the preferred technique in combination with transesophageal echocardiography, and is extremely sensitive in detecting and illustrating regurgitant flow from the left ventricle to the atrium during systole.

Through the use of Doppler techniques it is now widely recognized that all valves leak slightly, due to the displacement of blood from the normal motion of the valve during closure, and trivial or physiological regurgitation is frequently shown in normal patients. Physiological regurgitation,[54] which is most commonly defined with transesophageal echocardiography and color flow Doppler, is defined by small jets of flow reversal detected in close approximation to the mitral annular plane, usually during the early phase of systole, when the leaflets are closing. Pulsed Doppler sampling shows these jets usually within a 1 cm area about the annular plane. Single or multiple color flow jets with small jet areas and low flow velocities are imaged without significant turbulence or variance.

With transesophageal echocardiography and color flow Doppler, significant regurgitant flow jets are readily visualized, emanating from a closed mitral valve orifice as high velocity systolic jets of flow.[55–57] Regurgitant flow jets are easily recognized by their mosaic or green appearance produced by turbulence and variance maps recorded against the background of low velocity blood flow filling the atrium (Figure 4.3). Transesophageal echocardiography has a clear advantage over transthoracic imaging in mitral regurgitation. Eccentric regurgitant jets are easier to visualize from the multiple views provided by the esophageal window, and may be easily followed in their full extent throughout the atrium with minor changes in probe positioning. Generally, the regurgitant jets appear larger than they do from the transthoracic approach, with imaging from the esophageal window. The left atrium is physically closer to the transducer, which permits better resolution by taking full advantage of the transducer frequency and eliminating the acoustic shadowing from the valve apparatus that occurs in the apical windows with transthoracic imaging.

It is important to describe fully regurgitant flow jets when classifying mitral regurgitation by transesophageal echocardiography. Regurgitant jets are composed of an area of flow convergence on the ventricular surface of the regurgitant mitral orifice that narrows as it proceeds through the mitral orifice (vena contracta). The flow rapidly spreads out like a flame (maximal jet area) and mixes with blood flow in the left atrium. Regurgitant jet flow may be directed centrally into the left atrium, or may take an eccentric path as it originates from the regurgitant orifice.

DIASTOLIC MITRAL REGURGITATION

Mitral regurgitation or retrograde blood flow can occasionally be recorded during diastole as well as in systole, even though there is proper closure of the valve.[58–60] A positive pressure gradient develops between the left atrium and left ventricle due to improper timing of atrial-ventricular relaxation and contraction cycles. Doppler recordings of diastolic regurgitation consist of low volume, high velocity flow jets that diminish abruptly when the valve becomes completely competent during ventricular systole. Diastolic mitral regurgitation may be seen in cases of conduction disturbance as in atrioventricular block, atrial flutter, atrial fibrillation, in severe aortic regurgitation, or

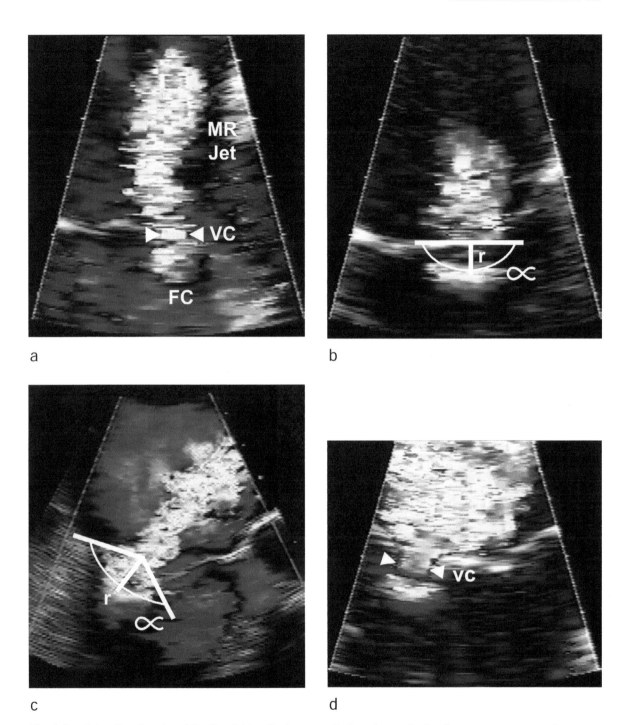

Fig. 4.3 Color flow Doppler of the flow jet in mitral egurgitation demonstrating flow conve gence and vena contracta, which may be utilized for deter mining the severity of mitral r egurgitation. (a) Typical central color flow jet of mitral r egurgitation extending into the body of the left atrium. (b) Enlar ged view of the flo convergence in a central dir ected jet, illustrating an angle of closur e of 180° as utilized in the pr oximal isovelocity sur face area (PISA) method. (c) When an eccentric mitral r egurgitant jet is detected the angle of leaflet closure may not be 180° and the angle must be cor rected and measur ed for proper utilization in the PISA method. (d) Enlar ged view of a mitral r egurgitant jet illustrating the pr oper point of measur ement (arrows) for the vena contracta method.

with decreased ventricular compliance and distensibility.

ESTIMATION OF THE SEVERITY OF MITRAL REGURGITATION

Measurement of regurgitant jet area

Doppler color flow mapping, in addition to identifying regurgitant jets, may also provide a semiquantitative method to estimate the volume of the regurgitant jet.[61–65] Planimetry of the cross-sectional jet area visualizes the extent of the maximal regurgitant signal. The maximal jet area must be optimally visualized by adjustment of the transducer, which improves by using the transesophageal approach, since jets do not need to be centrally oriented from the orifice to be seen adequately.[66] The sensitivity of this method, using transthoracic echocardiography rather than angiographic ventriculography, has been reported[67] to be about 86%, with a specificity of 100% and a correlation coefficient of 0.83. The severity is graded from mild to severe according to the jet area measured. Mild regurgitation has a jet area of less than 1.5 cm^2, moderate jet areas 1.5–3.0 cm^2, moderate to severe jet areas 3.0–4.5 cm^2, and severe regurgitation jets, more than 4.5 cm^2. Due to the technical factors involved in Doppler imaging, involving the spatial relations of flow jets, better results may not be possible with this method. The spatial distribution of the regurgitant jet imaged by color Doppler flow mapping is highly dependent on the velocity of the driving pressure transmitted from the left ventricle to produce regurgitation, rather than on the regurgitant volume. Under constant flow conditions *in vitro*, the spatial distribution of a regurgitant jet increases with increasing flow rate producing a larger regurgitant jet on color Doppler flow mapping, which leads to overestimation of the severity of regurgitation. Similarly, if the flow rate remains constant and the regurgitant jet orifice is modified,[68] the spatial distribution of the jet will decrease as the orifice size is increased, despite identical flow rate and regurgitant volume. In these situations, measurement of the jet area will underestimate the severity of mitral regurgitation.

The jet area depends not only on the regurgitant volume, but also on the regurgitant orifice and the velocity of blood flow.

There is wide variation in the spatial characteristics of regurgitant jets in patients with mitral regurgitation. Distortion of the spatial pattern of the regurgitant jet may occur, with collision of multiple and multi-directed jets or by jets directed towards and impacting the left atrial wall or Coanda effect,[69] all of which complicate the estimation of jet area. Pulmonary venous flow[70] directed towards the mitral regurgitant jet may produce smaller jet areas (through distortion and flattening) than may occur when the pulmonary venous flow is directed away from the regurgitant jet. The estimation of regurgitant areas can be modified by many hemodynamic variables, such as the level of the left atrial pressure, and by changes in heart rate, most pronounced in patients with acute severe mitral regurgitation. Considering all the factors that may influence the true measurements and calculations of mitral regurgitation, an experienced echocardiographer may be able to construct an accurate assessment of mitral regurgitation from visual impression alone.

To assess mitral regurgitation more precisely, the maximum jet area relative to the left atrial size can be determined also measuring the jet area in three orthogonal planes. With transthoracic imaging,[71] a ratio of the jet area to the left atrial area of less than 0.2 shows mild regurgitation, 0.2–0.4 moderate regurgitation, and greater than 0.4 severe regurgitation, as obtained with angiography. Unfortunately, these techniques have not increased the statistical correlation with angiography, supporting the fact that the Doppler method provides better information on the velocity of flow than on the regurgitant volume.

Many reports comparing transesophageal echocardiography with color flow Doppler and ventriculography have shown an excellent correlation between the two methods for quantifying mitral regurgitation.[72] With transesophageal echocardiography, the absolute jet area may be calculated with good results. Color Doppler mapping of the area of the regurgitant jet[73] is around 95% sensitive and 100% specific, with a predictive accuracy of 98%.

It has been suggested that the area calculation of only the mosaic portion (variance) of the regurgitant jet is sufficient to quantify severity.[74] A maximal mosaic area of less than 3 cm^2 showed mild regurgitation with a sensitivity of 96%, a specificity of 100%, and a predictive accuracy of 98%. A maximal mosaic jet area of greater than 6 cm^2 predicted severe regurgitation, with a specificity of 91%, a specificity of 100%, and a predicted accuracy of 98%.

Transesophageal echocardiographic comparison of the regurgitant jet area as a percentage of the left atrial area is accurate, despite limitations in visualizing the full atrial dimension.

Measurement of regurgitant volume and regurgitant fraction

Mitral regurgitant volumes can be calculated echocardiographically by comparing the difference between mitral and aortic stroke volumes, and expressing the regurgitant volume as a fraction of the total mitral inflow.[75,76]

Aortic outflow volume is derived from the product of aortic cross-sectional area multiplied by the flow velocity integral and heart rate. The aortic cross-sectional area is obtained by measuring the diameter of the aortic annulus just proximal to the point of insertion of the aortic cusps, and using $2\pi r^2$, assuming that the aortic orifice is circular. The aortic stroke volume is obtained by calculating the area under the flow velocity time integral curve. The aortic outflow can be obtained from the deep transgastric position at 0° or from the lower esophageal position at 0° using a five-chamber view. The aortic annulus diameter is usually best taken from the lower esophageal position at 135°–150°. This determination of aortic outflow by the pulse Doppler method is fairly accurate compared with the thermodilution technique.

The mitral inflow volume is calculated in a similar manner, but the mitral orifice probably should be considered elliptical instead of circular. The long axis of the mitral orifice can be measured in the transgastric view at about 90°, during mid-diastole. The short axis dimension can be taken from the transgastric short axis view at 0° to 15° to present the valve *en face* and again is measured at mid-diastole. The mitral valve area is calculated by: MVA = $(\pi/4) \times L \times S$. Pulsed Doppler measures the mitral inflow velocity in the lower esophageal position from 0° to 90° in four- or two-chamber views, placing the sample volume at the leaflet tips. With this method, using transthoracic echocardiography, a correlation coefficient of 0.92 has been obtained compared with angiographic methods.

Obviously, the measurement of the regurgitant volume in this manner is cumbersome and time-consuming. Accurate measurement of the aortic and mitral annulus is vital for adequate results, which should give multiplane transesophageal echocardiography an advantage since it gives more accurate results. In patients with atrial fibrillation and mitral regurgitation, numerous measurements must be taken of the flow velocity time integrals, averaged to compensate for variation in diastolic filling times.

Measurement of regurgitant orifice area

One of the first methods to calculate the effective regurgitant orifice area was described by the Mayo Clinic.[77] The effective regurgitant orifice area may be calculated by pulsed and continuous wave Doppler, as the ratio of regurgitant volume/regurgitant jet time-velocity integral. Mitral and aortic stroke volumes are estimated by pulsed wave Doppler, calculating the orifice flow for each (orifice area × velocity), and the regurgitant volume is calculated from the difference of the mitral inflow and aortic inflow. The time-velocity integral is obtained by continuous wave Doppler of the mitral regurgitant jet. The effective regurgitant orifice area obtained in this manner is strongly predictive of the severity of mitral regurgitation. Surgical observations have suggested that there is a marked difference between the mitral regurgitant orifice area of moderate and severe lesions (35±12 mm^2 and 75±33 mm^2, respectively, $p=0.009$), underlining the importance of this measurement.

Quantification of regurgitation from pulmonary venous flow patterns

Some authors suggest the use of the pulmonary venous flow patterns to predict the severity of mitral regurgitation. By definition, severe (4+) mitral regurgitation produces the systolic reflux of contrast media into the pulmonary veins during angiographic ventriculography. In animal models and patients, pulmonary venous flow patterns may be altered by regurgitant volume, left atrial compliance, left ventricular systolic and diastolic function, systolic blood pressure, and peripheral vascular resistance. Despite all of these factors, however, regurgitant volume is largely responsible for producing negative systolic pulmonary venous flow. Multiplane transesophageal echocardiography has provided an excellent non-invasive means to interrogate the pulmonary veins using pulsed wave and color flow Doppler to describe abnormal pulmonary venous flows (Figure 4.4). Recently, transesophageal echocardiographic Doppler studies have shown that increases in severity of mitral regurgitation produce characteristic pattern changes in pulmonary venous flow (Table 4.5).[78]

Normal pulmonary venous flow is pulsatile, and corresponds to the X and Y descent of the left atrial pressure curve. Normal flow emptying into the left atrium from either the right or left pulmonary vein is easily visualized by multiplane transesophageal echocardiography, and appears non-turbulent and reddish orange in color on standard color flow velocity maps. With pulsed wave Doppler, normal pulmonary venous flow appears as biphasic waves above the Doppler baseline, with forward flow recorded during systole and diastole. Occasionally, a small wave of reversed atrial flow is noted immediately after diastolic forward flow, corresponding to mitral valve closure. The peak velocity of the systolic integral is greater than the diastolic peak velocity, with a ratio of about 2:1. When recording pulmonary venous flow with pulsed Doppler, the sample volume must be placed at least 1–2 cm into the pulmonary vein to eliminate extraneous atrial flow turbulence near the orifice of

the vein or venous movement as a result of respiration. The angle of incidence of the Doppler sample can usually be made negligible by rotating the transducer of the multiplane probe. Discordant pulmonary venous flow has been described between the right and left pulmonary veins, so both veins should be sampled to ensure accurate results. It should also be noted that pulmonary venous systolic peak velocities and systolic flow integrals can increase in the left pulmonary vein in normal patients lying in the left lateral decubitus position.[79]

With varying degrees of mitral regurgitant volumes, pulmonary venous flow patterns have been described as normal, blunted, or reversed systolic flow, whereas diastolic forward flow generally remains the same.[78,80–84] Klein and colleagues[78] have found that 98% of patients with severe (4+) mitral regurgitation show systolic flow reversal, with a sensitivity of 93% and a specificity of 100% compared with other transesophageal echocardiographic color flow mapping methods. Patients who had moderate regurgitation (3+) had blunted systolic flow, with a sensitivity of 61% and a specificity of 97%. Patients with milder mitral regurgitation (2+ or 1+) had normal or equiphasic flow. Similarly, there were significant differences in peak systolic flow velocities and systolic/diastolic flow ratios between each grade of mitral regurgitation. Additionally, the presence of atrial fibrillation did not alter the significance of results in patients with different grades of mitral regurgitation. Discordant venous flow was seen between the right and left pulmonary veins, and was attributable to the direction and orientation of the mitral regurgitant jet, illustrating the importance of sampling both right and left pulmonary veins. In a follow-up study, the same group showed that pulmonary venous flow reflects the severity of mitral regurgitation on the left atrial pressure *a* and *v* waves.

Therefore, used with care, the transesophageal echocardiographic finding of reversed and blunted systolic flow is useful to differentiate clinically significant mitral regurgitation (4+ or 3+) from clinically insignificant

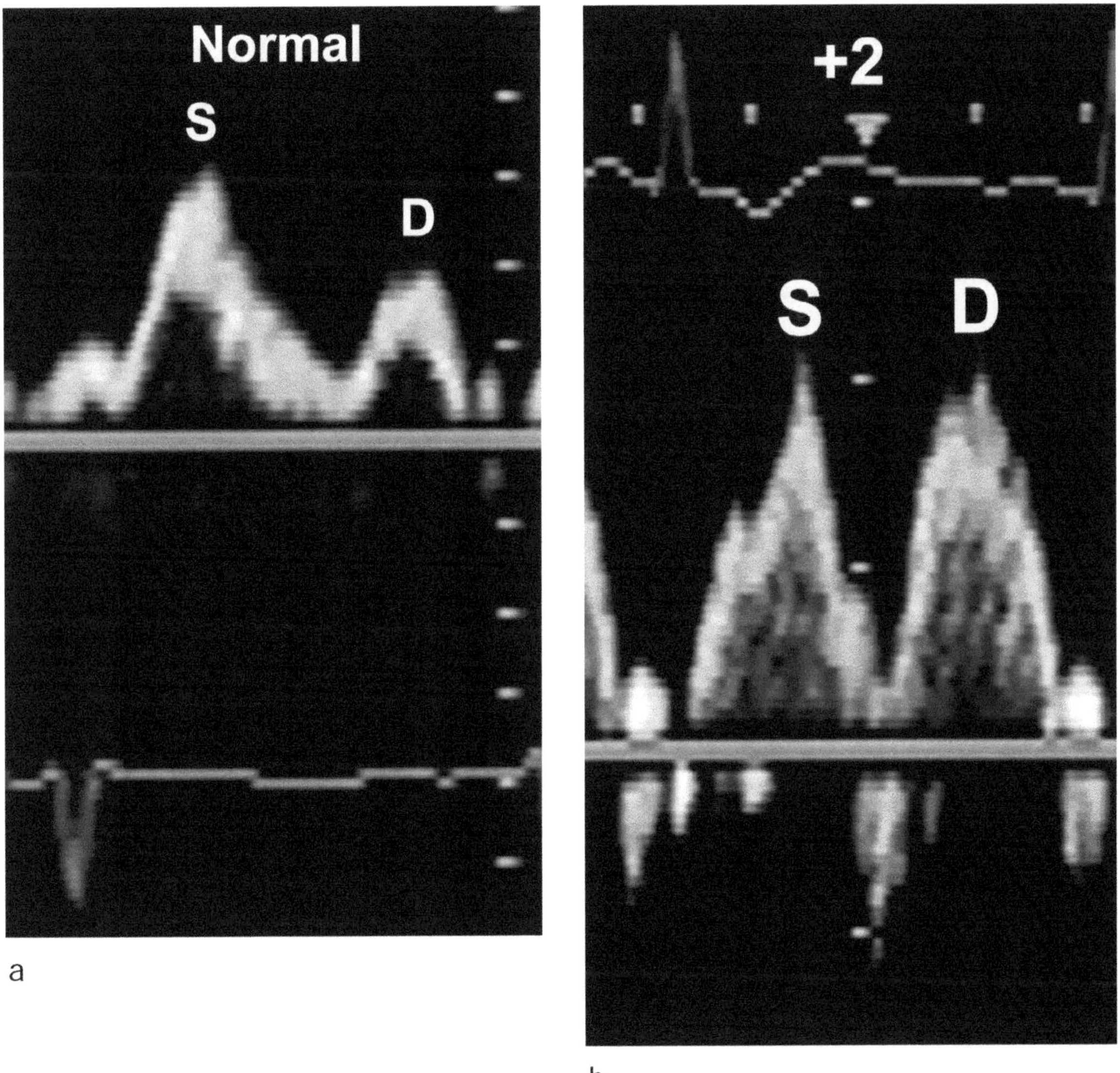

Fig. 4.4 Pulmonary venous flo . Pulsed Doppler pulmonar y venous flow patte ns recorded with mitral regurgitation. (a) Nor mal pulsed Doppler pulmonar y venous flow patte n, with systolic flow (S) componen greater than the diastolic flow (D) component. (b) In mild mitral egurgitation the systolic flow component i equal to the diastolic flow component

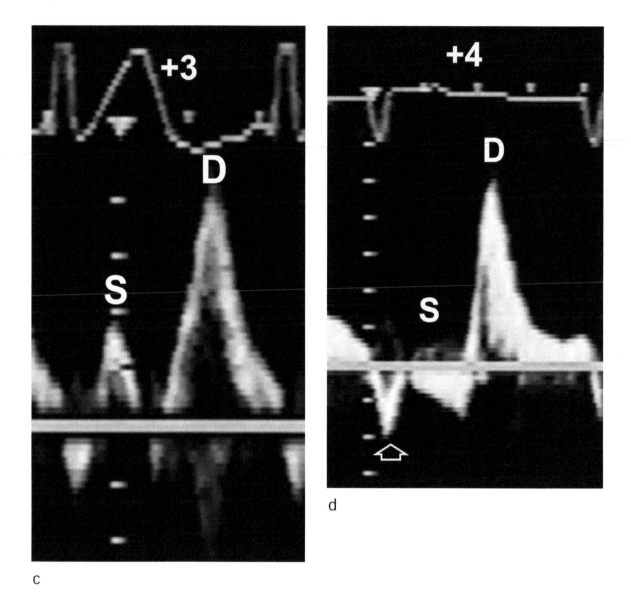

c

d

Fig. 4.4 (contd.)   (c) In moderate mitral r egurgitation the systolic for ward flow component becomes less tha the diastolic flow component and flow   eversal is detected. (d) In sever e mitral regurgitation forward systolic flow ceases and flow   eversal is noted during systole with for   ward flow only occu ring during diastole.

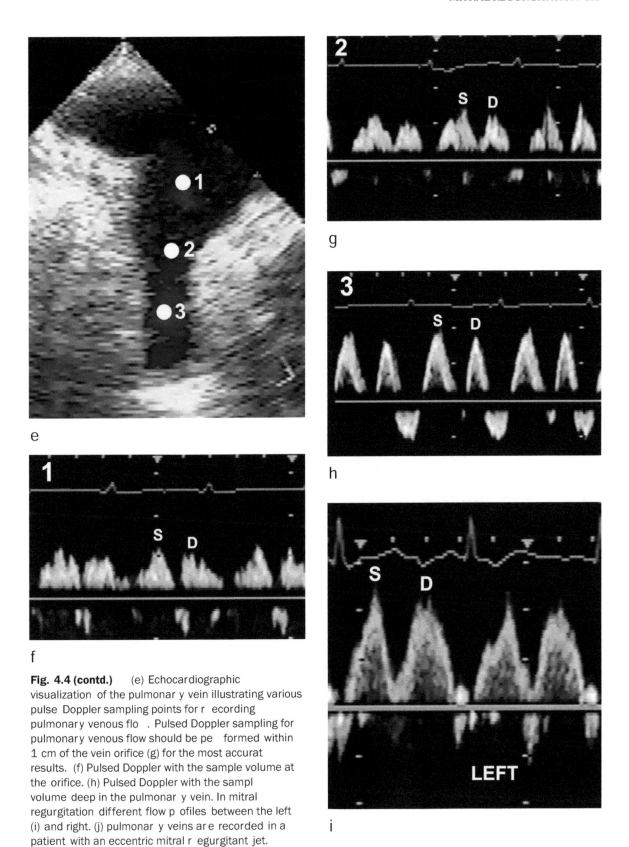

Fig. 4.4 (contd.) (e) Echocardiographic visualization of the pulmonary vein illustrating various pulse Doppler sampling points for recording pulmonary venous flo . Pulsed Doppler sampling for pulmonary venous flow should be pe formed within 1 cm of the vein orifice (g) for the most accurat results. (f) Pulsed Doppler with the sample volume at the orifice. (h) Pulsed Doppler with the sampl volume deep in the pulmonary vein. In mitral regurgitation different flow p ofiles between the left (i) and right. (j) pulmonary veins are recorded in a patient with an eccentric mitral r egurgitant jet.

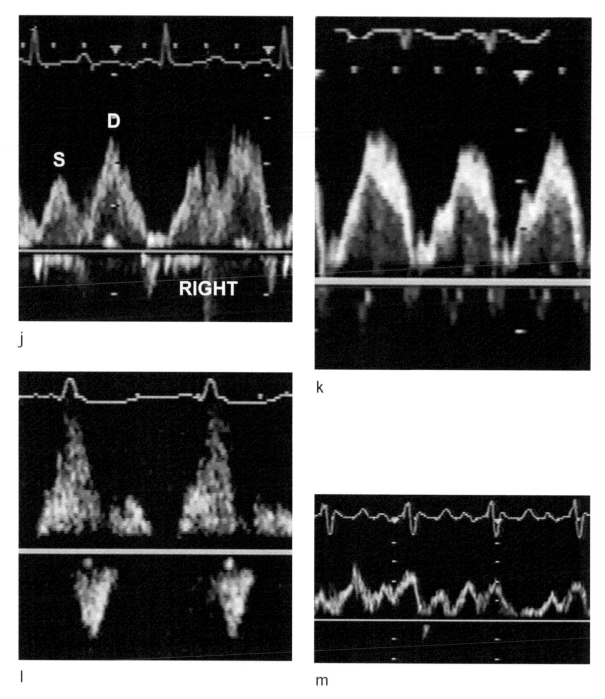

Fig. 4.4 (contd.)   The flow p ofile in (i) suggests nor mal-to-mild mitral r egurgitation and the pr ofile in (j) suggests mild-to-moderate mitral r egurgitation. This example underlines the impor tance of measuring both the right and left pulmonar y veins and illustrates the limitations of this method when evaluating the severity of mitral regurgitation. The pulmonar y venous flow p ofile may also be af fected by the underlying car diac rhythm. (k) Supraventricular tachycar dia. (l) Ventricular pacing. (m) Atrial flutte .

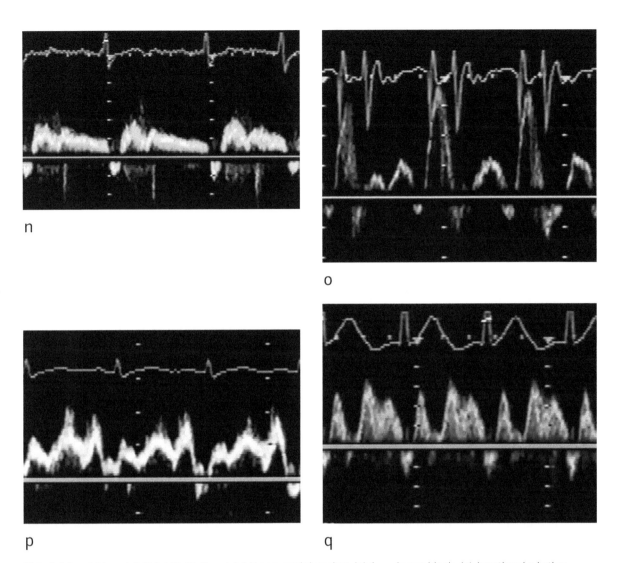

Fig. 4.4 (contd.) (n) Atrial fibrillation. (o) A-V sequential pacing. (p) 1 heart block. (q) Junctional r hythm.

Table 4.5	Pulmonary venous flow indices in mitral egurgitation			
Sellers MR grade	*1+*	*2+*	*3+*	*4+*
Patients (no.)	1	12	8	22
Peak systolic velocity (S) (cm/s)	44	37±20[†]	26±28*	14±20[‡]
Peak diastolic velocity (D) (cm/s)	53	53±22	52±26	61±18
Systolic/diastolic (S/D) ratio	0.8	0.8[†]	0.5*	0.3[‡]

* p<0.05 peak S, D, S/D ratio for 3+ versus 4+ mitral r egurgitation
† p<0.05 peak S, D, S/D ratio for 2+ versus 4+ mitral r egurgitation
‡ p<0.05 peak S, D, S/D ratio for 4+ versus (2+, 3+) mitral r egurgitation.

regurgitation (2+ or 1+), to further aid in the classification of mitral regurgitation.

Measurement of proximal jet width and vena contracta

Measurement with transesophageal echocardiography of the width of the proximal regurgitant jet just above the valve orifice is also promising.[85] When the width of the regurgitant jet orifice is greater than 5.5 mm, it correlates nicely with severe regurgitation on angiography and a regurgitant stroke volume of more than 60 ml. An advantage to the measurement of the jet width orifice is that it should not be susceptible to most of the physiological factors that plague measurements of the jet area. The vena contracta method assumes that the mitral regurgitant orifice does not change shape during systole, which may not be the case in patients with mitral valve prolapse.[86]

In a further refinement of this technique, measurement of the vena contracta portion of the regurgitant jet can be made quickly giving accurate results that are independent of hemodynamics and orifice geometry. The diameter of the vena contracta or narrowest extent of the regurgitant jet as it passes through the valve orifice may be measured in one or two orthogonal echocardiographic planes.[87–89] Studies have shown that the vena contracta width measured by transthoracic and transesophageal echocardiography correlates with the angiographic grading of mitral regurgitation.[90]

In a subsequent study,[89] vena contracta measurements by transthoracic echocardiography accurately predicted regurgitant volume (r = 0.85, SEE = 20 ml) and regurgitant orifice area (r = 0.86, SEE = 0.15 cm^2). In addition, the vena contracta width was the only independent predictor of the severity of mitral regurgitation by multivariate analysis when considering pulmonary venous flow reversal, maximal jet area, and left atrial size. A vena contracta width of 0.5 cm or more in the parasternal long-axis view was always associated with severe mitral regurgitation, a regurgitant volume of 60 ml, and a regurgitant orifice area of 0.4 cm^2. A vena contracta width of 0.3 cm or less was associated

usually with mild mitral regurgitation, and predicted a regurgitant volume of less than 60 ml and regurgitant orifice area of less than 0.4 cm^2.

Regurgitant volumes obtained by multiplane transesophageal echocardiography measurement of vena contracta width correlate nicely with regurgitant volumes obtained angiographically using the thermodilution technique.

Potential limitations of vena contracta width measurements are related to assumptions of the mitral orifice and validation in different clinical states. The mitral orifice is assumed to be circular or elliptical with this method, when it is usually irregular in shape. Another error may occur in assuming that the mitral regurgitant orifice is fixed and not dynamic. A technical consideration is that it is generally difficult to distinguish the narrowest flow zone corresponding to the vena contracta. Resolution of the vena contracta is highly dependent on the spatial resolution of the view and the echocardiographic equipment. At present, this method has not been validated for patients with coexistent aortic insufficiency or atrial fibrillation, but the vena contracta method should not be affected by the presence of aortic insufficiency.

Measurement of flow convergence (PISA)

Color flow Doppler mapping makes it possible to evaluate the acceleration of blood flow as it converges toward a regurgitant orifice. A zone of flow acceleration can be visualized proximal to the regurgitant orifice in almost all patients under transesophageal echocardiography, and it correlates well with the severity of mitral regurgitation.[91–94]

As blood flow accelerates toward the regurgitant orifice, concentric rings of isovelocity regions are produced in a radial fashion, decreasing in size as they approach the mitral orifice. Successive layers of isovelocity hemispheres are shown with color Doppler, and may be enlarged and enhanced with the zoom mode of the echocardiographic instrument. On velocity maps, aliasing layers of flow appear as alternating shades of red and blue, much like a rainbow. The velocity increases as flow converges on the mitral orifice, with the smallest hemisphere nearest the orifice having the highest velocity.

The zone of flow convergence proximal to a mitral regurgitant orifice is described mathematically as hemispherical. If all the blood flow within the convergence region passes through the regurgitant orifice, and the product of flow area times spatial velocity is constant at any position within the flow stream (law of continuity), then these data can be used to calculate the regurgitant flow rate. The flow rate Q (ml/sec) is equal to the velocity of blood flow multiplied by the cross-sectional area of the first isovelocity ring: $Q = 2\pi r^2 v$, where r is the radial distance of the first alias from the regurgitant orifice, $2\pi r^2$ is the area of the hemisphere at radial distance r, and v is the aliasing velocity in cm/sec at radial distance r.

The effective regurgitant orifice area can be calculated by dividing the flow rate Q by the maximal velocity of the mitral regurgitant jet through the orifice, as recorded with continuous wave Doppler. The regurgitant volume may be calculated by multiplying the effective regurgitant orifice area by the time velocity integral of the mitral regurgitant jet.

Many studies have been done in models and in clinical patients, to validate the utility of the flow convergence method for mitral regurgitation. These studies have addressed the potential limitations of flow convergence relating to the mathematical calculations, and the geometric assumptions made about the flow orifice and interaction of flow about the orifice.[94–102] When the proximity to the orifice causes the isovelocity surfaces to flatten out, the flow regions cannot be assumed to be hemispherical, and therefore it is necessary to lower color aliasing velocities, which increases the radius to allow for better measurement.[95]

Occasionally, mitral lesions produce an eccentrically placed regurgitant orifice in relation to the valve plane, which may distort the shape of the proximal flow convergence contour.[98,99] Clinically, with a flail or severely prolapsing posterior leaflet the flow convergence angle may be constrained by the posterior wall of the left ventricle. If the velocity contour in error is considered hemispherical,

the mitral flow rates are grossly overestimated by the flow convergence method. In this instance, the proximal flow contour can not be considered hemispherical and the flow equation must be corrected by the true convergence angle. There are two ways to correct for this: (1) involves measuring the true angle (a on the image sector) with a protractor and correcting the calculated regurgitant flow volume or regurgitant orifice area by multiplying by $\alpha/180$; or (2) substituting $2\pi r$ in the flow convergence by the true area of $\alpha = \tau + 2.\tan^{-1} d/r$, where d is the measured distance from the constraining wall to the radian of the regurgitant orifice. Good results have been obtained with both methods, eliminating the gross overestimation of regurgitant flow volumes.

The severity of mitral regurgitation can be described through the use of the regurgitant orifice area, since fundamentally its size is the major determinant of regurgitant volume and thus of regurgitant fraction. As validated by angiographic and echocardiographic methods,[100] a calculated regurgitant orifice area of more than 0.5 cm^2 correlates with severe (4+) mitral regurgitation, greater than 0.3 cm^2 but less than 0.5 cm^2 correlates with moderate (3+) regurgitation, and less than 0.1 cm^2 correlates with mild or trace regurgitation.

In an effort to reduce the time required for the flow convergence method, the Cleveland Clinic has simplified the formula by making various assumptions.[103] The regurgitant orifice area (ROA) may be simplified and calculated as $ROA = r^2/2$, where r is the distance of the aliasing contour when the aliasing velocity is set to 40 cm/s, and it is assumed that the pressure difference between the left ventricle and the left atrium in systole is 100 mmHg (as produced by a 5 m/s regurgitant jet).

PREDICTION OF VENTRICULAR FUNCTION AFTER SURGICAL CORRECTION

Left ventricular dysfunction is the most common cause of morbidity and mortality after the successful surgical correction of mitral regurgitation. Although the operative mortality for mitral repair or replacement has fallen in the

1990s, patients that present with left ventricular dysfunction still have a poor long-term prognosis. For this reason many asymptomatic patients are being considered as surgical candidates for the treatment of mitral regurgitation, to prevent the development of significant left ventricular dysfunction.[104–113]

The operative mortality for the surgical correction of mitral regurgitation is related to age and functional class.[107] The operative mortality for surgical correction of mitral regurgitation is 1.3% in patients less than 75 years old and 5.7% in patients over 75 years old. The operative mortality for mitral regurgitation is 9% for patients in functional classes III and IV, versus 1.5% for functional classes I and II. Mitral valvular repair has had a significant effect on the operative mortality of mitral regurgitation, with or without other cardiac surgery. In most institutions currently undertaking mitral valve repair for the treatment of organic mitral regurgitation, the operative mortality is approaching 0%.

Late survival after the surgical correction of mitral regurgitation is related to preoperative left ventricular function, and echocardiographic measurement of ejection fraction (EF) is an excellent predictor of late survival.[108] Late survival at 10 years is 32% with an echocardiographic EF of less than 50%. Survival is about 53% with an EF between 50 and 60%, and 72% survival can be expected with an EF of 60% or more. End-systolic ventricular enlargement is also an excellent echocardiographic predictor of poor left ventricular contractile reserve for the development of postoperative ventricular dysfunction. The demonstration of an end-systolic ventricular dimension after exercise of more than 40–45 mm with stress exercise echocardiography reliably predicts poor left ventricular function after valve repair.

PAPILLARY MUSCLE DYSFUNCTION

The papillary muscles contribute to the functional integrity of the mitral valve unit. Dysfunction of the papillary muscles may result in regurgitation, obstruction, or both. Transesophageal echocardiography has led to significant advances in the visualization and diagnosis of papillary muscle abnormalities. Papillary muscle dysfunction may be the result of morphological, positional, or functional changes due to acquired or congenital heart disease. In some patients there is severe calcification of the whole papillary muscle extending into the ventricular myocardium and/or the chordae tendineae, by contrast with the normal age-related changes of calcification of the head of the papillary muscle in elderly patients. Papillary muscle dysfunction can be catastrophic, such as in muscle rupture associated with acute myocardial infarction, or can be of lesser or unknown significance in many other clinical circumstances.

Papillary muscle enlargement occurs together with ventricular hypertrophy states.[113] In cases of hypertrophic cardiomyopathy, the papillary muscles may be hypertrophic to the extent that they cause mid-ventricular obstruction, especially when the ventricular cavity is small as occurs in low volume states. The location of the papillary muscles may also be an issue in hypertrophic cardiomyopathy, particularly when there is non-concentric left ventricular hypertrophy, and may produce systolic anterior motion (SAM) of the subvalvular apparatus.[114] SAM plus mitral insufficiency without the presence of septal hypertrophy has been shown using echocardiography to displace papillary muscles in dogs. Studies have also shown reduced papillary muscle fractional shortening due to the increased width of the papillary muscle, despite normal papillary muscle length.

MITRAL ANNULAR CALCIFICATION

Mitral annular calcification is frequently observed in patients with or without significant mitral valvular disease. Degenerative disease occurs frequently in the mitral annulus and the fibromuscular skeleton of the heart, either in association with other disease entities or as a consequence of aging. Annular calcification is common in the elderly without disease of the chordae or leaflets, especially in women over 70 years old.[115] Calcification of the mitral annulus is one of the most common abnormalities found at necropsy, occurring in 10% of necropsies in patients over 50 years old.[115–117] Mitral annular calcification is frequently associated with disorders that produce mitral regurgitation, such as myxomatous degeneration.[118] Mitral annular calcification is also common in several metabolic disorders involved with calcium deposition,[119] such as Hurler's syndrome,[120] Paget's disease, and bone dystrophy of chronic renal failure.[121]

Calcium deposition is commonly encountered in the loose connective tissue of the posterior aspect of the mitral annulus, especially near the central scallop of the posterior leaflet. In addition, degenerative calcium deposits may be found in the junction formed by the ventricular surface of the posterior leaflet and the posterior left ventricular wall (posterior submitral angle). When severe calcium deposition totally surrounds the annulus and extends into the posterior leaflet tissue and proximal ventricular myocardium, obstruction of the left ventricular inflow tract may occur.[122] Mitral annular calcification is usually limited to the posterior annulus, and extends medially and laterally towards the fibrous trigones. The anterior aspect of the annulus is usually unaffected, unless there is associated aortic sclerosis or calcific aortic stenosis that extends into the aorto-mitral fibrosa. When there is calcification of the medial margin of the annulus, the conduction system may be involved, resulting in conduction disturbances. When the width of the calcific annular band exceeds 5 mm, there is a significant increase in the incidence of conduction defects, atrial fibrillation, and heart failure.[123–125]

In patients with mitral annular calcification, transthoracic echocardiography has a sensitivity of 76% and a specificity of 94% compared with fluoroscopy.[126] Echocardiography is less sensitive if thickening of the annulus is due to sclerosis or fibrosis and not calcification. Transesophageal echocardiography is extremely helpful in moderate-to-severe cases of mitral annular calcification, since with transthoracic echocardiography the mitral valve leaflets and subvalvular apparatus may be overshadowed by the dense calcium deposits similar to the acoustic shadowing produced by a prosthetic valve. Extensive mitral annular calcification occasionally produces an irregular or raised margin in the annulus, to form a crevice or potential space between the annulus and atrial wall. These deformities of the annulus are associated with bacterial endocarditis and thrombus formation, and are more easily shown with transesophageal echocardiography. Extensive mitral annular calcification is associated with a greater incidence of cerebral and retinal embolism than age-matched controls.[124]

The deep transgastric views allow good visualization of the mitral valve unit without acoustic shadowing. The short axis and longitudinal transgastric views allow good visualization of the entire annulus to determine the full extent of annular involvement. The four-chamber and two-chamber lower esophageal views (0°–180°) allow full evaluation of the mitral valve and surrounding left ventricular myocardium to identify calcific extension to the leaflets and myocardial wall.

Echocardiographically, mitral annular calcification appears as highly reflective areas of increased echogenicity. Calcification may occur as single or multiple small discrete areas (1.5 mm or more), or as larger semicircular linear bands in the area of the annulus adjacent to the posterior mitral leaflet at the atrioventricular junction. Mitral annular calcification may extend into the posterior leaflet and render the leaflet immobile. When annular calcification extends and involves the body and tip of the anterior leaflet and chordae tendineae, left ventricular inflow obstruction may be produced, as shown with Doppler echocardiography.[122]

The echocardiographic identification of mitral annular calcification is extremely important in patients who present for mitral valve repair, as well as for mitral valve replacement, since annular calcification is not always readily appreciated by the cardiac surgeon. Paraprosthetic leaks are technically unavoidable during valve replacement in patients with severe mitral annular calcification. Small or large areas of calcification interfere with the ability to adequately suture or secure rigid prosthetic sewing rings to the fibrous skeleton.

In patients with significant annular calcification, mitral repair appears to be a better option than mitral replacement. Newer techniques in mitral repair allow for the near total debridement of the mitral annulus with good results.[127] Removing annular calcium enables easier suture placement with better tissue approximation, easier placement of the annuloplasty ring, less annular distortion (better geometry avoids regurgitation or obstruction), better leaflet mobility, and the theoretical advantage of allowing annular remodeling and restoring annular motion.

Case Studies

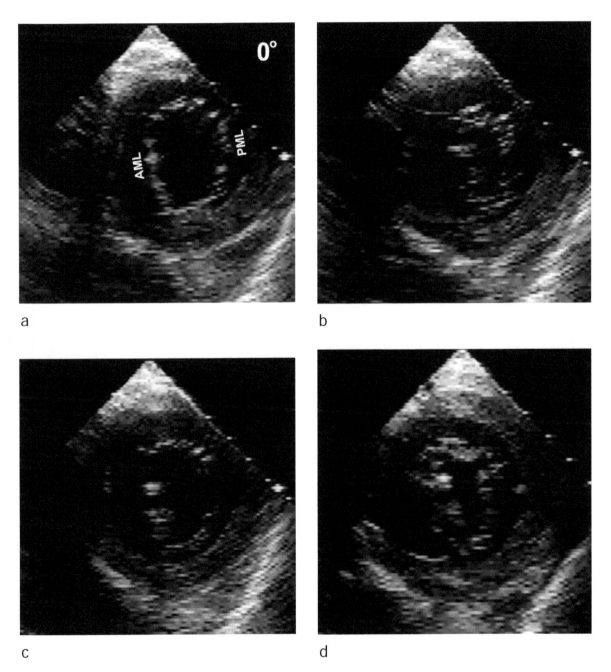

a

b

c

d

Case 4.1 Mitral annular dilatation. Shor t-axis echocardiographic images of the mitral valve r ecorded through diastole to systole. (a) Early diastole. (b) Mid diastole. (c) Atrial systole. (d) End diastole.

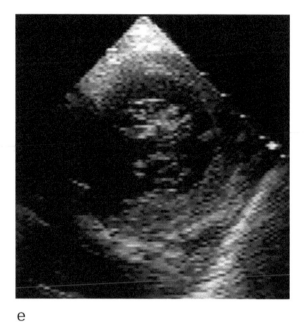

e

Case 4.1 (contd.)   (e) End systole. AML, anterior leaflet; PML, posterior leaflet

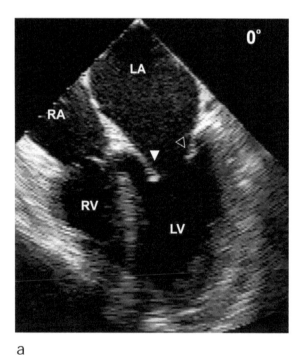

a

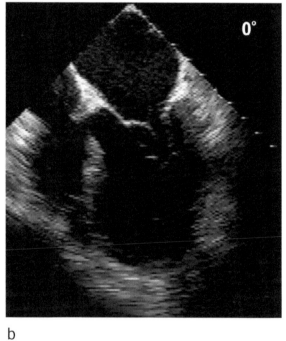

b

Case 4.2   Mitral annular dilatation. Four-chamber view fr om the lower esophageal window at 0°. Note mitral valve leaflet motion appears no mal in this view; anterior leaflet (solid a row) and posterior leaflet (open a row). The only noticeable abnor mality is mild annular dilatation. (a) Early diastole. (b) Mid diastole.

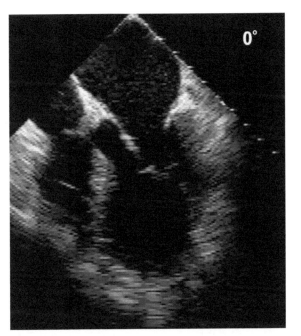

c

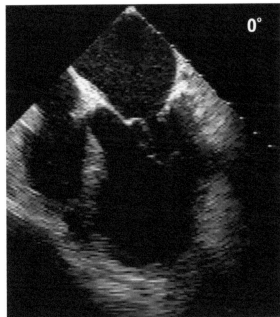

d

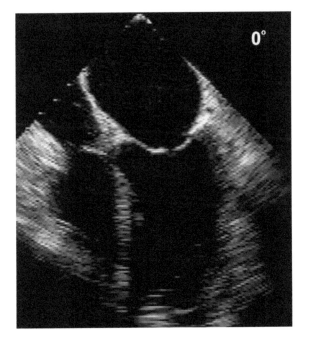

e

Case 4.2 (contd.) (c) Atrial systole. (d) End diastole. (e) End systole. RA, right atrium; LA, left atrium; RV, right ventricle; L V, left ventricle.

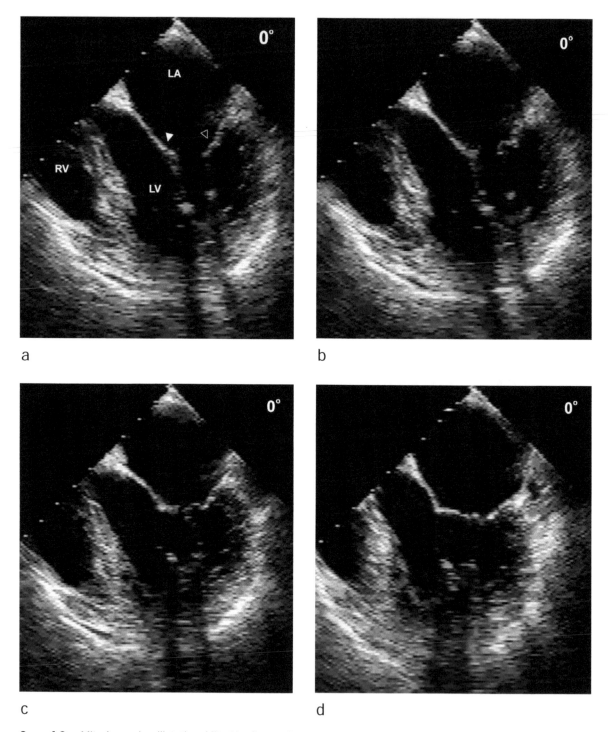

Case 4.3 Mitral annular dilatation. Mitral leaflet motion appears no mal, but the leaflets appear small durin closure in relation to the enlar ged mitral annulus. (a) Early diastole. (b) Mid diastole. (c) End diastole. (d) End systole.

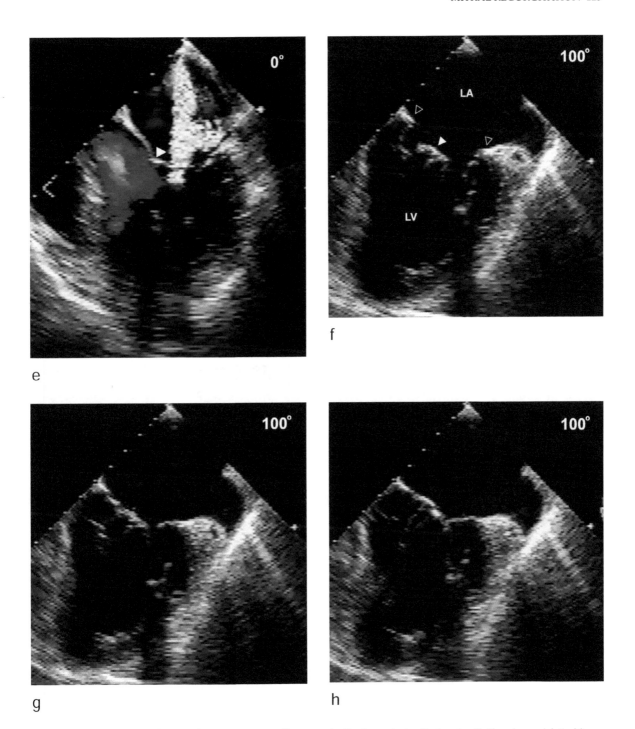

Case 4.3 (contd.) (e) Systolic frame demonstrating a centrally directed mitral regurgitation (arrow) jet with color flow Dopple . (f) Early diastole. (g) Mid diastole. (h) Systole.

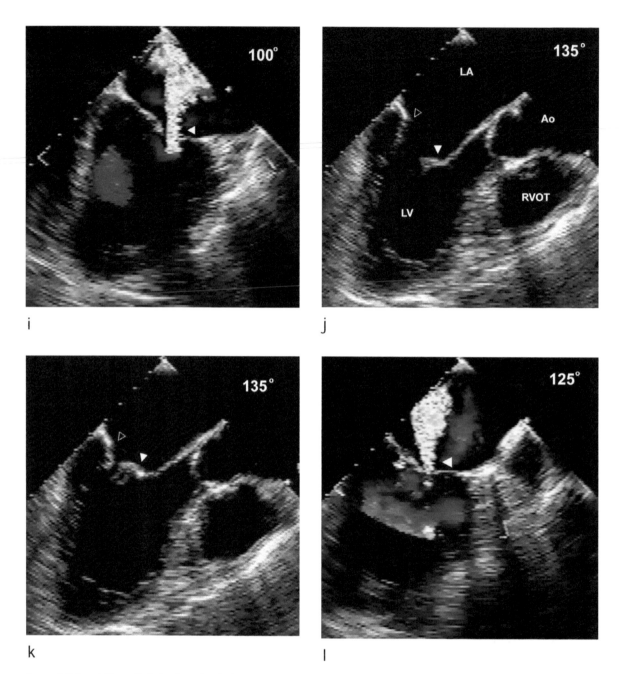

Case 4.3 (contd.) (i) Color Doppler during systole demonstrating a central mitral r egurgitant jet. (j) Diastolic frame at 125°. (k) Systolic frame at 125°. (l) Color Doppler during systole demonstrating a central mitral regurgitant jet. A, anterior leaflet (solid a row); P, posterior leaflet (open a row); LV, left ventricle; LA, left atrium; Ao, aor ta; RVOT, right ventricular outflow tract; V, right ventricle.

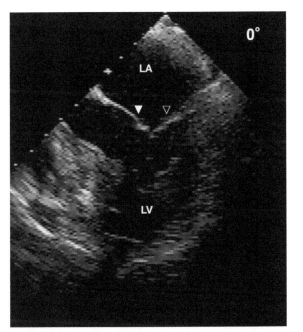

a

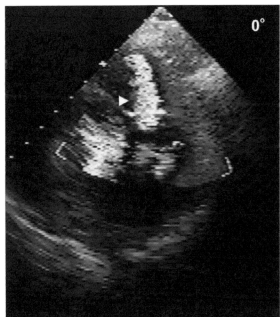

b

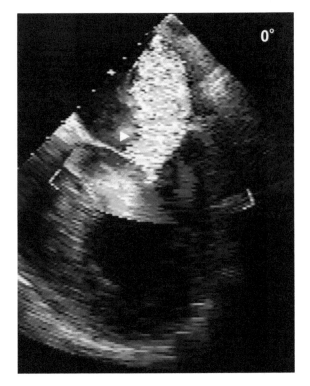

c

Case 4.4 Mitral annular dilatation. (a) Systolic frame demonstrating annular dilatation. (b) Mild mitral regurgitation (arrow). (c) Sever e mitral regurgitation (arrow) with phar macological provocation.

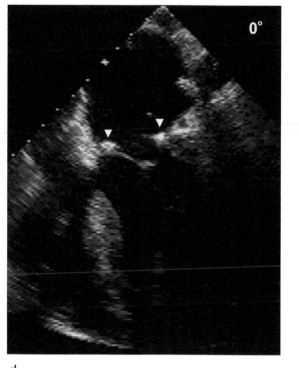

d

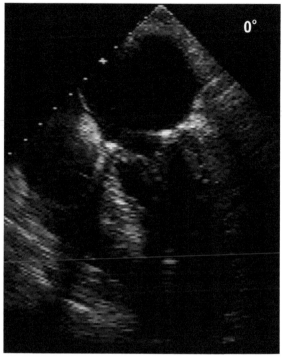

e

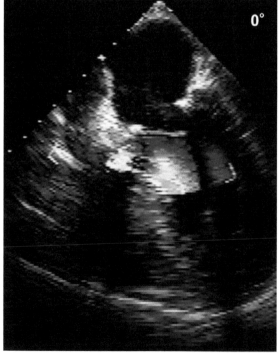

f

Case 4.4 (contd.) (d) Diastolic frame of mitral annuloplasty ring (arrows) following mitral repair. (e) Systolic frame following mitral repair. (f) Color flo Doppler recorded during systole with trace mitral regurgitation (arrow). LA, left atrium; LV, left ventricle; AML, anterior leaflet (solid arrow); PML posterior leaflet (open arrow).

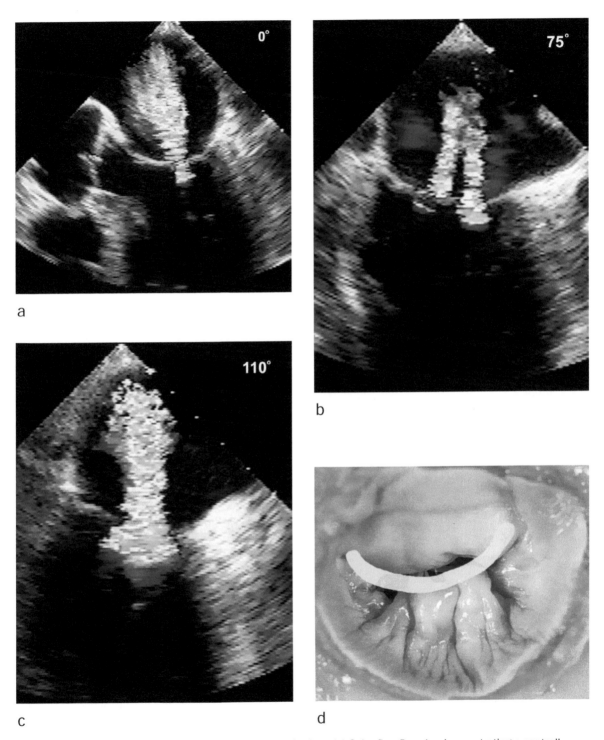

Case 4.5 Mitral annular dilatation and mitral r egurgitation. (a) Color flow Doppler demonstrating a centrall directed regur gitant jet with annular dilatation viewed at 0°. (b) When viewed at 75°, the centrally dir ected jet is demonstrated as two separate jets. With annular dilatation two r egurgitant jets ar e frequently seen originating from both cor ners of the valve. (c) A single r egurgitant jet is again visualized at 110°. (d) Anatomical specimen of the mitral valve illustrating the line of closur e. With annular dilatation, one or multiple jets can originate anywhere along the line of closur e most fr equently in the cor ners of the leaflets near th commissur es.

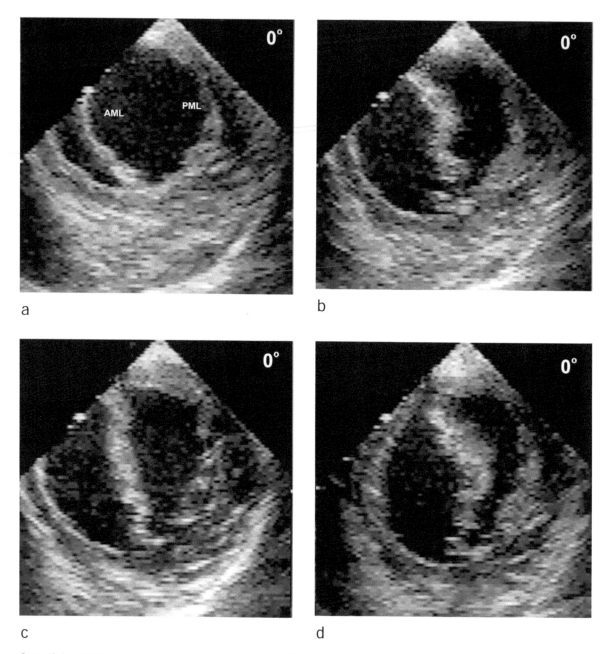

Case 4.6 Mitral valve prolapse. Short-axis echocardiographic images of the mitral valve recorded from diastole through systole. In all stages of the cardiac cycle the valve motion appears distorted and the valve opening more circular than with normal motion. This may also be attributed to annular dilatation, which frequently accompanies prolapse. Maximum valve opening occurs during early diastole and not during atrial systole. (a) Early diastole. (b) Mid diastole. (c) Atrial systole. (d) End diastole.

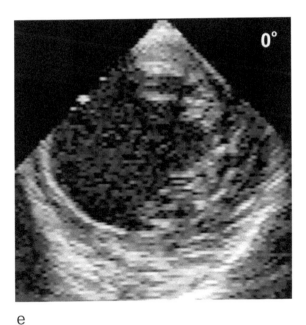

e

Case 4.6 (contd.)   (e) End systole. AML, anterior
leaflet; PML, posterior leaflet

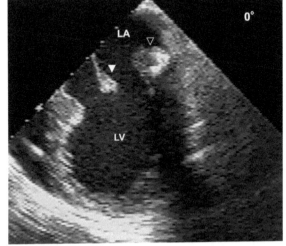

a

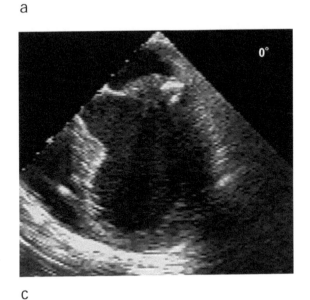

b

c

Case 4.7   Mitral valve prolapse. Views obtained from the lower esophageal window at 0° from diastole to
systole. (a) Early diastole. (b) End diastole. (c) Systole. The mitral valve appears thickened especially near the
leaflet tips throughout the cardiac cycle, consistent with myxomatous degenerative changes in the leaflet
tissue. In addition there is mild mitral annular calcification noted in the posterior annulus. LA, left atrium; V,
left ventricle.

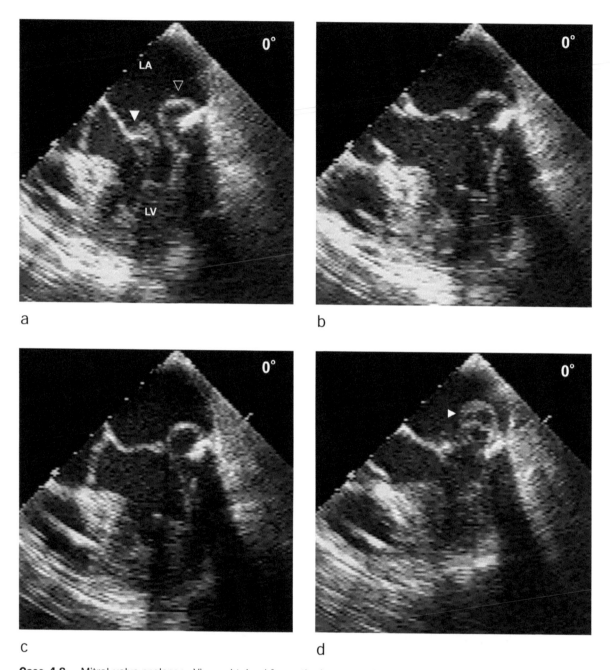

Case 4.8 Mitral valve pr olapse. Views obtained fr om the lower esophageal window at 0° from diastole to systole (a–d). The mitral leaflets appear markedly thickened in all views, with billowing of the leaflet tissue in the left atrium. The lack of leaflet coaption or p olapse of the posterior leaflet is demonstrated in the systoli frame (d). LA, left atrium; L V, left ventricle; AML, anterior leaflet (closed a row); PML, posterior leaflet (ope arrow).

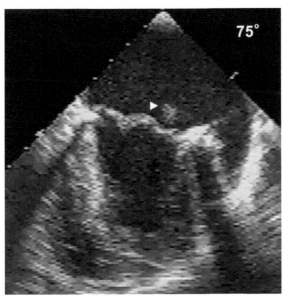

a

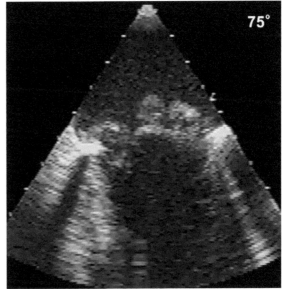

b

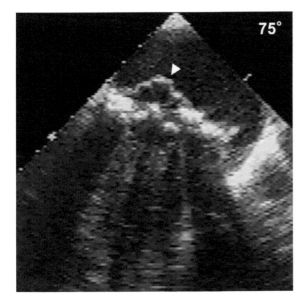

c

Case 4.9 Mitral valve prolapse. Views obtained from the lower esophageal window at 75° from diastole to systole (a–c), in the same patient as in Case 4.8. Marked billowing (arrows) of the posterior leaflet superimposed on the plane of the anterior mitral leaflet

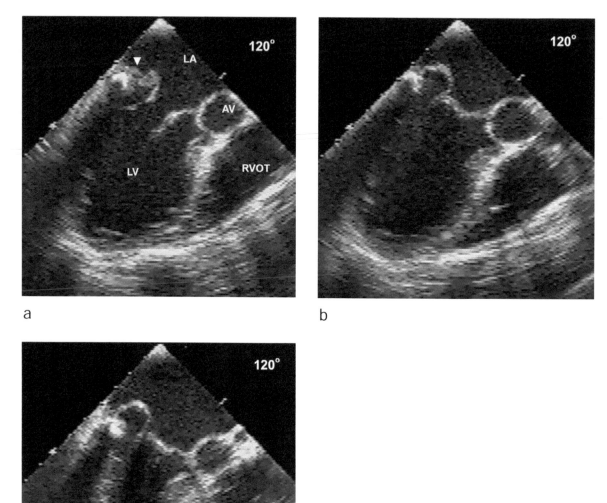

a

b

c

Case 4.10 Mitral valve prolapse. Views obtained from the lower esophageal window at 120° from diastole to systole (a–c), in the same patient as in Case 4.8. Marked billowing (arrows) of the posterior leaflet superimposed on the plane of the anterior mitral leaflet. LA, left atrium; V, left ventricle; RV, right ventricle.

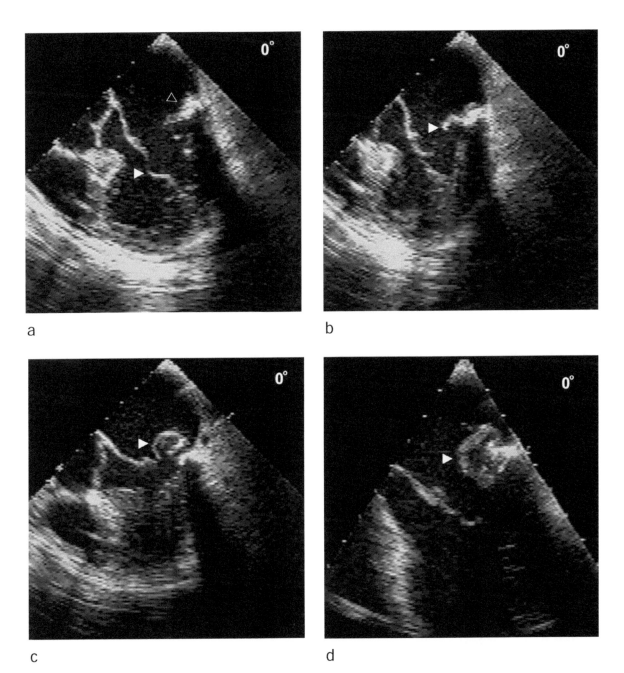

Case 4.11 Associated findings in mitral valve p olapse. (a) Mitral annular calcification (solid a row) and elongated redundant chordae of the anterior leaflet (open a row). (b–d) Ruptured chordae tendineae and flai posterior leaflet segment (a rows).

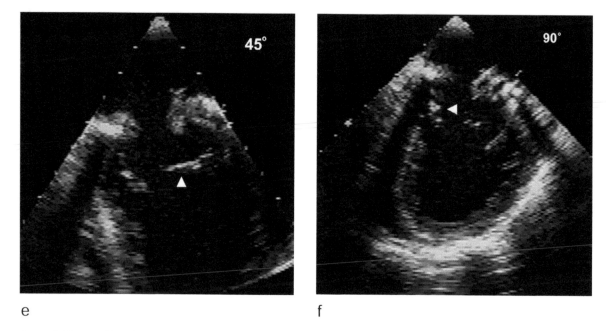

e f

Case 4.11 (contd.) (e) Ruptured chordae (arrow) noted in the left ventricle. (f) Calcified cho dae tendineae (arrow) of the posterior leaflet. LA, left atrium; V, left ventricle; A V, aortic valve; R VOT, right ventricular outflo tract.

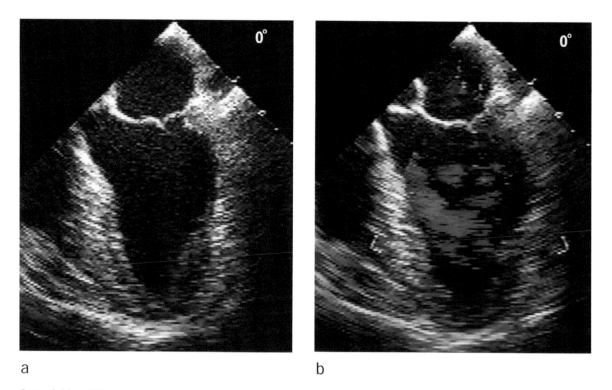

a b

Case 4.12 Mitral valve pr olapse with a r uptured anterior leaflet cho dae tendineae occur ring immediately following cardiopulmonar y bypass. (a) Systolic frame demonstrating valve closur e. (b) Color flow Dopple demonstrating mild r egurgitation.

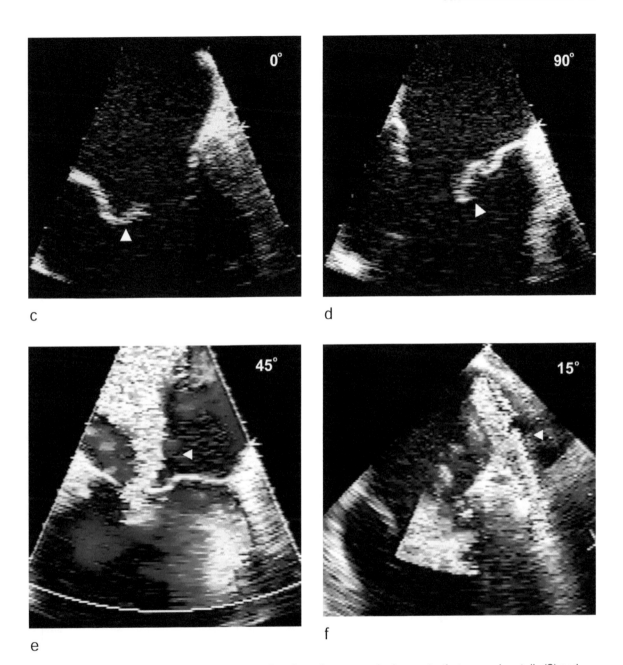

Case 4.12 (contd.) (c) Pulsed Doppler r ecording the pulmonar y vein demonstrating nor mal systolic (S) and diastolic (D) flow p ofiles. Immediately following weaning fr om cardiopulmonar y bypass, enlar ged views of the anterior mitral leaflet at 0 (d) and 90° (e) demonstrating a r uptured chorda (arrow). (f) Pulsed Doppler recording of the pulmonar y vein demonstrating systolic flow eversal (arrow) and predominance of diastolic flo , suggesting sever e regurgitation.

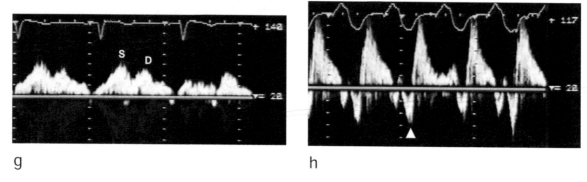

g   h

Case 4.12 (contd.) Color flow Doppler of a new posteriorly di ected mitral regurgitant jet at 45° (g) and 15° (h).

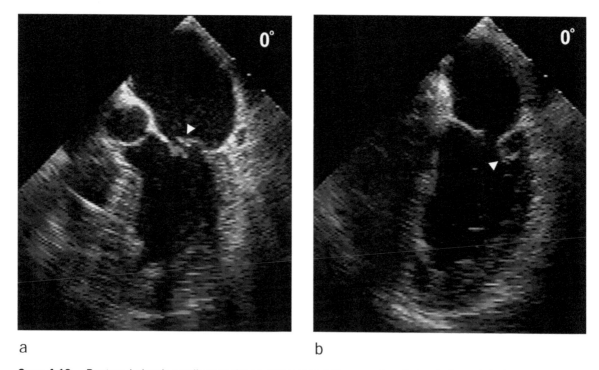

a   b

Case 4.13 Ruptured chorda tendinea to the posterior leaflet. The uptured chorda (arrow) is demonstrated freely moving from the left ventricle to the left atrium during the car diac cycle. Views obtained fr om systole to diastole (a–d) at 0°.

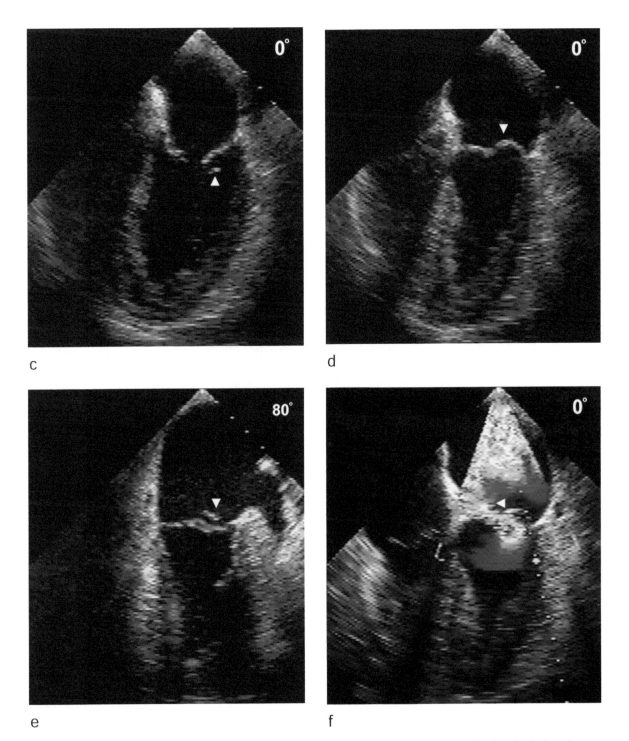

Case 4.13 (contd.)   (e) Systolic frame at 90° demonstrating the ruptured chorda prolapsing freely into the left atrium. (f) Color flow Doppler at 0 demonstrating an anterior directed mitral regurgitant jet (arrow).

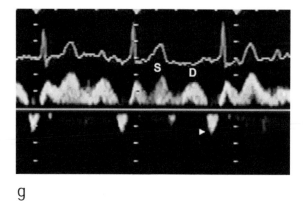

g

Case 4.13 (contd.)   (g) Pulsed wave Doppler recording of pulmonary venous flow demonstrating nearly normal pulmonary venous flow despite significant regurgitant jet. S, systolic flow; D diastolic flo .

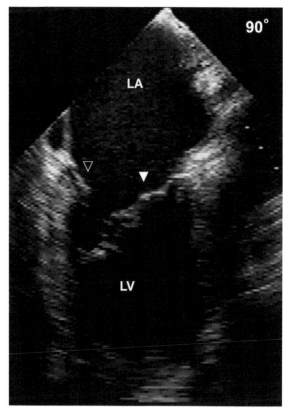

a

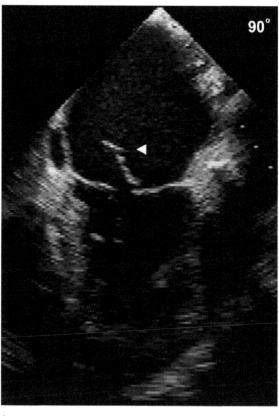

b

Case 4.14   Ruptured chorda tendinea. (a) Diastolic frame fr om the lower esophageal window at 90° demonstrates a lar ge left atrium and nor mal valve opening. (b) Systolic frame demonstrates the r   uptured chorda (arrow) projecting into the left atrium.

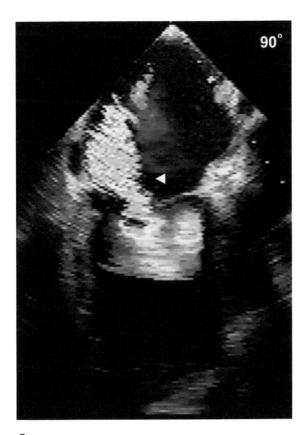

c

d

Case 4.14 (contd.) (c) Systolic frame with color flow Doppler yields moderate mitral r egurgitation (arrow). Although the jet appears to be dir ected posteriorly in this view , it is tempting to label the ruptured chorda to the anterior leaflet. However th ruptured chorda was attached to the posterior leaflet. (d) Gastric view at 90° demonstrates the ruptured chorda projecting into the left atrium. The gastric and deep transgastric views ar e extremely useful for evaluating the subvalvular apparatus when there are questions fr om the other views. LA, left atrium; LV, left ventricle; AML, anterior leaflet (close arrow); PML, posterior leaflet (open a row).

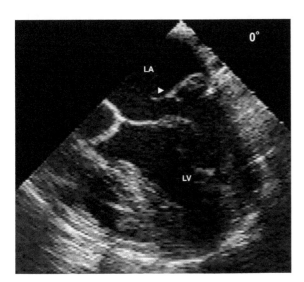

a

Case 4.15 Ruptured chorda tendinea with a flai posterior leaflet. o construct a mental thr ee-dimensional image, multiple views may be necessar y to demonstrate all of the associated pathology , especially when describing the abnor malities prior to mitral valve r epair. (a) Systolic frame fr om the lower esophageal window at 0° demonstrating a r uptured chorda and flail posterior leaflet (row).

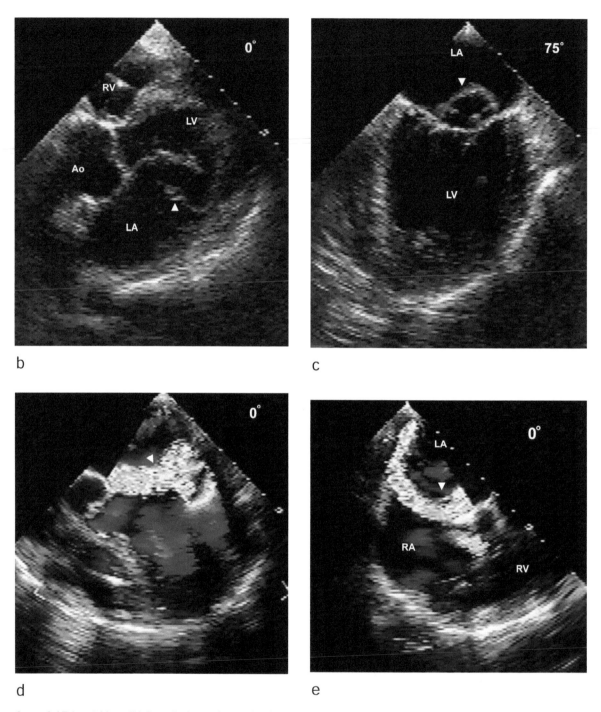

b

c

d

e

Case 4.15 (contd.) (b) Systolic frame fr om the deep transgastric window at 0° demonstrating the ruptured chorda. (c) Systolic frame fr om the lower esophageal window demonstrating marked billowing of the P2 or central scallop (ar row) of the posterior leaflet superimposed on a no mal anterior leaflet. (d) Color flow Doppl from the lower esophageal window at 0° demonstrating severe mitral regurgitation directed anteriorly towar ds the atrial septum. (e) Color flow Doppler after slight withdrawal and rightwa d rotation of the pr obe demonstrates the mitral r egurgitant jet hugging the atrial septum and wrapping ar ound the atrium.

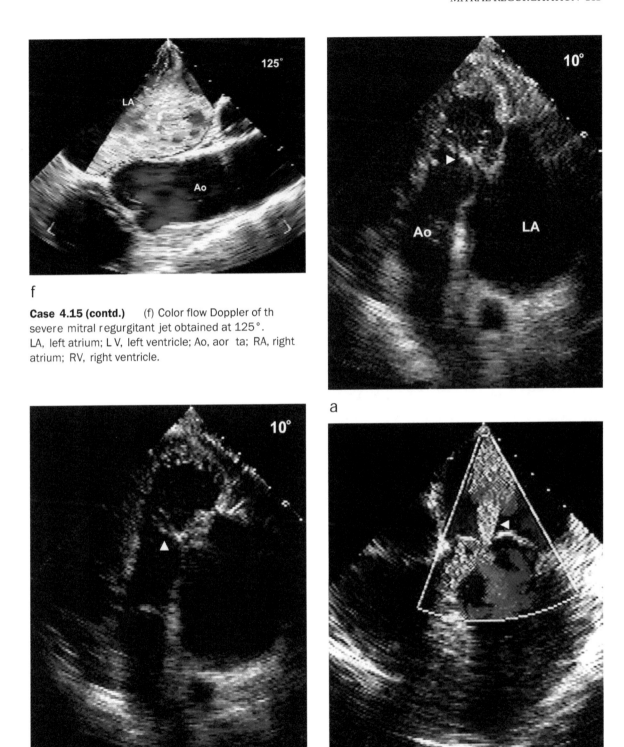

f

Case 4.15 (contd.) (f) Color flow Doppler of th
severe mitral regurgitant jet obtained at 125°.
LA, left atrium; L V, left ventricle; Ao, aor ta; RA, right
atrium; RV, right ventricle.

a

b   c

Case 4.16 Mitral valve prolapse and SAM. (a) End-diastolic frame from the deep transgastric window at 10°,
demonstrating elongated and thickened chordae (arrow). (b) Systolic frame demonstrating systolic anterior
motion or SAM (arrow). (c) Color flow Doppler from the lower esophageal window at 0° demonstrating billowing
and prolapse of the mitral valve leaflets with associated mitral regurgitation and accelerated and disturbed flo
in the left ventricular outflow tract.

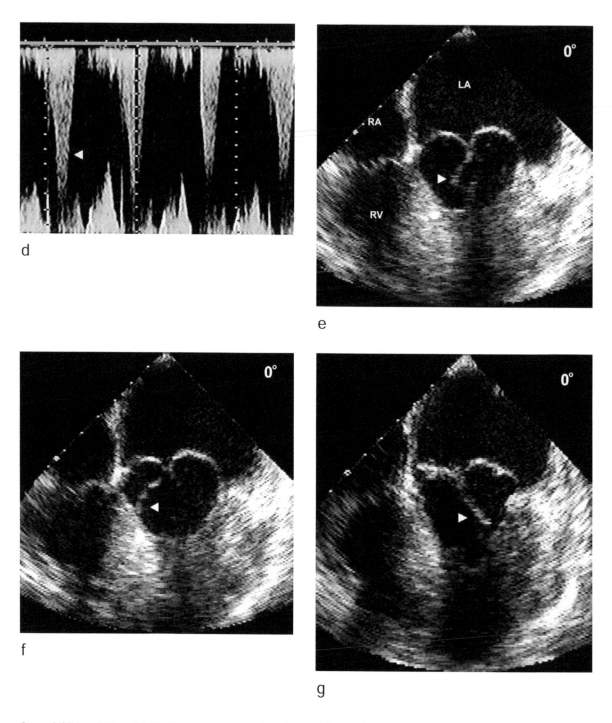

Case 4.16 (contd.) (d) Continuous wave Doppler obtained fr om the deep transgastric window demonstrating high velocity flow in the outflow tract. (e–h) Systolic frames obtained om the lower esophageal window at 0° with anteflexion of the p obe highlights the systolic motion of the chor dae tendineae thr oughout systole (arrows).

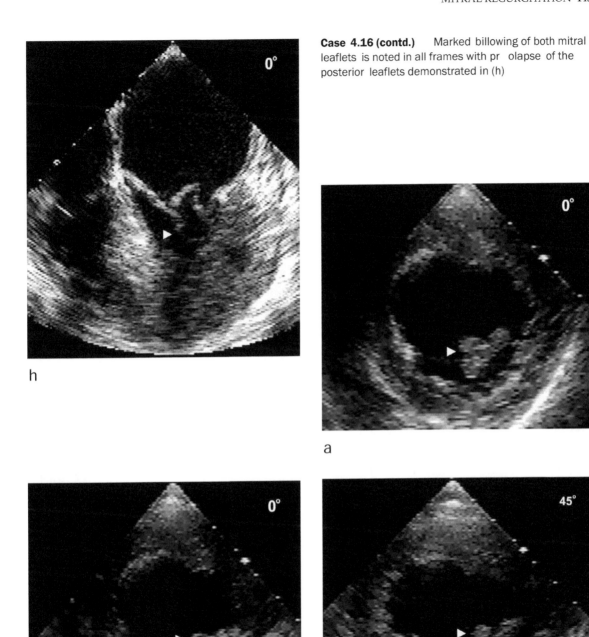

Case 4.16 (contd.) Marked billowing of both mitral leaflets is noted in all frames with pr olapse of the posterior leaflets demonstrated in (h)

Case 4.17 Ruptured papillar y muscle. (a) Diastolic frame fr om the shor t axis view at the mid ventricular level, 0°, demonstrates par tial rupture of the anterior papillar y muscle. (b) Systolic frame demonstrating partial rupture of the papillar y muscle. (c) Diastolic frame at 45° demonstrates the chaotic motion of the papillar y muscle.

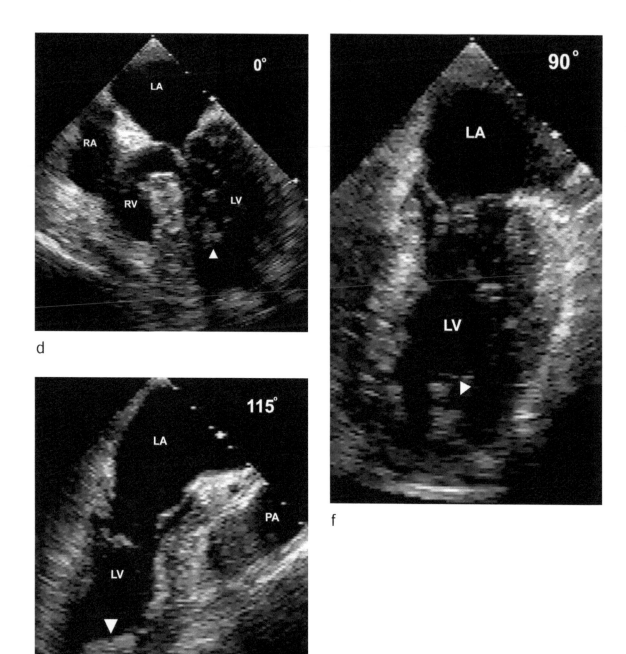

Case 4.17 (contd.) Systolic frame from the lower esophageal window at 0°. (d), 110° (e) and 90° (f) demonstrates multiple echodensities (ar row) near the papillary muscle.

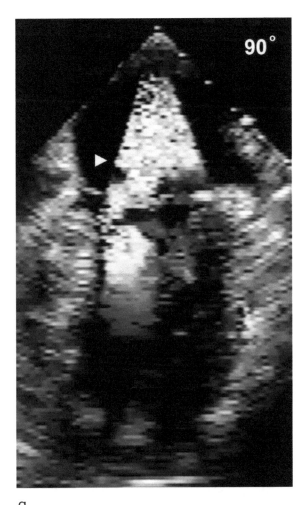

g

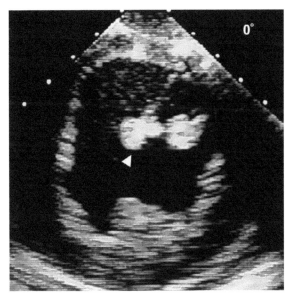

a

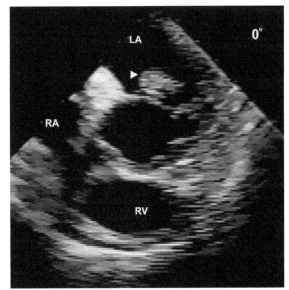

b

Case 4.17 (contd.) Although partial rupture of the papillary muscle usually produces dramatic mitral regurgitation (g), careful inspection of the papillary muscles must be performed in multiple views to document the defect. In addition to the papillary muscle abnormality, the anterior left ventricular wall was noted to be severely hypokinetic. Although partial rupture of a papillary muscle may be suggested by transthoracic imaging, the definitive diagnosis of partial rupture of a papillary muscle is made with TEE. LA, left atrium; LV, left ventricle; RA, right atrium; RV, right ventricle.

Case 4.18 Ruptured papillary muscle. (a) Mid-ventricular short-axis view demonstrates a freely floating posterior papillary muscle in diastole. (b) Systolic frame from the mid-esophageal window of the base of the heart demonstrates the papillary muscle (arrow) prolapsing into the left atrium above the mitral valve annular plane.

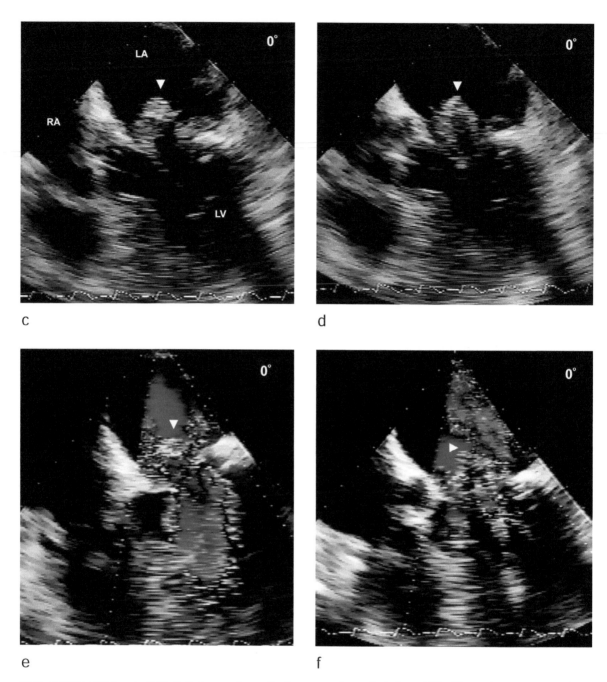

Case 4.18 (contd.) (c,d) Systolic frames from the lower esophageal window at 0° illustrating the ruptured papillary muscle (arrow) prolapsing through the mitral valve plane. (e,f) Color flow Doppler demonstrating mitral regurgitation associated with the ruptured papillary muscle.

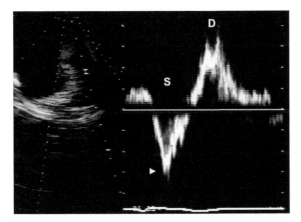

g

Case 4.18 (contd.)   (g) Pulsed wave Doppler of the left upper pulmonary vein demonstrating systolic (S) flow reversal (arrow) and diastolic (D) flo predominance suggesting severe mitral regurgitation. LA, left atrium; LV, left ventricle; RA, right atrium.

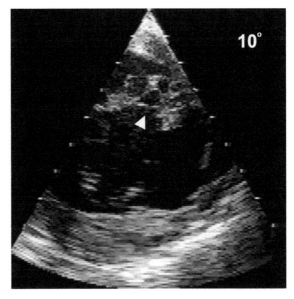

a

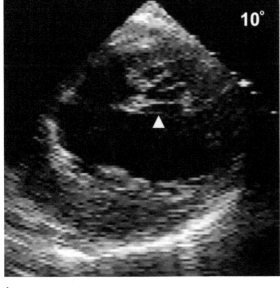

b

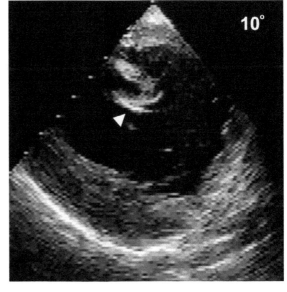

c

Case 4.19   Papillary muscle hemorrhage. (a–c) Short-axis views at the mid-ventricular level at 10° demonstrating hemorrhage of the posterior papillary muscle during the cardiac cycle. The papillary muscle appears enlarged with multiple cystic, echo-free areas within the confines of the papillary muscle.

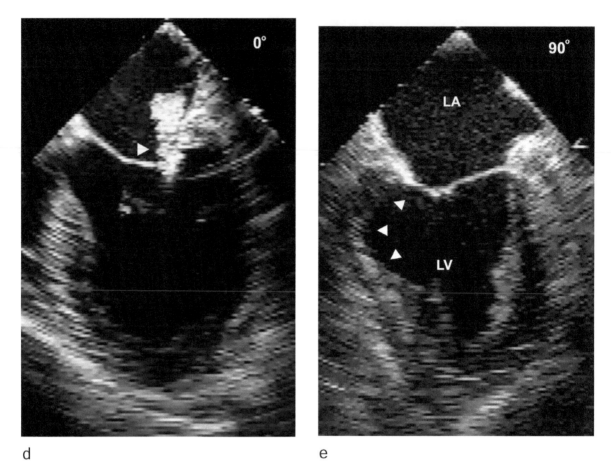

d   e

Case 4.19 (contd.)   (d) Color flow Doppler demonstrating mitral   egurgitation associated with the dysfunction of the papillar y muscle. (e) Systolic frame fr om the lower esophageal window at 90°   highlights a posterior wall infarction and small ventricular aneur ysm (arrows) of that ar ea. Papillar y muscle hemor rhage usually pr oduces mitral regurgitation through restriction of leaflet motion (type III) rather than by p   olapse of the leaflet a associated with r upture or par tial rupture of the papillar y muscle. As for par tial rupture of a papillar y muscle, the resolution provided with TEE is needed for a definitive diagnosis. LA, left atrium;   V, left ventricle.

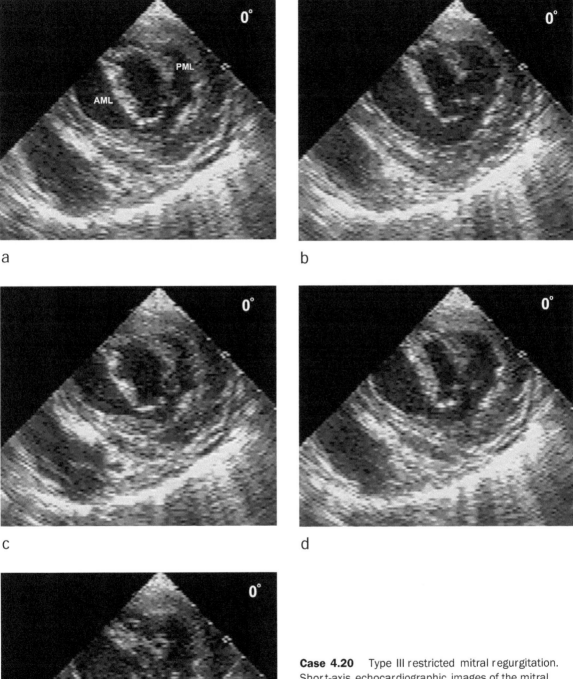

a

b

c

d

e

Case 4.20 Type III restricted mitral regurgitation. Shor t-axis echocardiographic images of the mitral valve recorded from diastole thr ough systole. (a) Early diastole. (b) Mid diastole. (c) Atrial systole. (d) End diastole. (e) End systole. Note that all leafle motion is pr oduced by the anterior leaflet, with th posterior leaflet emaining fixed and non-mobil during the entir e cardiac cycle. With type III r estricted motion, severe mitral r egurgitation usually does not occur until ther e is co-existent annular dilatation. AML, anterior leaflet; PML, posterior leafle

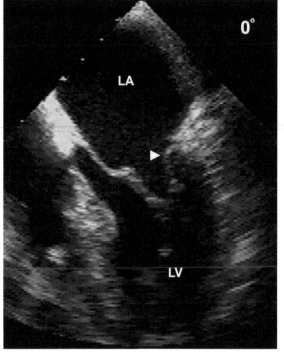

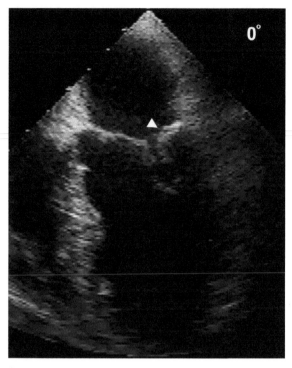

a

b

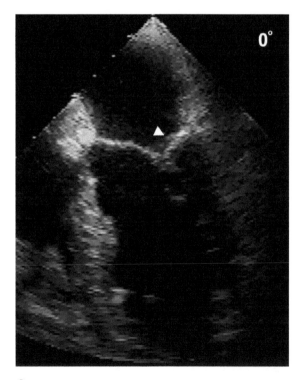

Case 4.21 Type III mitral r egurgitation. (a–c) Frontal views of the mitral valve obtained fr om the lower esophageal window at 0° from diastole to systole in the same patient as in Case 7.5. The anterior mitral leaflet is on the left and the posterio leaflet (arrow) is on the right. The posterior leaflet i thickened with mild calcification and is elatively immobile during the car diac cycle. LA, left atrium; LV, left ventricle.

c

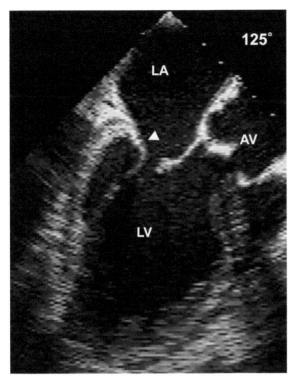

a

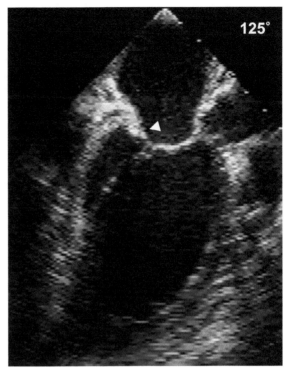

b

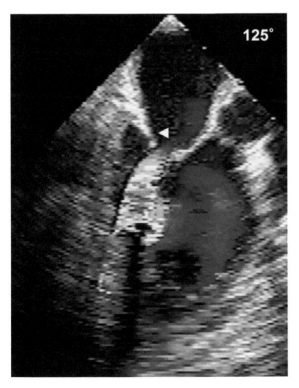

c

Case 4.22 Type III mitral r egurgitation. Mitral valve images obtained fr om the lower esophageal window at 125° in diastole (a) and systole (b), demonstrating an immobile, fixed posterior leaflet t oughout the cardiac cycle. (c) Color flow Doppler of the lef ventricular inflow tract depicting high velocity fl (arrow) across the mitral orifice suggesting a mil degree of obstr uction associated with the fixe leaflet.

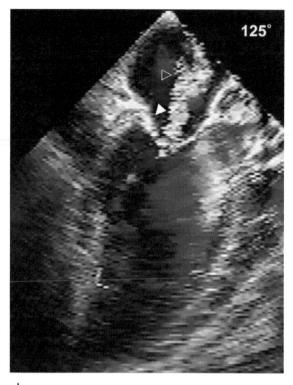

d

Case 4.22 (contd.) (d) Color flow Doppler durin systole demonstrating mitral r egurgitation (arrow). Restriction to the posterior leaflet may no necessarily be symmetrical or involve the entir e leaflet. Since ther e are three scallops and inter vention by two papillar y muscles fr om different regions of the myocar dium, only par t of the posterior leaflet may be involved, depending on the pathology responsible for the r estrictive process. It is important to view the entir e posterior leaflet i multiple views in or der to diagnosis type III motion. LA, left atrium; L V, left ventricle; A V, aortic valve.

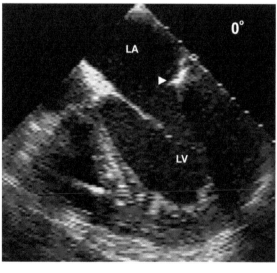

a

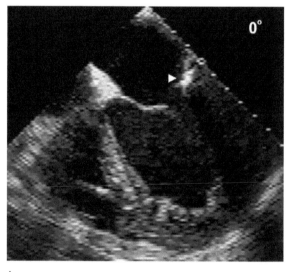

b

Case 4.23 Type III mitral r egurgitation. Mitral valve images obtained fr om the lower esophageal window at 0° in diastole (a), mid-diastole (b) and systole (c) demonstrating an immobile posterior leaflet (a row).

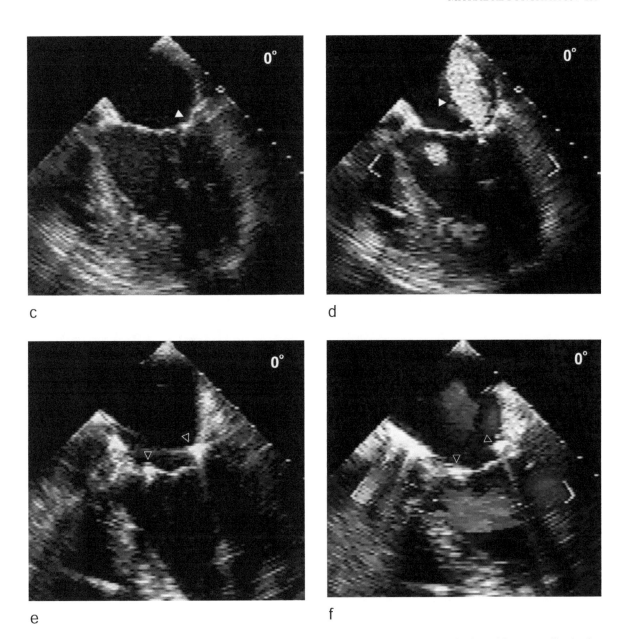

Case 4.23 (contd.)   (d) Color flow Doppler demonstrating significant mitral   egurgitation. Often, type III mitral regurgitation only requires an annuloplasty ring during r epair to eliminate the r egurgitation. Postoperative views in the same patient, (e) demonstrating a mitral annuloplasty ring (ar   rows), (f) color flow Doppler demonstratin the absence of mitral r egurgitation. LA, left atrium; L V, left ventricle.

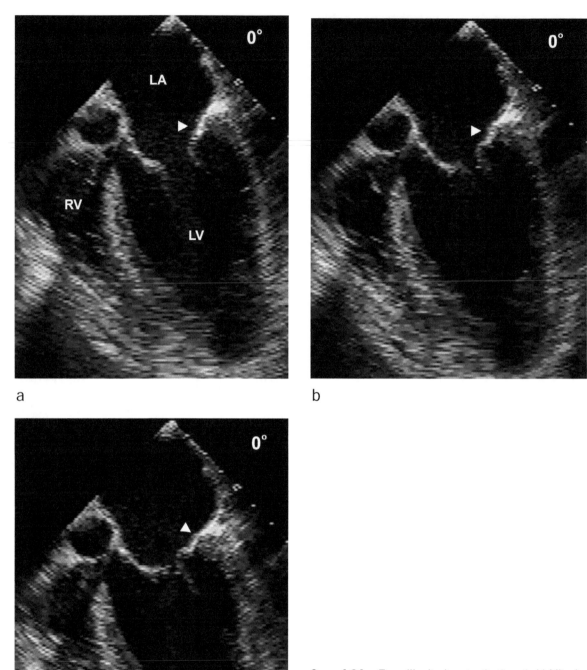

a

b

c

Case 4.24 Type III mitral r egurgitation. (a,b) Mitral valve images obtained fr om the lower esophageal window at 0°. The posterior leaflet is immobil throughout the car diac cycle. In systole (c) a small por tion of the leaflet p olapses past the anterior leaflet. At the time of sur gery there was a small flai segment, although the major pathology was restrictive.

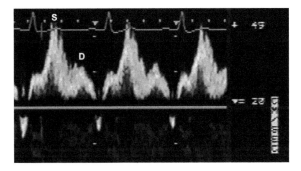

d

e

Case 4.24 (contd.) (d) Color flow Dopple demonstrating mitral regurgitation. (e) Pulsed wave Doppler of pulmonary venous flo . LA, left atrium; LV, left ventricle; R V, right ventricle; S, systolic; D, diastolic.

REFERENCES

1. Cosgrove DM, Stewart WJ. Current problems in cardiology: mitral valvuloplasty. 1989;14(7):353–416.
2. Peterson KL. Timing of cardiac surgery in chronic mitral valve disease: implications of natural history studies and left ventricular mechanics. Sem Thorac Cardiovasc Surg 1989;1:106–117.
3. Ling LH, Enriquez-Sarano M, Seward JB, et al. Clinical outcome of mitral regurgitation due to flail leaflet. N Engl J Med 1996;335:1417–1423.
4. Ling LH, Enriquez-Sarano M, Seward JB, et al. Early surgery in patients with mitral regurgitation due to flail leaflets. A long-term outcome study. Circulation 1997;96:1819–1825.
5. Sand ME, Naftel DC, Blackstone EH, Kirklin JW, Karp RB. A comparison of repair and replacement for mitral valve incompetence. J Thorac Cardiovasc Surg 1987;94:208–219.
6. Carpentier A. Cardiac valve surgery-the "French correction". J Thorac Cardiovasc Surg 1983;86:323–337.
7. Bonchek LI. Correction of mitral valve disease without valve replacement. Am Heart J 1982;104:865–868.
8. Antunes MJ, Colsen PR, Kinsley RH. Mitral valvuloplasty: a learning curve. Circulation 1983;68:II–70–75.
9. Cosgrove DM, Chavez AM, Lytle BW, et al. Results of mitral valve reconstruction. Circulation 1986;74:1–82–7.
10. Hellemans IM, Pieper EG, Ravelli ACJ, et al. Prediction of surgical strategy in mitral valve regurgitation based on echocardiography. Am J Cardiol 1997;79:334–338.
11. Stewart WJ, Currie PJ, Salcedo EE, et al. Intraoperative Doppler color flow mapping for decision-making in valve repair for mitral regurgitation. Technique and results in 100 patients. Circulation 1990;81:556–566.
12. Oki T, Fukuda N, Iuchi A, et al. Possible mechanisms of mitral regurgitation in dilated hearts: a study using transesophageal echocardiography. Clin Cardiol 1996;19:639–643.
13. Chandraratna PAN, Aronow WS. Mitral valve ring in normal vs. dilated left ventricle. Cross-

sectional echocardiographic study. Chest 1981;79:151–154.

14. Tsakiris AG, von Bernuth G, Rastelli GC, et al. Size and motion of the mitral valve annulus in anesthetized intact dogs. J Appl Physiol 1971;30:611–18.

15. Bulkley BH, Roberts WC. Dilatation of the mitral annulus: a rare cause of mitral regurgitation. Am J Med 1975;59:457–63.

16. Madu EC, Reddy RC, D'Cruz IA. Papillary muscle morphology and function in LV systolic dysfunction and dilated cardiomyopathy: a transesophageal echocardiographic study (abstr). J Am Soc Echocardiogr 1996;9:371A.

17. Sigfusson G, Ettedgui JA, Silverman NH, Anderson RH. Is a cleft in the anterior leaflet of an otherwise normal mitral valve an atrioventricular canal malformation? J Am Coll Cardiol 1995;26:508–15.

18. Creech O, Ledbeter MK, Reemtsma K. Congenital insufficiency with a cleft in the posterior leaflet. Circulation 1962;25:390.

19. DiSegni E, Edwards JE. Cleft anterior leaflet of the mitral valve with intact septa. A study of twenty cases. Am J Cardiol 1983;51:915.

20. DiSegni E, Bass JL, Lucas RV Jr, et al. Isolated cleft mitral valve: a variety of congenital mitral regurgitation identified by 2-dimensional echocardiography. Am J Cardiol 1983;51:927–31.

21. Becker AE, De Wit APM. Mitral valve apparatus. A spectrum of normality relevant to mitral valve prolapse. Br Heart J 1979;42:680–9.

22. Levine RA, Triulzi MO, Harrigan P, Weyman AE. The relationship of mitral annular shape to the diagnosis of mitral valve prolapse. Circulation 1987;75:756–67.

23. Levine RA, Handschumacher MD, Sanfilippo AJ, et al. Three-dimensional echocardiographic reconstruction of the mitral valve, with implications for the diagnosis of mitral valve prolapse. Circulation 1989;80:589–98.

24. Zuppiroli A, Rinaldi M, Kramer-Fox R, et al. Natural history of mitral valve prolapse. Am J Cardiol 1995;75:1028.

25. Boudoulas H, Kolibash AJ, Baker P, et al. Mitral valve prolapse and the mitral valve prolapse syndrome: a diagnostic classification and pathogenesis of symptoms. Am Heart J 1989;118:796–817.

26. Joh Y, Yoshikawa J, Yoshida K, et al. Transesophageal echocardiographic finding of mitral valve prolapse. J Cardiol 1989;19(suppl 21):85–95.

27. Titus JL, Edwards J. Mitral insufficiency other than rheumatic, ischemic, or infective: Emphasis on mitral valve prolapse. Sem Thorac Cardiovasc Surg 1989;1:118–28.

28. Pini R, Greppi B, Kramer-Fox R, et al. Mitral valve dimensions and motion and familial transmission of mitral valve prolapse with and without mitral leaflet billowing. J Am Coll Cardiol 1988;12:1423–31.

29. Turabian M, Chan K-L. Rupture of mitral chordae tendineae resulting from blunt chest trauma: diagnosis by transesophageal echocardiography. Can J Cardiol 1990;6:180–2.

30. Alam M, Sun I. Superiority of transesophageal echocardiography in detecting ruptured mitral chordae tendineae. Am Heart J 1991;121:1819–21.

31. Roth SL, Friedman GH, Bodenheimer MM, Chasanoff H. Redundant loops of chordae tendineae: a new potential cardiac source of embolism detected by transesophageal echocardiography. J Am Coll Cardiol 1994;22:75A.

32. Hozumi T, Yoshikawa J, Yoshida K, et al. Direct visualization of ruptured chordae tendineae by transesophageal two-dimensional echocardiography. J Am Coll Cardiol 1990;16:1315–19.

33. Schlueter M, Kremer P, Hanrath P. Transesophageal 2-D echocardiographic feature of flail mitral leaflet due to ruptured chordae tendineae. Am Heart J 1984;108:609–10.

34. Himelman RB, Kusumoto F, Oken K, et al. The flail mitral valve: echocardiographic findings by precordial and transesophageal imaging and Doppler color flow imaging. J Am Coll Cardiol 1991;17:272–9.

35. Louie EK, Langholz D, Mackin WJ, et al. Transesophageal echocardiographic assessment of the contribution of intrinsic tissue thickness to the appearance of a thick mitral valve in patients with mitral valve prolapse. J Am Coll Cardiol 1996;28:465–71.

36. Stewart WJ, Currie PJ, Salcedo EE, et al. Evaluation of mitral leaflet motion by echocardiography and jet direction by Doppler color flow mapping to determine the mechanism of

mitral regurgitation. J Am Coll Cardiol 1992;20:1353–1361.

37. Eliot RS, Edwards JE. Pathology of rheumatic fever and chronic valvular disease. In: Hurst JW (ed). The Heart (3rd edn) New York: McGraw-Hill, 1974.

38. McDonald L, Dealy JB, Rabinowitz M, et al. Clinical, physiological and pathological findings in mitral stenosis and regurgitation. Medicine 1957;36:237.

39. Perloff JK, Roberts WC. The mitral apparatus functional anatomy of mitral regurgitation. Circulation 1972;46:227.

40. Davies MJ, Moore BP, Brainbridge MB. The floppy mitral valve study of incidence, pathology and complications in surgical, necropsic and forensic material. Br Heart J 1978;40:468.

41. Guthrie RG, Edwards JE. Pathology of the myxomatous mitral valve. Nature, secondary changes and complications. Minn Med 1976;59:637.

42. Mintz GS, Victor MF, Kotler MN, et al. Two-dimensional echocardiographic identification of surgically correctable complications of acute myocardial infarction. Circulation 1981;64:91–6.

43. Come PC, Riley MF, Weintraub R, et al. Echocardiographic detection of complete and partial papillary muscle rupture during acute myocardial infarction. Am J Cardiol 1985;56:787–789.

44. Sakai K, Nakamura K, Hosoda S. Transesophageal echocardiographic findings of papillary muscle rupture. Am J Cardiol 1991;68:561–563.

45. Manning WJ, Waksmonski CA, Boyle NG. Papillary muscle rupture complicating inferior myocardial infarction: identification with transesophageal echocardiography. Am Heart J 1995;129:191–193.

46. Moursi MH, Bhatnagar SK, Vilacosta I, et al. Transesophageal echocardiographic assessment of papillary muscle rupture. Circulation 1996;94:1003–1009.

47. Cerza RF. Echocardiography of papillary muscle hemorrhage. J Cardiothor Vasc Anesth 1994;8:446–447.

48. Hauser A, Rathod K, McGill J, et al. Blood cysts of the papillary muscle. Am J Cardiol 1983;51:612–613.

49. Fishbein MC. Mitral insufficiency in coronary artery disease. Sem Thorac Cardiovasc Surg 1989;1:129–132.

50. Voci P, Bilotta F, Catetta Q, et al. Papillary muscle perfusion pattern. A hypothesis for ischemic papillary muscle dysfunction. Circulation 1995;91:1714–1718.

51. Kaul S, Sponitz WD, Glasheen WP, Touchstone DA. Mechanism of ischemic mitral regurgitation: an experimental evaluation. Circulation 1991;84:2167–2180.

52. Madu EC, D'Cruz IA. The vital role of papillary muscles in mitral and ventricular function: Echocardiographic insights. Clin Cardiol 1997;20:93–98.

53. Byram MT, Roberts WC. Frequency and extent of calcific deposits in purely regurgitant mitral valves: analysis of 108 operatively excised valves. Am J Cardiol 1983;52:1059–1061.

54. Akamatsu S, Uematsu H, Yamamoto M, et al. Evaluation of physiological mitral regurgitant flow with transesophageal Doppler echocardiography (abstr). Jpn Circulation J 1989;53:663.

55. Omoto R, Kyo S, Matsumura M, et al. Evaluation of biplane color Doppler transesophageal echocardiography in 200 consecutive patients. Circulation 1992;85:1237–1247.

56. Matsumara M, Kyo S, Shah P, et al. A new look at mitral valve pathology with bi-plane color Doppler transesophageal probe (abstr). Circulation 1989;80 suppl 2:II–579.

57. Yoshida K, Yoshikawa J, Yamaura Y, et al. Assessment of mitral regurgitation by biplane transesophageal color Doppler flow mapping. Circulation 1990;82:1121–1126.

58. Schnittger I, Appleton CP, Hatle LK, Popp RL. Diastolic mitral and tricuspid regurgitation by Doppler echocardiography in patients with atrioventricular block: new insight into the mechanism of atrioventricular valve closure. J Am Coll Cardiol 1988;11:83.

59. Rokey R, Murphy DJ Jr, Nielsen AP, et al. Detection of diastolic atrioventricular valvular regurgitation by pulse Doppler echocardiography and its association with complete heart block. Am J Cardiol 1986;57:692.

60. Clyne CA, Cuenoud HF, Pape LA. Diastolic mitral regurgitation occurring with complete atrioventricular block detected by Doppler color flow mapping. Echocardiography 1989;6:543.

61. Sadoshima J-I, Koyanagi S, Sugimachi M, et al. Evaluation of the severity of mitral regurgitation by transesophageal Doppler flow echocardiography. Am Heart J 1992;123:1245–1251.

62. Cooper JW, Nanda NC, Philpot EF, Fan P. Evaluation of valvular regurgitation by color Doppler. J Am Soc Echocardiogr 1989; 2:56–66.

63. Wang SS, Rubenstein JJ, Goldman, Sidd JJ. A new Doppler-echocardiography method to quantify regurgitant volume. J Am Soc Echocardiogr 1992;5:107–114.

64. Walker PG, Oyre S, Pedersen EM, et al. A new control volume method for calculating valvular regurgitation. Circulation 1995;92:579–586.

65. Kleinman JP, Czer LSC, DeRobertis M, et al. A quantitative comparison of transesophageal and epicardial color Doppler echocardiography in the intraoperative assessment of mitral regurgitation. Am J Cardiol 1989;64:1168–1172.

66. Enriquez-Sarano M, Tajik AJ, Bailey KR, Seward JB. Color flow imaging compared with quantitative Doppler assessment of severity of mitral regurgitation: influence of eccentricity of jet and mechanism of regurgitation. J Am Coll Cardiol 1993;21:1211–1219.

67. Miyatake K, Izumi, Okamoto M, et al. Semiquantitative grading of severity of mitral regurgitation by real-time two dimensional Doppler flow imaging technique. J Am Coll Cardiol 1986;7:82–88.

68. Shiota T, Jones M, Teien DE, et al. Dynamic change in mitral regurgitant orifice area: Comparison of color Doppler echocardiographic and electromagnetic flowmeter-based methods in a chronic animal model. J Am Coll Cardiol 1995;26:528–536.

69. Sahn DJ. Instrumentation and physical factors related to visualization of stenotic and regurgitant jets by Doppler color flow mapping. J Am Coll Cardiol 1988;12:1354–1365.

70. Mizushige K, Shiota T, Paik J, et al. Effects of pulmonary venous flow direction on mitral regurgitation jet area as imaged by color Doppler flow mapping. An in vitro study. Circulation 1995;19:1834–1839.

71. Helmcke F, Nanda NC, Hsiung MC, et al. Color Doppler assessment of mitral regurgitation with orthogonal planes. Circulation 1987;75:175–183.

72. Castello R, Lenzen P, Aquirre F, Labovitz A. Variability in the quantitation of mitral regurgitation by Doppler color flow mapping: comparison of transthoracic and transesophageal studies. J Am Coll Cardiol 1992;20:433–438.

73. Smith MD, Harrison MR, Pinton R, et al. Regurgitant jet size by transesophageal compared with transthoracic Doppler color flow imaging. Circulation 1991;83:79–86.

74. Castello R, Lenzen P, Aguirre F, Labovitz A. Quantitation of mitral regurgitation by transesophageal echocardiography with Doppler color-flow mapping: correlation with cardiac catheterization. J Am Coll Cardiol 1992;19:1516–1521.

75. Enriquez-Sarano M, Bailey KR, Seward JB, et al. Quantitative Doppler assessment of valvular regurgitation. Circulation 1993;87:841–848.

76. Rokey R, Sterling LL, Zoghbi WA, et al. Determination of regurgitant fraction in isolated mitral or aortic regurgitation by pulsed Doppler two-dimensional echocardiography. J Am Coll Cardiol 1986;7:1273–1278.

77. Enriquez-Sarano M, Seward JB, Bailey KR, Tajik AJ. Effective regurgitant orifice area: a noninvasive Doppler development of an old hemodynamic concept. J Am Coll Cardiol 1994;23:443–451.

78. Klein AL, Obarski TP, Stewart J, et al. Transesophageal Doppler echocardiography of pulmonary venous flow: a new marker of mitral regurgitation severity. J Am Coll Cardiol 1991;18:518–526.

79. Tanabe K, Yoshitomi H, Oyake N, et al. Effects of supine and lateral recumbent positions on pulmonary venous flow in healthy subjects evaluated by transesophageal Doppler echocardiography. J Am Coll Cardiol 1994;24:1552–1557.

80. Teien DE, Jones M, Shiota T, et al. Doppler evaluation of severity of mitral regurgitation: relation to pulmonary venous flow patterns in an animal study. J Am Coll Cardiol 1995;25:264–268.

81. Passafini A, Shiota T, Depp M, et al. Factors influencing pulmonary venous flow velocity patterns in mitral regurgitation: an in vitro study. J Am Coll Cardiol 1995;26:1333–1339.

82. Klein AL, Obarski TP, Calafiore PC, et al. Reversal of systolic flow in pulmonary veins by

transesophageal Doppler echocardiography predicts severity of mitral regurgitation (abstr). J Am Coll Cardiol 1990;15:74A.

83. Klein AL, Tajik AJ. Doppler assessment of pulmonary venous flow in healthy subjects and in patients with heart disease. J Am Soc Echocardiogr 1991;4:379–392.

84. Castello R, Pearson AC, Lenzen P, Labovitz AJ. Effect of mitral regurgitation on pulmonary venous velocities derived from transesophageal echocardiography color-guided pulse Doppler imaging. J Am Coll Cardiol 1991;17:1499–1506.

85. Tribouilloy C, Shen WF, Quere JP, et al. Assessment of severity of mitral regurgitation by measuring regurgitating jet width at its origin with transesophageal Doppler color flow imaging. Circulation 1992;85:1248–1253.

86. Baumgartner H, Schima H, Kuhn P. Value and limitations of proximal jet dimensions for the quantitation of valvular regurgitation: an in vitro study using Doppler flow imaging. J Am Soc Echocardiogr 1991;4:57–66.

87. Mele D, Vandervoort P, Palacios I, et al. Proximal jet size by Doppler color flow mapping predicts severity of mitral regurgitation. Clin Stud Circ 1995;91:746–754.

88. Hall SA, Brickner E, Willet DL, et al. Assessment of mitral regurgitation severity by Doppler color flow mapping of the vena contracta. Circulation 1997;95:636–642.

89. Simpson IA, Sahn DJ. Hydrodynamic investigation of a hemodynamic problem: a review of the in vitro evaluation of mitral insufficiency by color Doppler flow mapping. J Am Soc Echocardiogr 1989;2:67–72.

90. Grayburn PA, Fehske W, Omran H, et al. Multiplane transesophageal echocardiographic assessment of mitral regurgitation by Doppler color flow mapping of the vena contracta. Am J Cardiol 1994;74:912–917.

91. Recusani F, Bargiggia GS, Yoganathan AP, et al. A new method for quantification of regurgitant flow rate using color Doppler flow imaging of the flow convergence region proximal to a discrete orifice: an in vitro study. Circulation 1991;83:594–604.

92. Utosonomiya T, Ogawa T, Tang HA, et al. Doppler color flow mapping of the proximal isovelocity surface area: a new method for measuring volume flow rate across a narrowed orifice. J Am Soc Echocardiogr 1991;4:338–348.

93. Giesler MO, Stauch M. Color Doppler determination of regurgitant flow: from proximal isovelocity surface areas to proximal velocity profiles. Echocardiography 1992;9:51–62.

94. Geisler M, Grossmann G, Schmidt A, et al. Color Doppler echocardiographic determination of mitral regurgitant flow from the proximal velocity profile of the flow convergence region. Am J Cardiol 1993;71:217–224.

95. Deng Y-B, Matsumoto M, Wang X-F, et al. Estimation of mitral valve area in patients with mitral stenosis by the flow convergence region method: selection of aliasing velocity. J Am Coll Cardiol 1994;24:683–689.

96. Enriquez-Sarano M, Miller FA, Hayes SN, et al. Effective mitral regurgitant orifice area: clinical use and pitfalls of the proximal isovelocity surface area method. J Am Coll Cardiol 1995;25:703–709.

97. Enriquez-Sarano M, Sinak LJ, Tajik AJ, et al. Changes in effective regurgitant orifice throughout systole in patients with mitral valve prolapse. A clinical study using the proximal isovelocity surface area method. Circulation 1995;92:2951–2958.

98. Pu M, Vandervoort PM, Griffin BP, et al. Quantification of mitral regurgitation by the proximal convergence method using transesophageal echocardiography. Clinical validation of a geometric correction for proximal flow constraint. Circulation 1995;92:2169–2177.

99. Pu M, Vandervoort PM, Greenberg NL, et al. Impact of wall constraint on velocity distribution in proximal flow convergence zone. Implications for color Doppler quantification of mitral regurgitation. J Am Coll Cardiol 1996;27:706–713.

100. Vandervoort PM, Rivera JM, Mele D, et al. Application of color Doppler flow mapping to calculate effective regurgitant orifice area: an in vitro study with initial clinical observations. Circulation 1993;88:1150–1156.

101. Shiota T, Sinclair B, Ishii M, et al. Three-dimensional reconstruction of color Doppler flow convergence regions and regurgitant jets: an in vitro quantitative study. J Am Coll Cardiol 1996;27:1511–1518.

102. Simpson IA, Shiota T, Gharib M, Sahn D. Current status of flow convergence for clinical applications: is it a leaning tower of "PISA"? J Am Coll Cardiol 1996;27:504–509.

103. Thomas JD. How leaky is that mitral valve? Simplified Doppler methods to measure regurgitant orifice area. Circulation 1997;95:548–550.

104. Stoddard MF, Prince CR, Dillon S, et al. Exercise-induced mitral regurgitation is a predictor of morbid events in subjects with mitral valve prolapse. J Am Coll Cardiol 1995;25:693–699.

104a. Enriquez-Sarano M, Avierinos JF, Messika-Zeitoun D, et al. Quantitative determinants of the outcome of asymptomatic mitral regurgitation. N Engl J Med 2005;352(9):875–83.

105. Kontos GJ, Schaff HV, Gersh BJ, Bove AA. Left ventricular function in subacute and chronic mitral regurgitation. Effect on function early postoperatively. J Thorac Cardiovasc Surg 1989;98:163–169.

106. Starling MR. Effects of valve surgery on left ventricular contractile function in patients with long-term mitral regurgitation. Circulation 1995;92:811–818.

107. Enriquez-Sarano M, Schaff HV, Orszulak TA, et al. Valve repair improves the outcome of surgery for mitral regurgitation. A multivariate analysis. Circulation 1995;91:1022–1028.

108. Enriquez-Sarano M, Tajik AJ, Schaff HV, et al. Echocardiographic prediction of left ventricular function after correction of mitral regurgitation: results and clinical implications. J Am Coll Cardiol 1994;24:1536–1543.

109. Goldman ME, Mora F, Guarino T, et al. Mitral valvuloplasty is superior to valve replacement for preservation of left ventricular function: an intraoperative two-dimensional echocardiographic study. J Am Coll Cardiol 1987;10:568–575.

110. Rahko PS, Berkoff HA. Echocardiographic comparison of cardiac size and function before and after surgery for isolated mitral valve repair versus mitral valve replacement. Acta Cardiolog 1990;3:189–194.

111. Enriquez-Sarano M, Schaff HV, Orszulak TA, et al. Congestive heart failure after surgical correction of mitral regurgitation. A long-term study. Circulation 1995;92:94–96.

112. Corin WJ, Sutsch G, Murakami T, et al. Left ventricular function in chronic mitral regurgitation: preoperative and postoperative comparison. J Am Coll Cardiol 1995;25:113–121.

113. Madu EC, Reddy RC, D'Cruz IA. Transesophageal echocardiography assessment of papillary muscle anatomy and contraction in patients with and without left ventricular hypertrophy. J Am Coll Cardiol 1996;27(suppl A):350A.

114. Levine RA, Vlahakes GJ, Lefebvre X, et al. Papillary muscle displacement cause systolic anterior motion of the mitral valve. Experimental validation and insights into the mechanism of subaortic obstruction. Circulation 1995;91:1189–1195.

115. Pomerance A. Pathological and clinical study of calcification of the mitral valve ring. J Clin Pathol 1970;23:354–360.

116. Roberts WC. Morphological features of the normal and abnormal mitral valve ring. Am J Cardiol 1983;51:1005–1028.

117. Pomerance A, Davies MJ. The pathology of the heart. Oxford: Blackwell Scientific Publication, 1975.

118. Criley JM, Lewis K, Humphries JO, Ross RS. Prolapse of the mitral valve; clinical and cineangiographic findings. Br Heart J 1966;28:488–496.

119. Schieken R, Kerber RE, Ionasescu W, Zellweger H. Cardiac manifestations of the mucopolysaccharidoses. Circulation 1975;52:700–705.

120. Harrison CV, Lennox B. Heart block in osteitis deformans. Br Heart J 1948;10:167–173.

121. Nestico PF, Depace NL, Morganroth J, et al. Mitral annular calcification: clinical pathophysiology and echocardiographic review. Am Heart J 1984;107:989–996.

122. Hammer WJ, Roberts WC, deLeon AC Jr. "Mitral stenosis" secondary to combined "massive" mitral annular calcific deposits and small, hypertrophied left ventricles: hemodynamic documentation in four patients. Am J Med 1978;64:371–376.

123. Mellino M, Salcedo EE, Lever HM, et al. Echocardiographic quantified severity of mitral annulus calcification. Am Heart J 1982;103:222–225.

124. DeBono DP, Warlow CP. Mitral annulus calcification and cerebral or retinal ischemia. Lancet 1979;2:383–385.

125. Meltzer RS, Martin RP, Robbins BS, Popp RL. Mitral annular calcification: clinical and echocardiographic features. Acta Cardiol (Brux) 1980;35:189–202.

126. Wong M, Tei C, Shah PM. Sensitivity and specificity of two-dimensional echocardiogra-phy in the detection of valvular calcification. Chest 1983;84:423–427.

127. Asmar BE, Acker M, Couetil JP, et al. Mitral valve repair in the extensively calcified mitral valve annulus. Ann Thorac Surg 1991;52:66–69.

5

Mitral Valve Endocarditis

Infective endocarditis   •   Non-bacterial endocarditis   •   Indications for transesophageal echocardiography in endocarditis

INFECTIVE ENDOCARDITIS

Infective endocarditis is caused by a microbial infection of the endocardial lining of the heart, and may be difficult to diagnose and treat. It generally results in permanent damage, even with successful antibiotic treatment. The characteristic lesion of infective endocarditis is a vegetation. Transesophageal echocardiography is the diagnostic procedure of choice and is the gold standard for detection of mitral valve vegetations.[1-6] Transthoracic echocardiography reliably detects vegetations about 3mm in size.[7] In a study comparing transesophageal echocardiography with transthoracic echocardiography for detecting vegetations sized 2–5 mm, monoplane transesophageal echocardiography showed a sensitivity of 90% compared with 58% for transthoracic echocardiography.[8] The diagnosis of infective endocarditis is still primarily a clinical diagnosis, since pathological studies show that up to 50% of patients who die of acute endocarditis do not have vegetations.[9] However, Shively and colleagues[10] suggested that the absence of the characteristic abnormalities by transesophageal echocardiography indicate a low probability of disease in a patient with intermediate pre-test likelihood of endocarditis.

Mitral valve vegetations impair the functional integrity of the mitral valve apparatus through destruction of the annulus, leaflets, or chordae. With transthoracic echocardiography, vegetation size and appearance are highly variable. They may be nodular, or resemble irregular echogenic masses attached to one or both of the valve leaflets or, occasionally, to the chordae tendineae. With multiplane transesophageal echocardiography, vegetation morphology may be better defined and vegetations can be categorized as nodular, globular, shaggy, frond-like, polypoid, or tubular.[11-14] When vegetations appear tubular they may be confused with senescent valvular thickening, papillomas, or papillary fibroelastomas of the mitral valve that frequently appear as thin, multiple hairlike projections on the leaflet margins or chordal structures. Vegetations may be sessile or pedunculated, and may be as large as 40 mm in diameter. Placing the M-mode cursor on the vegetation in the zoom mode, sessile vegetations may show fine vibratory movements. Vegetations move in concert with the leaflet when firmly adherent to it, but are almost independent of valve motion or chaotic when pedunculated. Pedunculated vegetations usually appear larger with multiplane transesophageal echocardiography, and are frequently noted to prolapse between the left ventricular outflow tract and left atrial cavity during the cardiac cycle.[15,16] Even with transesophageal echocardiography, it may not be easy to distinguish vegetation from small ruptured chordae and prolapsing leaflet with myxomatous degeneration. With transesophageal echocardiography, vegetations may be distinguishable from senescent valvular thickening, discrete calcifications, or annular calcification as relatively fixed, symmetrical, or variably hyper-refractile masses. Vegetations usually occur on previously deformed valves, but depending on the offending bacterial organism, vegetations may be produced on normal valves or may spread to produce satellite vegetations. The size or morphology of vegetations bears no correlation with the location or specific causative organism.[8,14,17] Newer or acute vegetations may appear less dense or hypo-refractile in echogenicity compared with chronic lesions that appear more echodense and less mobile, but this finding is clearly subjective.[18–20]

Vegetations usually occur on the atrial surface of the leaflet tips, where they prevent the normal coaptation and approximation of the leaflets during systole and cause mitral regurgitation. In abnormal mitral valves, vegetations may occur at friction sites or jet lesions, such as the body of the leaflets and atrial wall, the basal surface of the ventricular septum, or on chordae showing systolic anterior motion.[16] Complications of vegetations in infective endocarditis of the mitral valve may produce perforation in the body of the leaflet, or result in ruptured chordae, flail or prolapsing leaflets, or disruption of the mitral annulus from a perivalvular abscess.[21] Perivalvular abscesses appear as distinct echodense (signifying purulent debris) or echolucent (sterile cavity) areas near the annular ring or annular attachment of the leaflet, and are found in about 20–30% of patients in surgical or necropsy studies.[22,23] Careful scanning with multiplane transesophageal echocardiography is ideal to identify perivalvular abscess and to distinguish abscess from lipomatous tissue, which may be frequently observed in the region of the annulus and the primum area of the atrial septal wall that is not generally echolucent. With color Doppler, flow jets may appear moving in and out of the echolucent area with systolic expansion or diastolic collapse. Subaortic extension of aortic valve endocarditis may affect the anterior mitral leaflet, leading to an aneurysm or perforation of the leaflet.[24–29] Echocardiographically, an aneurysm of the leaflet appears as a bulge in the leaflet during systole and diastole, and is an ominous sign since there appears to be a high rate of rupture.

There is a 25% embolization rate with mitral valve endocarditis. Rohmann and colleagues[17] found that mitral valve vegetations were an independent predictor of embolic complications with multivariate analysis, especially in vegetations larger than 10 mm. Mobility of the vegetation has also been associated with an increased risk of embolization and death in endocarditis. In cases of native mitral valve endocarditis, 85% of large vegetations are mobile when visualized with TEE, in contrast only 48% of small vegetations (less than 10 mm) demonstrate mobility.[8] Embolic episodes are more common with mobile vegetations (38%) than sessile vegetations (19%).[8] The visualization of spontaneous echocontrast or smoke on transesophageal echocardiography is also a risk factor for embolization, prolonged vegetation healing, and surgical intervention, under multivariate analysis.[30–33]

Serial examination during treatment of infective endocarditis with transesophageal echocardiography shows that vegetations may regress or grow larger.[30–33] In a study of vegetation size during treatment, only 39% of vegetations decreased in size, with 47% not significantly changing and 14% of vegetations increasing in size. A significant increase in vegetation size after two weeks of effective antibiotic therapy is a medical therapeutic failure for infectious endocarditis.

NON-BACTERIAL ENDOCARDITIS

Transesophageal echocardiography has sparked a considerable interest in the recognition of non-bacterial endocarditis.[34–39] Non-bacterial vegetations are more common in left-sided cardiac valves, especially the mitral valve. Non-bacterial thrombotic endocarditis has been associated with malignancy (marantic endocarditis), uremia, and connective tissue disorders. Non-bacterial vegetations usually appear as small, sessile, and verucous lesions on the valve leaflets. Prominent valvular vegetations may be shown in patients with lupus erythematosus who have high anticardiolipin (anti-phospholipid) antibody titers.[37] In the antiphospholipid syndrome, vegetations can be either primary, occurring in the absence of an underlying disorder, or secondary, in association with lupus erythematosus. Libman-Sacks endocarditis has been identified in about one-third of patients with primary involvement, and in increased frequency in patients with systemic lupus erythematosus and high anti-phospholipid antibody titers compared with patients with low titers. Although Libman-Sacks vegetations have been found in 35–65% of lupus patients in early necropsy studies, they are usually clinically silent or show only minor hemodynamic abnormalities.[34] Libman-Sacks lesions are described in pathological studies as sterile fibrofibrinous vegetations 3–4 mm in size that may develop anywhere on the endocardial surface, with a propensity for the ventricular surface of the mitral valve. Healed Libman-Sacks lesions show a fibrous plaque pathologically, sometimes with focal calcification. In extensive lesions or with corticosteroid therapy, healing may produce valve dysfunction as a result of valve deformities secondary to marked scarring or thickening. Libman-Sacks lesions may serve as a nidus for bacterial endocarditis or valve thrombi. Vegetations are frequently diagnosed by transesophageal echocardiography in patients with systemic lupus erythematosus. In an analysis of lupus patients with transesophageal echocardiography, valvular lesions were found in 61%, predominantly as valvular thickening in 51%, or as leaflet masses or vegetation in 43%. The lesions produced hemodynamics for regurgitation in 25%, and stenosis in 4% of patients.[38]

Echocardiographically, vegetations appear as thickening or masses of varying size and shape, with irregular borders and echodensity, firmly attached to the valve surface of the leaflet body or margins. Vegetations show relatively little motion. Roldan and colleagues[38] reported that on serial transesophageal echocardiographic examinations done almost 2.5 years apart, valvular abnormalities frequently resolved, appeared for the first time, or persisted but changed in appearance or size between the two studies. Mild or moderate valvular regurgitation did not progress to become severe, and new stenoses did not develop. Neither the presence of valvular disease nor changes in the echocardiographic findings were temporally related to the duration, activity, or severity of lupus, or to its treatment. The presence of valvular lesions is related to increased morbidity and mortality.

Echocardiographic analysis in the Antiphospholipid Antibodies in Stroke Study Group disclosed mitral valve abnormalities in 22.2% of patients with cerebral ischemic events and high antiphospholipid antibody titers.[39] Antithrombotic therapy is indicated for secondary prevention in patients with antithrombotic associated valvular disease who have already had a thromboembolic event.

INDICATIONS FOR TRANSESOPHAGEAL ECHOCARDIOGRAPHY IN ENDOCARDITIS

The indications of transesophageal echocardiography in suspected mitral valve endocarditis are a negative transthoracic echocardiogram in the setting of persistent bacteremia, without another obvious detected source of infection. If transthoracic echocardiography is diagnostic for vegetation and regurgitation is adequately defined, a transesophageal echocardiogram is usually not necessary and does not supply additional information, especially if there are no complications and the patient is clinically stable and responding to therapy. If these conditions are not met, transesophageal echocardiography is especially helpful in the diagnosis of mitral valve endocarditis (Table 5.1). Serial examinations either by transesophageal echocardiography or transthoracic echocardiography should be done to follow the vegetation

---

Table 5.1   Indications for transesophageal echocar diography (TEE) in endocar ditis

Initial baseline study (diagnostic)
Strong clinical suspicion with negative or poor images on transthoracic echo
Clinical picture different from transthoracic echo finding
Suspected prosthetic valve endocar ditis

During course of therapy (2 to 4 weeks)*
Evaluate vegetation size and appearance on therapy
Evaluate abscess or valve destr uction noted on baseline study
Rule out new complications

*TEE is often not necessar y even if it was the baseline study , if the transthoracic image quality was adequate and TTE findings are interpretable in view of the initial TEE findings

Acute complications
Change in clinical pictur e
Worsening hemodynamics
Persistently positive blood cultur es

---

size, suspected access formation, to assess intracardiac hemodynamics and left ventricular function. Transthoracic echocardiography usually enables assessment of regurgitation and cardiac hemodynamics even if the specific vegetation is not seen. Subsequent examinations may be done on a weekly basis by transthoracic echocardiography and every two weeks by transesophageal echocardiography if that was the diagnostic study. With the clinical presentation of new physical signs, complications, or hemodynamic instability, transesophageal echocardiography should be performed in all patients with mitral valve endocarditis.

Case Studies

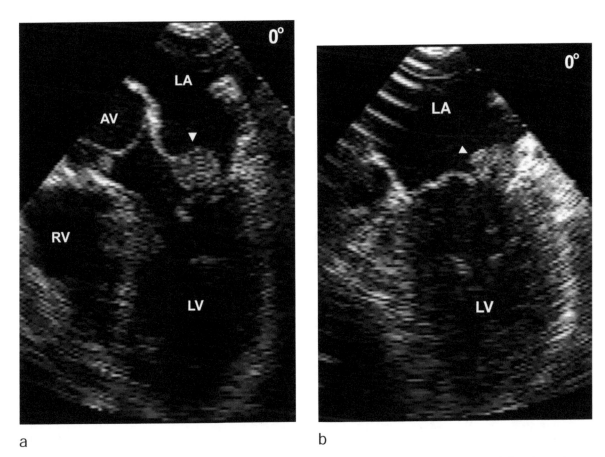

a   b

Case 5.1   Mitral valve vegetation. A medium sized multilobular , *Staphylococcus aureus* vegetation (arrow) attached to the posterior leaflet as   ecorded from the lower esophageal window at 0° during the car diac cycle (a–e). (f) Enlar ged view of the vegetation (ar row). Although visualized in multiple views the vegetation was rather sessile and did not exhibit excessive motion. LA, left atrium; L   V, left ventricle; A V, aortic valve; R V, right ventricle.

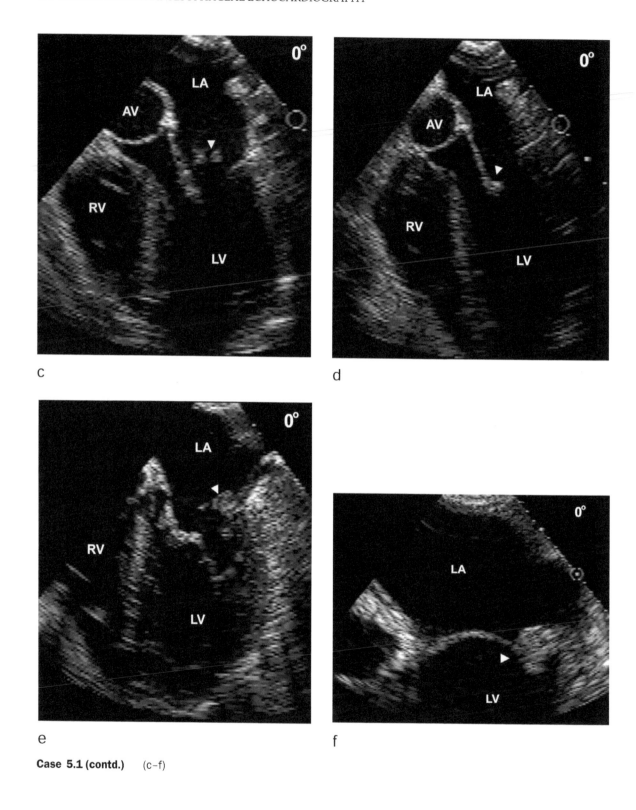

Case 5.1 (contd.) (c–f)

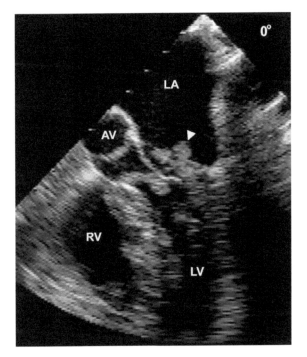

a

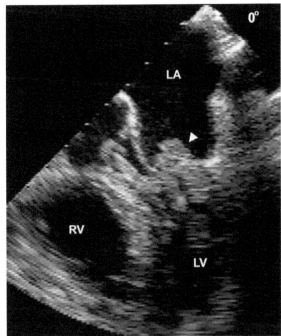

b

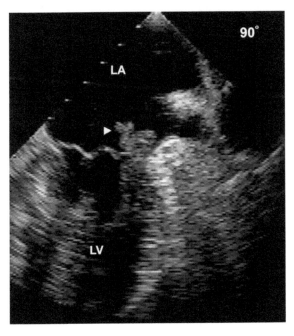

c

Case 5.2   Mitral valve vegetation. A lar ge
multilobular vegetation (ar rows) attached
predominately to the anterior leaflet with segment
noted on the atrial and ventricular sur face of the
leaflet. During the car diac cycle the vegetation flippe
in and out of the left ventricular outflow tract. Viewin
the vegetation fr om 0° to 135° (a–e) gives full
appreciation of the size and mobility of the
vegetation. LA, left atrium; L V, left ventricle;
AV, aortic valve; R V, right ventricle; R VOT, right
ventricular outflow tract; Ao, ao   ta.

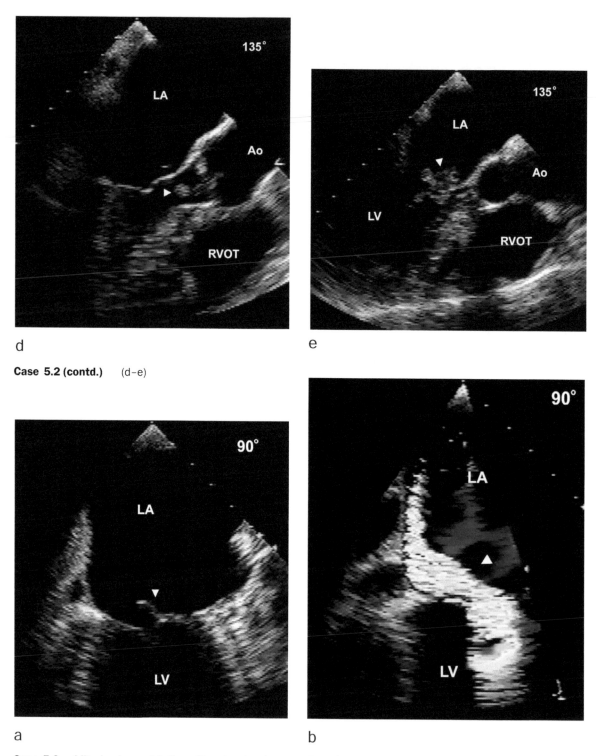

d

e

Case 5.2 (contd.)   (d–e)

a

b

Case 5.3   Mitral valve vegetation with extensive destruction of the mitral apparatus. (a) Flail anterior leaflet (arrow) producing severe mitral regurgitation (b) with a posterior directed color flow jet recorded at 90°. Visualization of the vegetation (arrow) from the lower esophageal window at 0° (c) and 90° (d). (e) Color flow Doppler demonstrating disturbed flow (arrow) in the area of the vegetation. LA, left atrium; LV, left ventricle; RV, right ventricle; RA, right atrium.

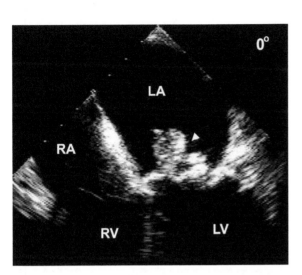

c

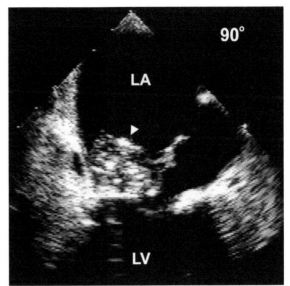

d

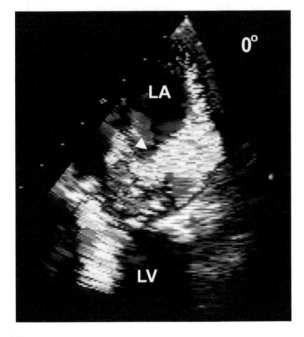

e

Case 5.3 (contd.)   (c–e)

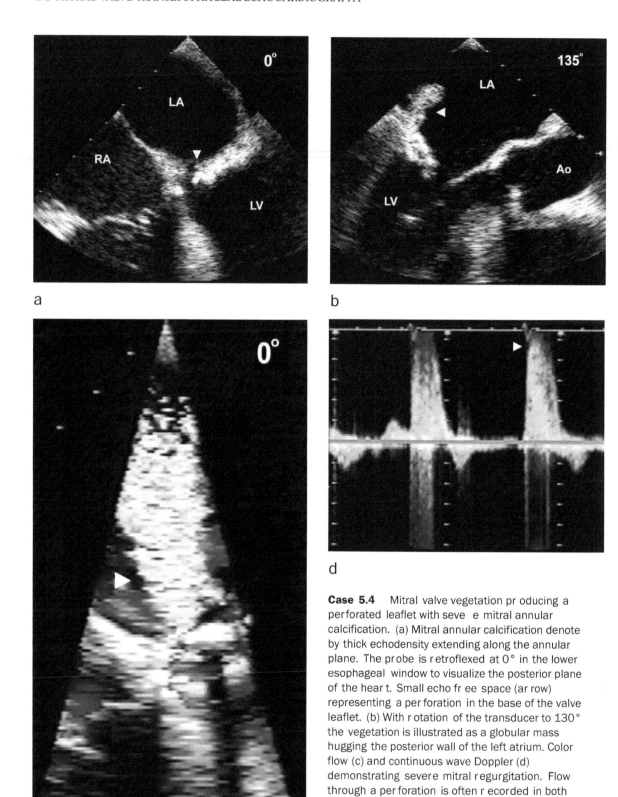

a

b

c

d

Case 5.4 Mitral valve vegetation pr oducing a perforated leaflet with seve e mitral annular calcification. (a) Mitral annular calcification denote by thick echodensity extending along the annular plane. The pr obe is r etroflexed at 0° in the lower esophageal window to visualize the posterior plane of the hear t. Small echo fr ee space (ar row) representing a per foration in the base of the valve leaflet. (b) With r otation of the transducer to 130° the vegetation is illustrated as a globular mass hugging the posterior wall of the left atrium. Color flow (c) and continuous wave Doppler (d) demonstrating severe mitral r egurgitation. Flow through a per foration is often r ecorded in both phases of the car diac cycle in a to and fr o manner. LA, left atrium; L V, left ventricle; RA, right atrium; Ao, aorta.

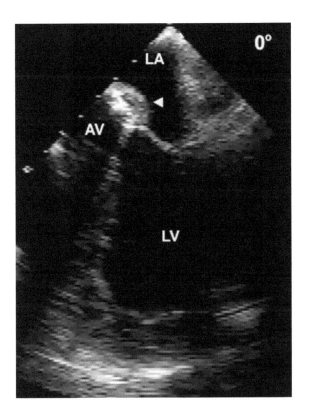

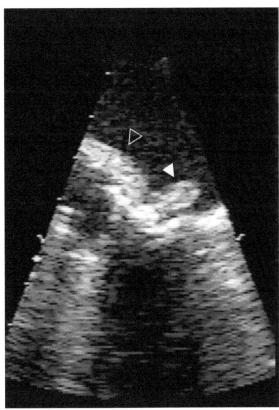

a   b

Case 5.5   Mitral valve vegetation with an annular abscess. (a) Small annular abscess (ar   row) visualized near the aorto-mitral fib osa from the lower esophageal view at 0°. (b) Slight r   etroflexion of the pr obe demonstrates a small vegetation (ar row) in close pr oximity to the abscess in an enlar   ged view. (c) Color flow Dopple demonstrates a mitral r egurgitant jet emanating fr om the same ar ea as the vegetation and the abscess, which is not allowing apposition of the leaflets near the a   ea of the posterior commissur   e. (d,e) Rotating the transducer to appr oximately 90° demonstrates the full extent of the abscess and the vegetation (ar   row). (f) Enlarged view of the vegetation (ar   row). LA, left atrium; L V, left ventricle; LAA, left atrial appendage.

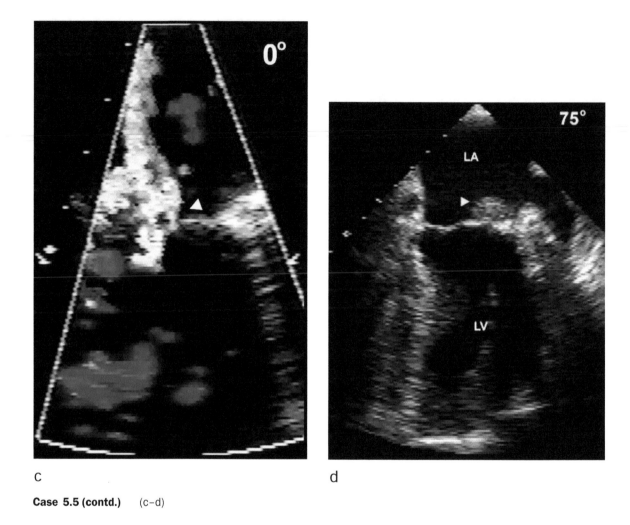

c

d

Case 5.5 (contd.) (c–d)

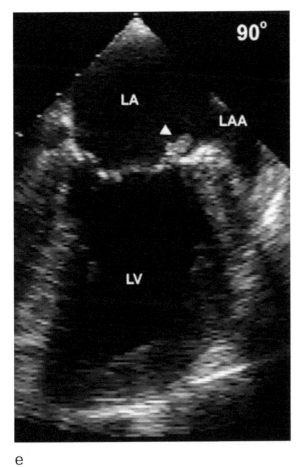

e

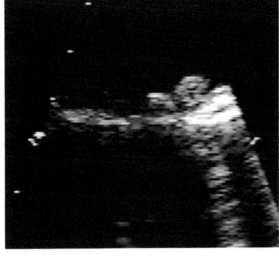

f

Case 5.5 (contd.)   (e–f)

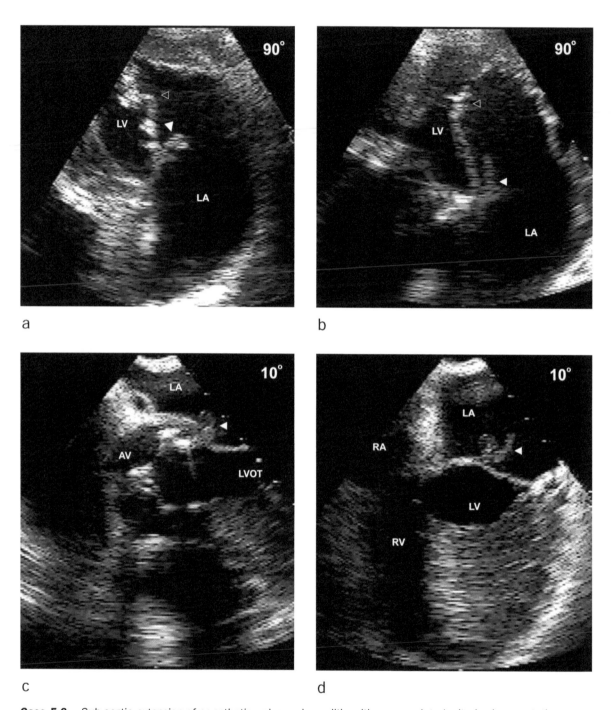

Case 5.6 Sub-aortic extension of prosthetic valve endocarditis with an associated mitral valve vegetation. Careful scanning with multiplane TEE is ideal for identifying perivalvular abscesses. Deep transgastric view at 0° demonstrates a mobile vegetation attached to the anterior leaflet during (a) systole and (b) diastole Vegetation (open arrow); Chordae (solid arrow). In the lower esophageal view at 10° (c,d) an aortic prosthetic valve is seen with an associated small annular abscess. With rotation of the transducer to 45° the same vegetation demonstrated in (a) and (b) is seen.

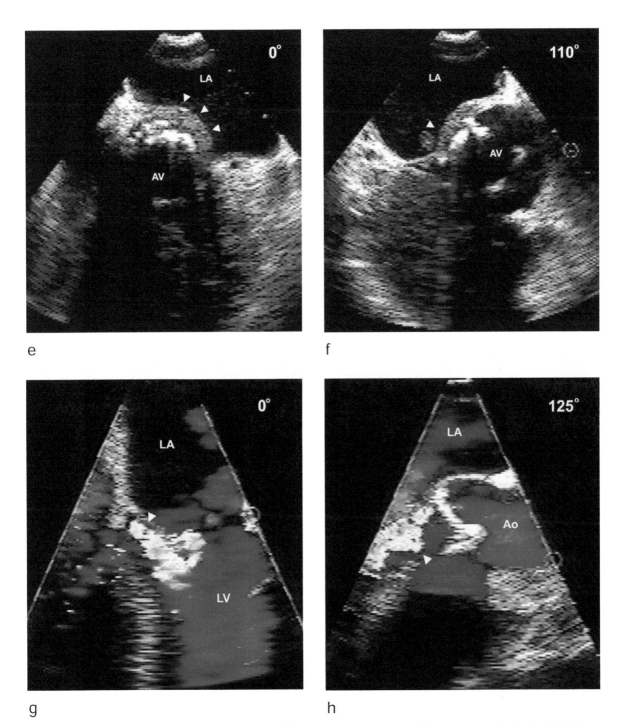

Case 5.6 (contd.)   (e) At 0° the abscess (ar row) is seen wrapping ar ound the aor tic prosthetic ring. (f) With further rotation of the transducer to 110° the abscess and the vegetation ar e demonstrated in close pr oximity to each other. Aortic regurgitation is demonstrated with color flow Doppler at 0   (g) and 125° (h). LA, left atrium; LV, left ventricle; RA, right atrium; R V, right ventricle; Ao, aor ta; AV, aortic valve; LVOT, left ventricular outflow tract.

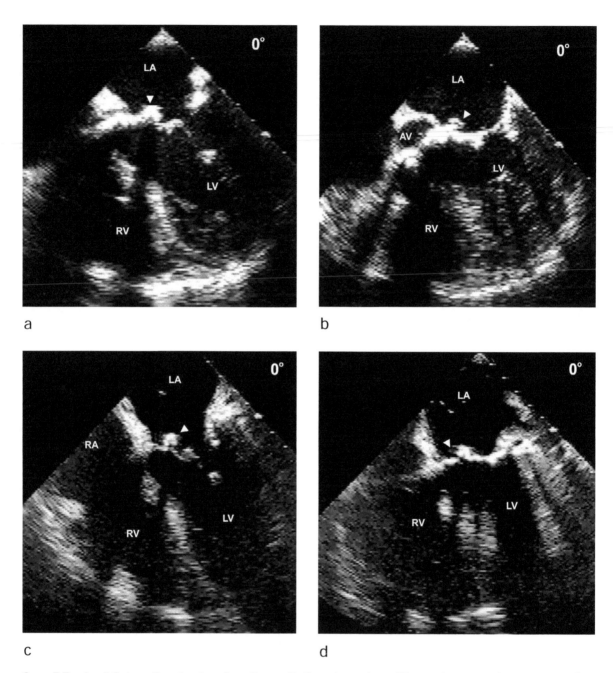

Case 5.7 (a–d) Sub-aortic extension of aortic prosthetic valve endocarditis causing a mycotic aneurysm of the mitral valve which appears as a bulge in the anterior mitral leaflet expanding and contracting during systol through diastole.

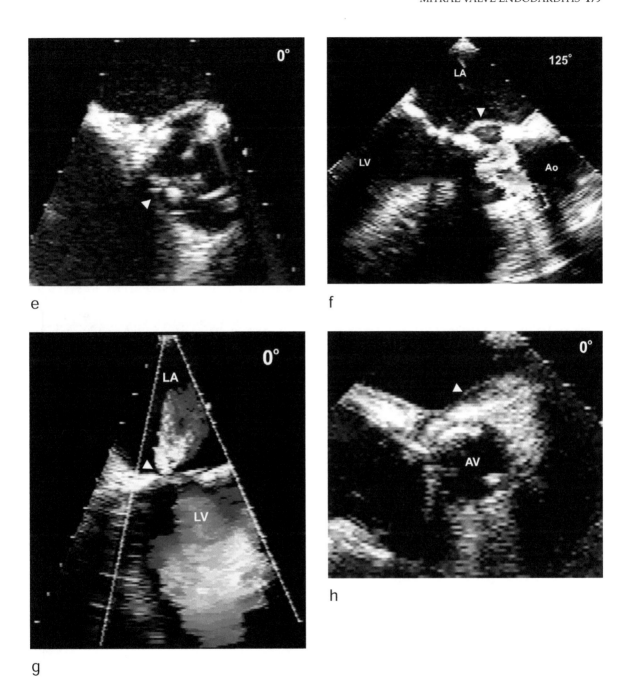

Case 5.7 (contd.)   (e) Small vegetation (ar row) associated with a pr osthetic aortic valve. (f) Color flo
Doppler demonstrating flow into an ao   tic annular abscess at 125°   during systole. (g) At 0°   a color flow je
(arrow) is demonstrated in the left atrium demonstrating per   foration. During diastole color flow does no
demonstrate flow into the abscess cavity at 0   (h) or 125° (i).

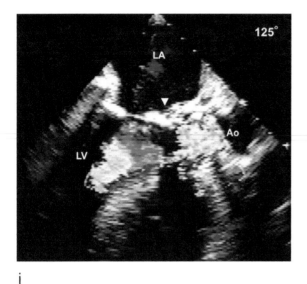

i

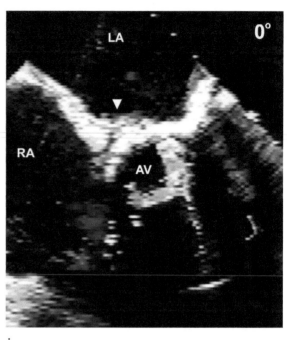

j

Case 5.7 (contd.) (j) Enlarged view demonstrating a collapsed abscess cavity during diastole. LA, left atrium; LV, left ventricle; RA, right atrium; R V, right ventricle; AV, aortic valve; Ao, aor ta.

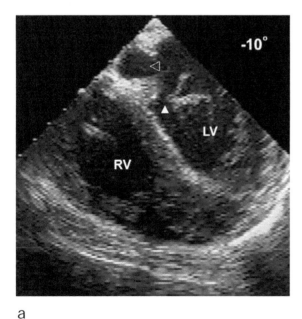

a

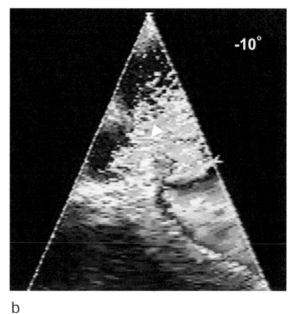

b

Case 5.8 Mitral valve endocar ditis producing a per forated leaflet with an annular abscess. (a) View of th mitral valve with the pr obe in the gastr oesophageal junction at appr oximately −10°. The posterior aspect of the mitral valve annulus is seen with a small submitral aneur ysm (open ar row). A per foration is visualized in the mitral leaflet (closed a row) with vegetative debris noted near the per foration. (b) Color flow Dopple demonstrates flow (a row) in the aneur ysm and thr ough the per foration.

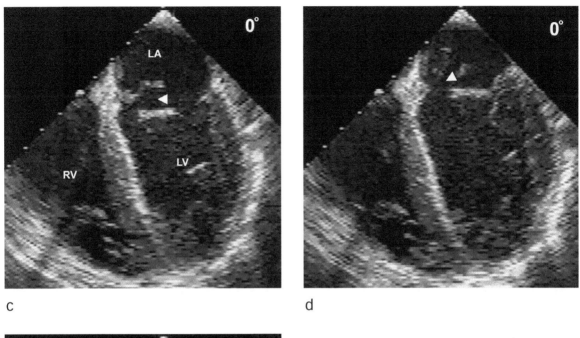

c

d

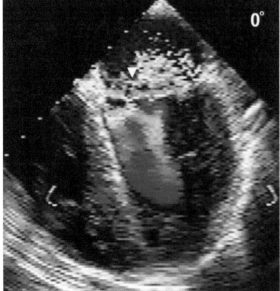

e

Case 5.8 (contd.) Views obtained from the lower esophageal window at 0° demonstrate mobility of the vegetation during diastole (c) and systole (d), and color flow Doppler demonstrates flow (row) through the perforation (e). LA, left atrium; L V, left ventricle; RV, right ventricle.

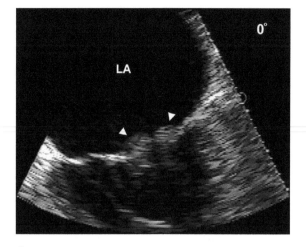

a

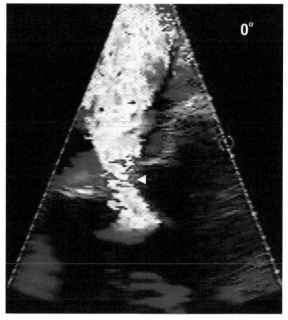

b

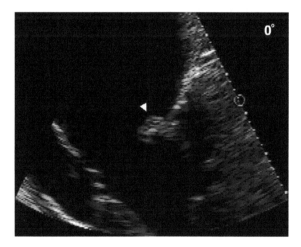

c

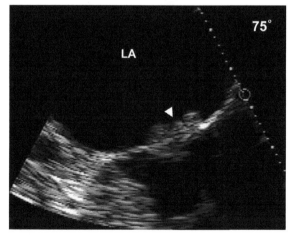

e

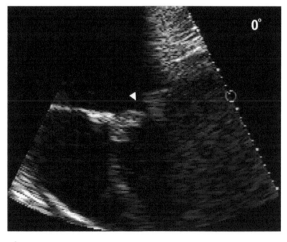

d

Case 5.9 Non-bacterial endocarditis in a patient with lupus erythematosus; the TEE indication was to rule out a cardiac source of embolus. (a) Thickening of both leaflet tips is seen (arrows). (b) Significant mitral regurgitation is demonstrated by color flow Doppler. Angulation of the probe, with enlarged views visualizes the posterior leaflet (c) and anterior leaflet (d), both leaflets (e,f) with thickening and shaggy echoes noted on the leaflet margin. It is not unusual to see this picture of "kissing vegetations" on both leaflet margins in non-bacterial endocarditis. LA, left atrium; LV, left ventricle.

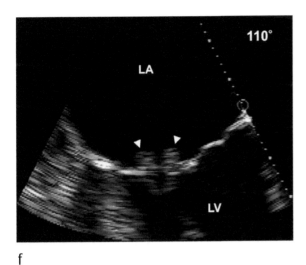

Case 5.9 (contd.)

f

REFERENCES

1. Erbel R, Rohmann S, Drexler M, et al. Improved diagnostic value of echocardiography in patients with infective endocarditis by transesophageal approach. A prospective study. Eur Heart J 1988;9:45–53.
2. Daniel WG, Shroder E, Mugge A, Lichtlen PR. Transesophageal echocardiography in infective endocarditis. Am J Card Imaging 1988;2:78–85.
3. Daniel WG, Schroder E, Nonnast-Daniel B, Lichtlen PR. Conventional and transesophageal echocardiography in the diagnosis of infective endocarditis. Eur Heart J 1987;8(suppl J):287–292.
4. Klodas E, Edwards WD, Khandheria BK. Use of transesophageal echocardiography for improving detection of valvular vegetations in subacute bacterial endocarditis. J Am Soc Echocardiogr 1989;2:386–389.
5. Birmingham GD, Rahko PS, Ballantyne F III. Improved detection of infective endocarditis with transesophageal echocardiography. Am Heart J 1992;123:774–781.
6. Khandheria BK. Suspected bacterial endocarditis: to TEE or not to TEE. J Am Coll Cardiol 1993;21:222–224.
7. Martin RP, Meltzer RS, Chia BL, et al. Clinical utility of two dimensional echocardiography in infective endocarditis. Am J Cardiol 1980;46:379–385.
8. Mugge A, Daniel WG, Frank G, Lichtlen PR. Echocardiography in infective endocarditis: reassessment of prognostic implications of vegetation size determined by the transthoracic and the transesophageal approach. J Am Coll Cardiol 1989;14:631–638.
9. Sochowski RA, Chan K-L. Implications of negative results on a monoplane transesophageal echocardiographic study in patients with suspected infective endocarditis. J Am Coll Cardiol 1993;21:216–221.
10. Shively BK, Gurule FT, Roland CA, et al. Diagnostic value of transesophageal compared with transthoracic echocardiography in infective endocarditis. J Am Coll Cardiol 1991;18:391–397.
11. Taams MA, Gussenhoven EJ, Bos E, et al. Enhanced morphological diagnosis in infective endocarditis by transesophageal echocardiography. Br Heart J 1990;63:109–113.
12. Dillion JC, Feigenbaum H, Konecke LL, et al. Echocardiographic manifestations of valvular vegetations. Am Heart J 1973;86:698–704.
13. Roy P, Tajik AJ, Giuliani ER, et al. Spectrum of echocardiographic findings in bacterial endocarditis. Circulation 1976;53:474–482.
14. Sanfilippo AJ, Picard MH, Newell JB, et al. Echocardiographic assessment of patients with infectious endocarditis: prediction of risk for complications. J Am Coll Cardiol 1991;18:1191–19.
15. Job FP, Lethen H, Franke S, et al. Benefit of bi- or multiplane versus monoplane TEE for the assessment of endocarditic lesions (abstr). J Am Coll Cardiol 1993;21:488A.

16. Schwinger ME, Tunick PA, Freedberg RS, Kronzon I. Vegetations on endocardial surfaces struck by regurgitant jets: diagnosis by transesophageal echocardiography. Am Heart J 1990;119:1212–1215.

17. Rohmann S, Erbel R, Gorge G, et al. Clinical relevance of vegetation localization by transesophageal echocardiography in infective endocarditis. Eur Heart J 1992;13:446–452.

18. Stafford A, Wann LS, Dillion JC, et al. Serial echocardiographic appearance of healing bacterial endocarditis. Am J Cardiol 1979;44:754–760.

19. Stratton JR, Werner JA, Pearlman AS, et al. Bacteremia and the heart: serial echocardiographic findings in 80 patients with documented or suspected bacteremia. Am J Med 1982; 73:851–858.

20. Tak T, Rahimtoola SH, Kumar A, et al. Value of digital image processing of two-dimensional echocardiograms in differentiating active from chronic vegetations of infective endocarditis. Circulation 1988;78:116–123.

21. Stewart JA, Silimperi D, Harris P, et al. Echocardiographic documentation of vegetative lesions in infective endocarditis: clinical implications. Circulation 1980;61:374–380.

22. Buchbinder NA, Roberts WC. Left-sided valvular active infective endocarditis: a study of forty-five necropsy patients. Am J Med 1972;53:20–35.

23. Arnett EN, Roberts WC. Valve ring abscess in active infective endocarditis: frequency, location, and clues to clinical diagnosis from the study of 95 necropsy patients. Circulation 1976;54:140–145.

24. Nomeir A-M, Downes TR, Cordell AR. Perforation of the anterior mitral leaflet caused by aortic valve endocarditis: diagnosis by two-dimensional, transesophageal echocardiography and color flow Doppler. J Am Soc Echocardiogr 1992;5:195–198.

25. Ballal RS, Mahan EF III, Nanda NC, Sanyal R. Aortic and mitral valve perforation: diagnosis by transesophageal echocardiography and Doppler color flow imaging. Am Heart J 1991;121:214–217.

26. Daniel WG, Mugge A, Martin RP, et al. Improvement in the diagnosis of abscesses associated with endocarditis by transesophageal echocardiography. N Engl J Med 1991;324: 795–800.

27. Massey WM, Samdarshi TE, Nanda NC, et al. Serial documentation of changes in a mitral valve vegetation progressing to abscess rupture and fistula formation by transesophageal echocardiography. Am Heart J 1992;124:241–248.

28. Afridi I, Apostolidou MA, Saad RM, Zoghbi WA. Pseudoaneurysms of the mitral-aortic intervalvular fibrosa: dynamic characterization using transesophageal echocardiographic and Doppler techniques. J Am Coll Cardiol 1995;25:137–145.

29. Bansal RC, Graham BM, Jutzy KR, et al. Left ventricular outflow tract to left atrial communication secondary to rupture of mitral-aortic intervalvular fibrosa in infective endocarditis: diagnosis by transesophageal echocardiography and color flow imaging. J Am Coll Cardiol 1990;15:449–504.

30. Rohmann S, Erbel R, Darius H, et al. Prediction of rapid versus prolonged healing of infective endocarditis by monitoring vegetation size. J Am Soc Echocardiogr 1991;4:465–474.

31. Vuille C, Nidorf M, Weyman AE, Picard MH. Natural history of vegetations in successfully treated endocarditis (abstr). J Am Coll Cardiol 1993;21:200A.

32. Rohmann S, Erbel R, Darius H, et al. Influence of antibiotics on vegetation size in infective endocarditis: a comparative study (abstr). J Am Coll Cardiol 1993;21:391A.

33. Meric M, Castello R, Ofili EO, et al. Transesophageal echocardiography in infective endocarditis: prognostic implications of vegetation size and mobility (abstr). J Am Coll Cardiol 1993;21:391A.

34. Hojnik M, George J, Ziporen L, Shoenfeld Y. Heart valve involvement (Libman-Sacks endocarditis) in the antiphospholipid syndrome. Circulation 1996;93:1579–1587.

35. Blanchard DG, Ross RS, Dittrich HC. Nonbacterial thrombotic endocarditis: assessment by transesophageal echocardiography. Chest 1992;102:954–956.

36. Lopez JA, Ross RS, Fishbein MC, Siegel RJ. Nonbacterial thrombotic endocarditis: a review. Am Heart J 1987;113:773–784.

37. Nihoyannopoulos P, Gomez PM, Joshi J, et al. Cardiac abnormalities in systemic lupus erythematosus: association with raised anticardiolipin antibodies. Circulation 1990;82:369–375.

38. Roldan CA, Shively BK, Crawford MH. An echocardiographic study of valvular heart disease associated with systemic lupus erythematosus. N Engl J Med 1996;335:1424–1430.

39. Barbut D, Borer JS, Wallerson D, et al. Anticardiolipin antibody and stroke: possible relation of valvular heart disease and embolic events. Cardiology 1991;79:99–109.

6

Congenital Mitral Disease

Papillary muscle abnormalities • Chordal anomalies • Leaf et anomalies • Annular anomalies

Developmental abnormalities of one or more components of the mitral valve constitute congenital mitral valve disease as an isolated finding or in combination with other congenital malformations of the heart. Congenital mitral valvular disease may result in stenosis, incompetence, or both. Occasionally, congenital mitral valvular disease, with minor hemodynamic abnormalities, can go undetected or be confused with other forms of acquired disease and not be discovered until the patient is a young adult. In our experience it is not unusual for a young patient, presenting for assessment of mitral stenosis before valvuloplasty or for the feasibility of surgical repair of mitral valve prolapse, to have congenital abnormalities discovered by transesophageal echocardiography.

To better understand congenital mitral disease in the young adult, it is helpful to be familiar with the specific congenital abnormalities that may occur for each component of the mitral unit (Table 6.1)[1], rather than trying to label a specific syndrome based on image recognition.[2–4] By the time the congenital patient reaches adulthood the lesion has degenerated (wear and tear), and does not always appear as initially described, which generates confusion and perhaps an incorrect diagnosis with transthoracic echocardiography. Also, evaluating congenital mitral disease by its component parts may offer the patient an opportunity for repair rather than valve replacement, which is usually the first choice.[5–9]

Table 6.1   Congenital lesions of the mitral valvular unit

Valvular apparatus	Abnormality
Annulus	Dilatation – deformity
Commissur e	Fusion
	Double orific
Leaflet	Cleft
	Agenesis
Chordae	Absent
	Fusion
	Elongation
Papillar y muscle	Malposition
	Elongation
	Arcade
	Parachute valve

PAPILLARY MUSCLE ABNORMALITIES

Congenital abnormalities of the papillary muscles include the malposition of the muscles in the ventricular cavity, elongation of the muscles, accessory muscles, a single muscle with or without an accessory muscle, or muscles associated with extensive fibrotic tissue.

The parachute mitral valve is probably the most recognized congenital papillary muscle abnormality.[10,11] In the parachute valve there is only one, long papillary muscle, usually the posteromedial muscle which originates closer to the ventricular apex. If an anterolateral muscle is present, it is an accessory muscle, and is small with shortened, thickened chordae, usually aberrantly connected to the ventricle. The leaflets are normal at birth, and by adulthood may become thickened as a result of degenerative changes or the development of excessive leaflet tissue. All chordae emanate from the leaflets and converge into the single papillary muscle, which narrows the inflow tract, restricts normal leaflet motion, and produces an eccentric orifice opening. In this manner, stenosis or obstruction to flow is produced in the subvalvular region as flow is directed into a posteriorly oriented inflow tract towards the closely grouped and crowded chordae tendineae. Secondarily, regurgitation may occur due to the restricted leaflet motion interfering with the approximation of the leaflets during systole.[12] These findings, especially the visualization of one centrally placed papillary muscle in the transgastric short axis view of the left ventricle, are easily identified with transesophageal echocardiography.

Mitral arcade may also be occasionally seen in the young adult.[13] Transesophageal echocardiography in mitral arcade shows a bridge of fibrous tissue in between the papillary muscles that directly attaches to the anterior leaflet. The commissures are rudimentary and therefore distinct separation is not seen. The anterior leaflet may be rudimentary with a normal posterior leaflet. The chordae are short and thickened, giving the appearance that the papillary muscles extend directly to the leaflets. The papillary muscles are large and elongated, and may

be displaced anteriorly. These lesions predominantly produce regurgitation, and secondarily produce obstruction of flow.

The posterior placement of two hypertrophied papillary muscles may also cause subvalvular stenosis.[14] On transgastric short axis views, the papillary muscles are obviously thickened and abnormally placed in the left ventricular cavity with a small posterior interpapillary muscle dimension. Rotation of the transducer to 90° shows the chordae to be thickened, and anomalous thick muscular bands are common. Hypoplastic papillary muscles may occur, often in groups of three or more with thickened chordae, and may cause subvalvular obstruction.[15,16]

CHORDAL ANOMALIES

Congenital chordal anomalies may cause mitral insufficiency or stenosis.[6,14] Chordae may be fused or totally absent in congenital mitral stenosis. Chordae may be abnormally placed to the whole body of the anterior leaflet instead of just to the free edge, in a pattern similar to that of the posterior leaflet. Chordae may be elongated and may result in significant leaflet prolapse.

LEAFLET ANOMALIES

Leaflet clefts may occur mainly in the anterior leaflet and rarely in the posterior leaflet as previously described, with or without an AV canal defect.[17-22] In the isolated cleft of the anterior leaflet, an additional smaller leaflet may be formed by an accessory commissure with or without accessory chordal attachment, which produces mitral insufficiency. Careful scanning is required to avoid confusion with myxomatous degeneration and a ruptured posterior leaflet or a perforated leaflet.

The orifice formed by the mitral leaflets may be narrowed by agenesis of the leaflets, absence of the commissures, or congenital thickening or fibrosis of the leaflets, which appears similar echocardiographically to rheumatic stenosis without the presence of calcification.[23]

Congenital mitral insufficiency may be caused by hypoplastic leaflets that appear as small, fibrous, stubby leaflets. One or both commissures may be absent, producing multiple orifices.[14,23,24]

ANNULAR ANOMALIES

The mitral annulus may be dilated congenitally due to deficiency of the commissural tissue, usually in association with other anomalies of the valve unit.[14] The mitral annulus may be small, as an isolated finding with obstruction or without obvious obstruction in association with coarctation of the aorta.[10,23] Supravalvular rings may be present, consisting of thick fibrous rings on the left atrial side of the annulus, with the normal connections to the left atrium.[25] Nonobstructive rings may present as an incidental finding during transesophageal echocardiography, in association with other anomalies of the mitral unit.[24]

Case Studies

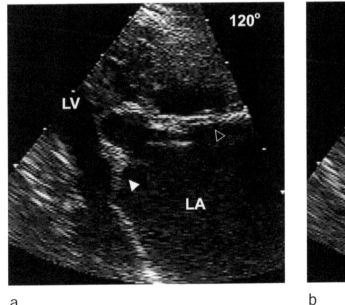

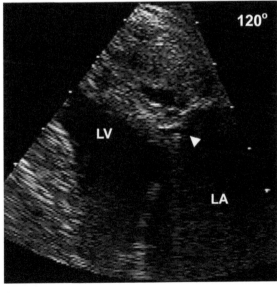

a b

Case 6.1 Parachute mitral valve. Deep transgastric view of the subvalvular apparatus during diastole (a) and systole (b). Chordae tendineae appear to be attached from only one papillary muscle that originates from the ventricular apex.

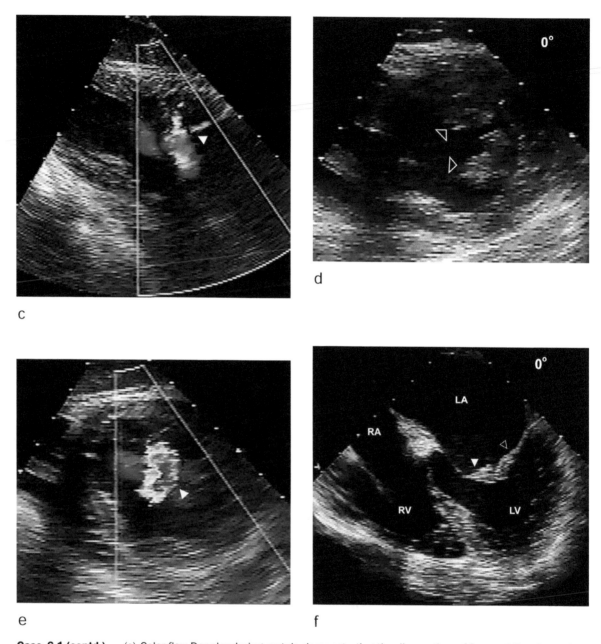

Case 6.1 (contd.)   (c) Color flow Doppler during systole demonstrating the di ection of for ward flow (a row) through the mitral apparatus. (d) Shor t-axis view of the left ventricle at the mid-ventricular level. The papillar   y muscles are grouped tightly together and originate fr om the inferior wall. (e) Color flow Doppler demonstratin flow during systole. (f) Thickening of the mitral valve leaflets   tips is demonstrated during systole.

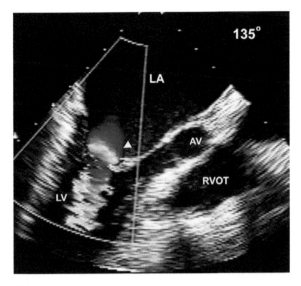

g

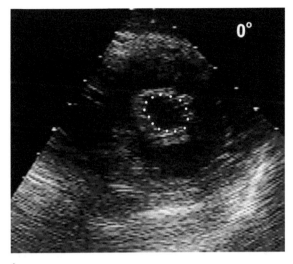

h

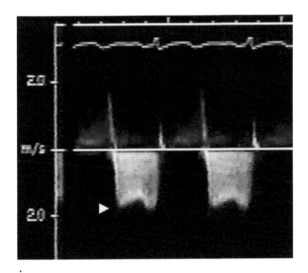

i

Case 6.1 (contd.) (g) Restricted opening of the mitral valve leaflets demonstrated by diastoli doming and high velocity color flow th ough the mitral valve orifice. (h) Sho t axis demonstrating the restricted valve ar ea of the mitral valve.
(i) Continuous wave Doppler of the left ventricular inflow tract demonstrating a 2 m/sec flow velocit across the mitral valve. LA, left atrium; L V, left ventricle; AL, anterior leaflet; PL, posterior leafle

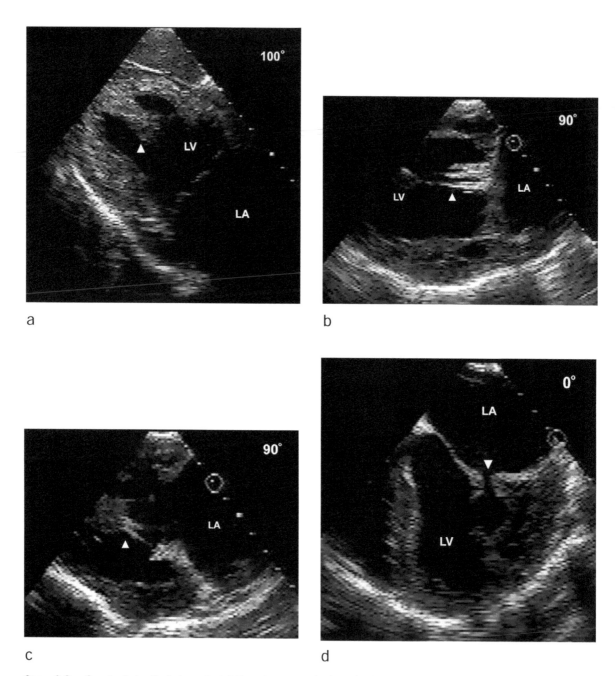

Case 6.2 Congenital mitral stenosis. (a) Deep transgastric view obtained at 100° demonstrates an abnormally placed papillary muscle emanating from the ventricular apex. In the longitudinal gastric views at 90° in systole (b) and (c) diastole abnormal chordal orientation is noted with the single papillary muscle-giving rise to both leaflets. During diastole the limited range of chordal motion is demonstrated due to restricted leaflet opening. (d) Marked thickening of both leaflets is noted, and with angulation of the probe (e) excessive tissue associated with the posterior leaflet and prolapse (arrow) is demonstrated. (f) Color flow Dopple demonstrates severe mitral regurgitation (arrow). (g) Restricted and abnormal motion of the anterior leaflet i demonstrated. LA, left atrium; LV, left ventricle; RV, right ventricle; AV, aortic valve.

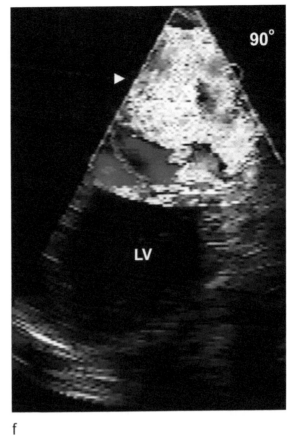

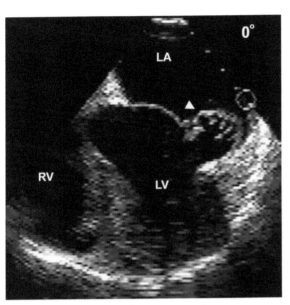

e

f

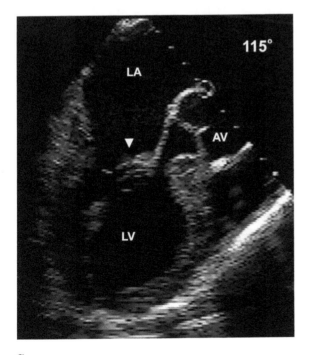

g

Case 6.2 (contd.)   (e–g)

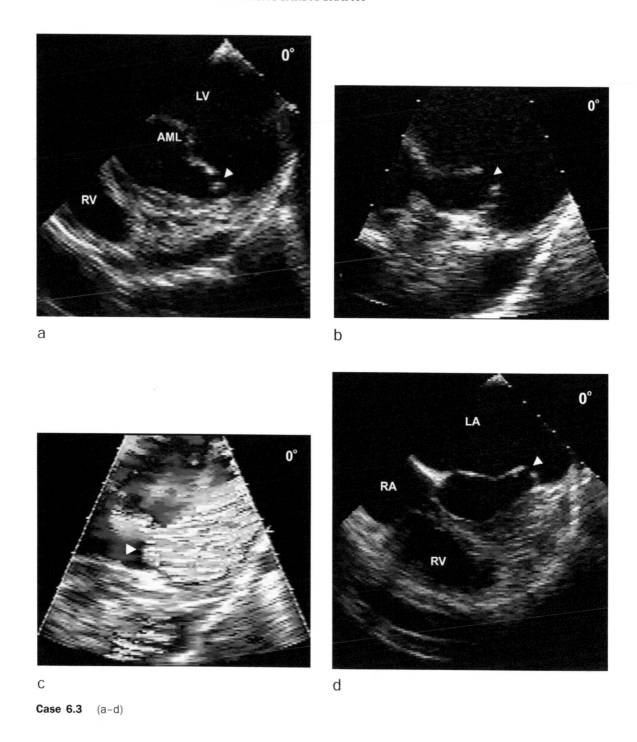

a

b

c

d

Case 6.3 (a–d)

e

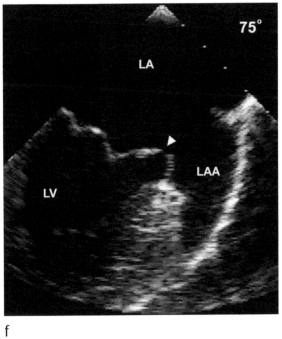

f

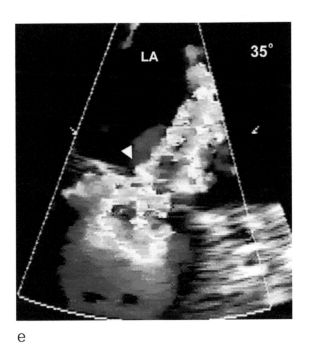

g

Case 6.3 (contd.)   (e–g)

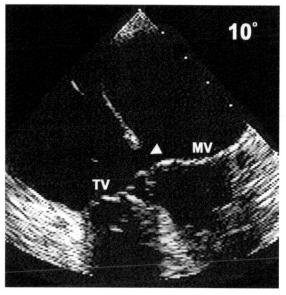

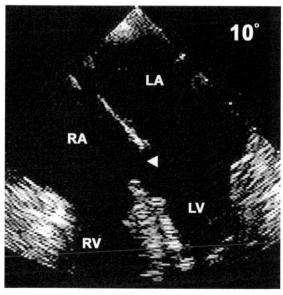

a

b

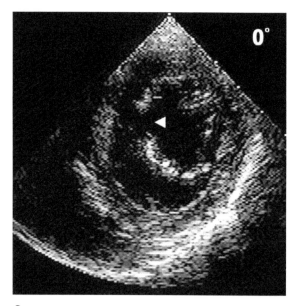

c

Case 6.4   Ostium primum atrial septal defect. (a) Four-chamber view at 10° demonstrating an ostium primum atrial defect as a lack of continuity of the atrial septum with the superior por tion of the cardiac crux. The usual of fset of the tricuspid and mitral valve is missing – both the tricuspid and mitral valve annulus lie in the same plane due to the defect in systole. (b) Diastolic frame in the same view . Cleft defects of the atrioventricular valves ar e frequently associated with ostium primum defects, ar e frequently associated with significant egurgitation and are readily demonstrated with multiplane transesophageal echocardiography (TEE). (c) In the shor t-axis transgastric view at 0° a cleft (ar row) is demonstrated in the anterior mitral leaflet

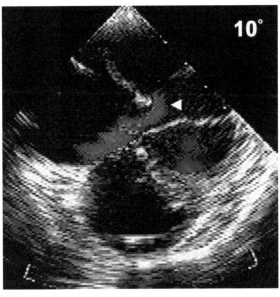 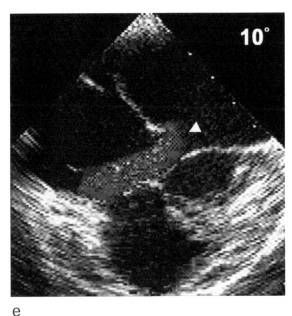

d   e

Case 6.4 (contd.) (d,e) Color Doppler frames fr om the four-chamber view demonstrating atrial shunt flow in left-to-right direction. TV, tricuspid valve; MV , mitral valve. LA, left atrium; RA, right atrium; L V, left ventricle; RV, right ventricle.

REFERENCES

1. Carpentier A. Cardiac valve surgery the "French correction". J Thorac Cardiovasc Surg 1983; 86:323–337.

2. Grenadier E, Sahn DJ, Valdes-Cruz LM, et al. Two-dimensional echocardiography Doppler study of congenital disorders of the mitral valve. Am Heart J 1984;107:319.

3. Smallhorn J, Tommasini G, Deanfield J, et al. Congenital mitral stenosis. Anatomical and functional assessment by echocardiography. Br Heart J 1981;45:527.

4. Vitarelli A, Landolina G, Gentile R, et al. Echocardiographic assessment of congenital mitral stenosis. Am Heart J 1984;108:523.

5. Chauvaud S, Perier P, Touati G, et al. Long-term results of valve repair in children with acquired mitral valve incompetence. Circulation 1986;74:1104–1109.

6. Coles JG, Williams WG, Watanabe T, et al. Surgical experience with reparative techniques in patients with congenital mitral valvular anomalies. Circulation 1987;76(suppl 111):111–117.

7. Stellin G, Bortolotti U, Mazzucco A, et al. Repair of congenitally malformed mitral valve in children. J Thorac Cardiovasc Surg 1988;95:480–485.

8. Curcio CA, Cronje SL. Partial atrioventricular canal in an adult: mitral valve repair by reverse implantation of a Carpentier ring. J Thorac Cardiovasc Surg 1987;94:444–445.

9. Levy MJ, Varco RL, Lillehei CW, Edwards JE. Mitral insufficiency in infants, children and adolescents. J Thorac Cardiovasc Surg 1963;45:434.

10. Shone JD, Sellers RD, Anderson RC, et al. The developmental complex of "parachute mitral valve", supravalvular ring of left atrium, subaortic stenosis, and coarctation of aorta. Am J Cardiol 1963;11:714.

11. Macartney FJ, Scott O, Ionescu MI, Deverall PB. Diagnosis and management of parachute mitral valve and supravalvar mitral ring. Br Heart J 1974;36:641.

12. Glancy DL, Chang MY, Dorney ER, Roberts WC. Parachute mitral valve. Further observations and associated lesions. Am J Cardiol 1971;27:309.

13. Layman TE, Edwards JE. Anomalous mitral arcade. A type of congenital mitral insufficiency. Circulation 1967;35:389.

14. Carpentier A, Branchini B, Cour JC, et al. Congenital malformations of the mitral valve in children. Pathology and surgical treatment. J Thorac Cardiovasc Surg 1976;72:854–866.

15. Castaneda AR, Anderson RC, Edwards JE. Congenital mitral stenosis resulting from anomalous arcade and obstructing papillary muscles. Report of correction by use of ball valve prosthesis. Am J Cardiol 1969;24:237.

16. Ruckman RN, Van Praagh R. Anatomic types of congenital mitral stenosis: report of 49 autopsy cases with consideration of diagnosis and surgical implications. Am J Cardiol 1978;42:592–601.

17. Sigfusson G, Ettedgui JA, Silverman NH, Anderson RH. Is a cleft in the anterior leaflet of an otherwise normal mitral valve an atrioventricular canal malformation? J Am Coll Cardiol 1995;26:508–515.

18. Creech O, Ledbeter MK, Reemtsma K. Congenital insufficiency with a cleft in the posterior leaflet. Circulation 1962;25:390.

19. DiSegni E, Edwards JE. Cleft anterior leaflet of the mitral valve with intact septa. A study of twenty cases. Am J Cardiol 1983;51:915.

20. DiSegni E, Bass JL, Lucas RV Jr, et al. Isolated cleft mitral valve: a variety of congenital mitral regurgitation identified by 2-dimensional echocardiography. Am J Cardiol 1983;51:927–931.

21. Wenink ACG, Gittenberger-de Groot AC, Brom AG. Developmental considerations of mitral valve anomalies. Int J Cardiol 1986;11:85.

22. Berghuis J, Kirklin JW, Edwards JE, Titus JL. The surgical anatomy of isolated congenital mitral insufficiency. J Thorac Cardiovasc Surg 1964; 47:791.

23. Collins-Nakai RL, Rosenthal A, Castaneda AR, et al. Congenital mitral stenosis. A review of 20 years' experience. Circulation 1977;56:1039.

24. Snider AR, Roge CL, Schiller NB, Silverman NH. Congenital left ventricular inflow obstruction evaluated by two-dimensional echocardiography. Circulation 1980;61:848–855.

25. Anabtawi IN, Ellison RG. Congenital stenosing ring of the left atrioventricular canal (supravalvular mitral stenosis). J Thorac Cardiovasc Surg 1965;49:994.

7

Mitral Valve Repair

Mitral valve repair techniques • Intraoperative echocardiographic evaluation of the mitral valve
after repair

It is helpful for the echocardiographer to have a cursory understanding of the techniques of mitral repair, to collect all of the information that will be needed by the cardiac surgeon. Carpentier and Duran have developed most of the techniques used in mitral valve repair, with some modifications by other institutions.[1–25] For this short review, the techniques of Carpentier will be highlighted.

MITRAL VALVE REPAIR TECHNIQUES

Mitral reconstructive surgery requires optimum exposure and visualization of the mitral leaflets and subvalvular apparatus. A median sternotomy is done and the left atrium is opened longitudinally from the patient's right side, posterior to the interatrial groove beneath both vena cavae, anterior to the right superior and inferior pulmonary veins (Figure 7.1). The heart is held open with special self-retaining retractors. The surgeon visualizes the mitral valve through the left atrium with a perspective similar to the transgastric short axis view at the base of the heart, with the echo image rotated 90° clockwise. Inspection of the mitral valve (Table 7.1) suggests obvious enlargement or deformity of the annulus, prolapse or overriding of the leaflets, jet lesions, or

foci of infection.[26] An asymmetric line of closure suggests leaflet prolapse or restriction. Thickening of the leaflets and restriction is apparent by their lack of pliability. Mobility of the leaflets is checked with the use of nerve hooks wrapped around the chordae at their marginal insertion, to retract gently the leaflet edges in an open and closed maneuver assessing normal, prolapse, or restricted motion. Prolapse and elongation of the chordae can be assessed by retracting corresponding segments for both leaflets with nerve hooks, observing the difference between the two leaflets (Figure 7.2). The P1 segment of the posterior leaflet (the posterior leaflet segment closest to the anterior commissure) usually serves as a normal reference point for comparison of other leaflet areas, since this segment is least prone to prolapse. Direct surgical observation in this manner is usually better than echocardiography in identifying the specific segment of leaflet pathology.

The distribution of lesions in patients with degenerative disease has been described by the Cleveland Clinic for 458 surgical patients.[27] Ruptured chordae tendineae to the mitral leaflets is certainly the most common finding in surgical patients with degenerative prolapse. Posterior chordal ruptures occurred in 41% of patients, with anterior chordal rupture in 10%,

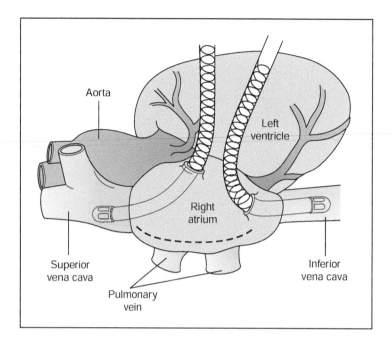

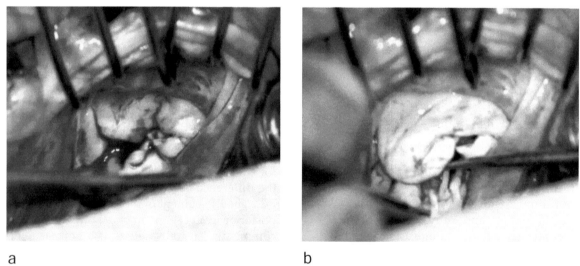

a   b

Fig. 7.1   Diagram depicting the surgical exposure of the heart during mitral valvular repair from the surgeon's perspective. Surgical exposure of the left atrium (LA) and mitral valve is provided by a surgical incision extending from the superior (SVC) and inferior vena cava (IVC), adjacent to the interatrial groove situated in the posterior aspect of the right atrium (RA), anterior to the insertion of the right pulmonary veins (PV). LV, left ventricle; Ao, aorta. (a–g) Photographs during various stages of a mitral valve repair. (a) Initial exposure of the mitral valve. (b) Evaluation of the anterior mitral leaflet. (c) Evaluation of the posterior mitral leaflet with prolapse of the central scallop due to a ruptured chorda. (d) Excision of the central scallop of the posterior leaflet. (e) Re-approximation of the posterior leaflet with a sliding repair. (f) View of the repaired posterior leaflet before ring placement. (g) Finished mitral repair with annuloplasty ring sewn in place.

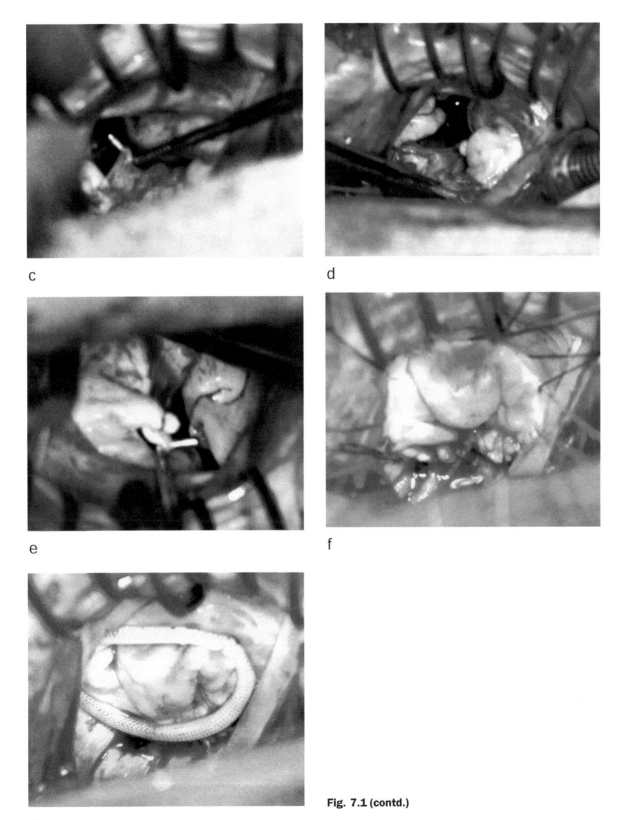

c

d

e

f

g

Fig. 7.1 (contd.)

Table 7.1   Anatomic lesions for valve repair

Lesion	Number	%
Annulus dilatation/deformation	171	87.6
Posterior leaflet prolapse	111	56.9
Anterior leaflet prolapse	78	40.0
Chordal elongation	128	65.6
Chordal rupture of anterior leaflet	29	14.8
Chordal rupture of posterior leaflet	98	50.2
Commissural fusion	11	5.2
Chordal fusion	16	8.2
Papillary muscle rupture	2	1.1

and anterior and posterior chordal rupture in 4%.

The type of pathology that is observed dictates the mitral reparative technique used. To achieve successful surgery, all abnormalities of the mitral apparatus must be repaired. Frequently, the mitral pathology will require more than one technique to obtain a satisfactory and complete repair (Table 7.2).[26]

Surgical repair of a ruptured chorda to the posterior leaflet involves resecting the excessive leaflet tissue along with the ruptured and

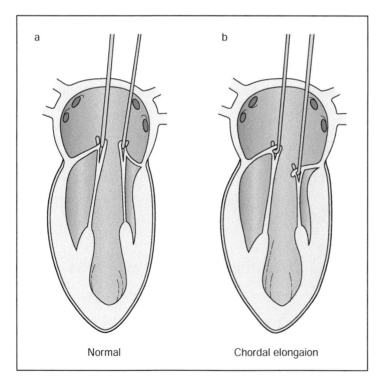

a   b

Normal   Chordal elongaion

Fig. 7.2   Diagram illustrating the surgical technique for testing chordal length. Chorda hooks are utilized to apply traction on different leaflet segments in order to demonstrate differences in chordal length contributing to leaflet prolapse. Although commonly performed in mitral valve evaluation during surgical repair, the limitations of this technique are obvious, especially when the heart is collapsed on cardiopulmonary bypass.

Table 7.2   Mitral reparative technique*

Procedure	Number	%
Carpentier ring annuloplasty	185	95.5
Resection of posterior leafle	121	62.0
Resection of anterior leafle	37	18.9
Chordal shortening	89	45.6
Leaflet mobilization	10	5.1
Associated commissurotomy	11	5.2
Papillary muscle reimplantation	2	1.1
Tricuspid annuloplasty	32	16.4

*Average number of techniques per patient = 2.35.

elongated chords. In cases requiring less than 25% resection of the total leaflet, and when there is not excessive height to the remaining posterior leaflet, a simple quadrangular resection can be done (Figure 7.3). Two perpendicular incisions are made from the leaflet margins to the annulus, on either side of the involved segment. The leaflet segment is removed by an incision along the base of the leaflet following the border of the annulus. The associated chordae are then cut near their origin at the tips of the papillary muscles. Resection is completed by surgical plication of the annulus and approximating the remaining two edges of the remnant posterior leaflet with intermittent sutures, so the knots are on the ventricular side of the leaflets.

In cases requiring up to 60% leaflet resection, or when there is excess tissue of the posterior leaflet, a sliding leaflet technique is required

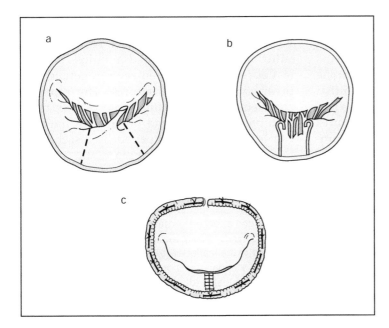

Fig. 7.3 Posterior leafle quadrangular resection. Surgical repair of a ruptured chord to the posterior leaflet (a) involves resecting the excessive leaflet tissue along with th ruptured and elongated chords. In cases requiring less than 25% resection of the total leaflet and whe there is not excessive height to the remaining posterior leaflet, a simpl quadrangular resection can be performed (b). Following resection of the leaflet tissue (c) the emaining leaflet tissue is sewn together and an annuloplasty ring is placed.

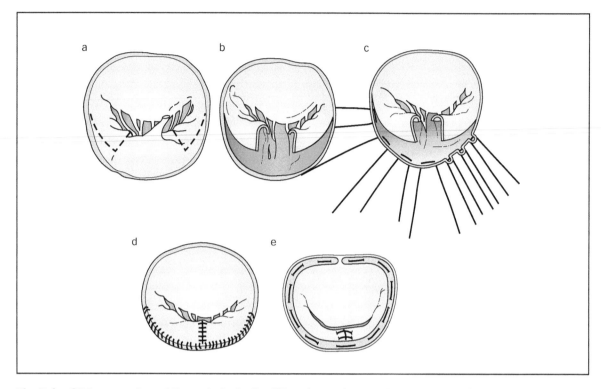

Fig. 7.4 Sliding resection of the posterior leaflet. When the e is excessive posterior leaflet tissue and/o ruptured chordae involving a lar ge resection (up to 60%) a sliding r epair is per formed to decr ease leafle height and allow r eduction of the annulus. (a) Ar ea of the posterior leaflet to be esected. (b) Leaflet tissu removed. (c) Annular ring r eduction sutures in place utilized to plicate the posterior annulus. (d) Reattachment of the posterior leaflet. (e) Final epair after annuloplasty ring placement.

(Figure 7.4). This involves incisions similar to a quadrangular resection, with the addition of two triangular resections at the base of the posterior leaflet remnants to correct for excess tissue height. All secondary and basal chordae are removed from the leaflet remnants so that they are free of restriction and tension when they are approximated later. Mattress sutures are passed through the annulus, which circumferentially decreases the annulus by compressing the posterior aspect of the annulus, bringing the leaflet remnants into approximation. Each leaflet remnant is then reattached by suturing to the compressed annulus. The two leaflet remnants are then sewn together with inverted, interrupted sutures. The repair is completed by the insertion of a prosthetic ring.

Ruptured chordae and prolapse of the anterior leaflet are never repaired by resection, so that the integrity and length of the anterior

Fig. 7.5 Diagram illustrating chor dal transfer. Chor dae may be transfer red from one segment of the same ▶ leaflet or from the opposite leaflet to epair a r uptured chorda tendinea. (a) Ruptur e chorda tendinea of the anterior mitral leaflet. (b) Longitudinal view of the uptured chorda and attached nor mal secondar y chordae in close approximation to the r uptured chorda. (c) The r uptured chorda is sur gically removed and a neighboring secondar y chorda is excised at its leaflet inse tion and transfer red to the leaflet edge, p oviding leaflet suppo t in order to pr event prolapse of that segment. In some cases when a secondar y chord from the same leaflet ma not be sufficient to transfe , a cor responding chorda from the posterior leaflet (d) may be excised an transfer red to the anterior leaflet. (e) The posterior leaflet is then epaired (f) after the chor da is r emoved and transfer red similarly to a posterior leaflet esection. The r epair is then completed with an annuloplasty ring.

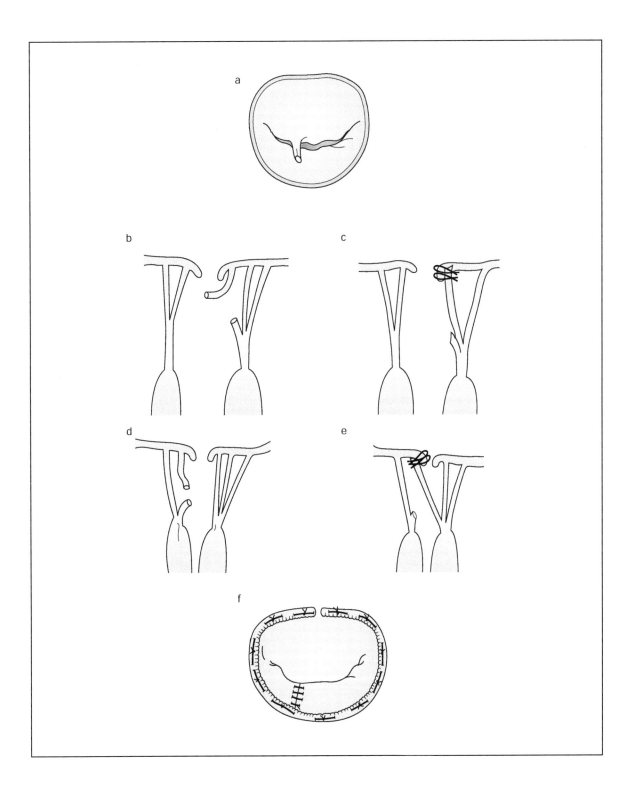

leaflet is preserved to ensure proper closure against the opposing posterior leaflet. Anterior chordal ruptures are repaired by secondary chordal transfer or transposition of chordae. In secondary chordal transfer, normal secondary chordae from the anterior leaflet close to the ruptured chorda leaflet are removed and reattached to the margin of the leaflet to act as a primary chorda (so as to spread out the existing chordae to provide leaflet integrity). Marginal or primary chordae are the most important and must be spaced about every 5 mm along the leaflet edge. Secondary chordae are of less importance and may be sacrificed to replace marginal chords. Transposition of chordae is performed by transferring chordae from the posterior leaflet to the anterior leaflet (Figure 7.5). Secondary chordae are removed from the posterior leaflet by resecting a small triangular portion from the free edge of the posterior leaflet, directly opposite the lesion of the anterior leaflet. The posterior leaflet segment and attached chordae are sutured to the anterior leaflet edge, and the posterior leaflet is repaired if necessary.

When there is chordal rupture of both leaflets it usually is a result of one leaflet chorda rupturing due to strain from rupture of the opposite leaflet chorda. This usually involves using both secondary chordal transfer and transposition of chordae. When chordae rupture near the commissures it usually involves the anterolateral commissure, and the commissure is reconstructed by transplanting chordae and surgically making a new commissure "magic suture" stitch.

In 30% of patients, the chordae are just elongated, and are not ruptured. In these instances, a shortening plasty may be done, which entails folding a small portion of the chorda on itself and burying that portion into an incision made longitudinally, creating a trough in the papillary muscle from which it originates (Figure 7.6). Chordae may be shortened in small groups by this method, and multiple groups may need to be shortened. Occasionally, prolapsed segments with elongated chordae may be corrected by chordal transfer techniques.

When chordae are thickened, areas of thickening can be trimmed or shaved. When chordae are fused they can be split or debrided with a scalpel or rongeur.[28–30] In fusion of the centrally placed chordae, fenestration or removal of triangular wedges of tissue is performed. When retraction of the posterior leaflet occurs, secondary and tertiary chordae may be removed to permit better pliability of the leaflet. In cases of subvalvular stenosis, the chordae may need to be shaved to the level of the papillary muscles, and occasionally the papillary muscles may

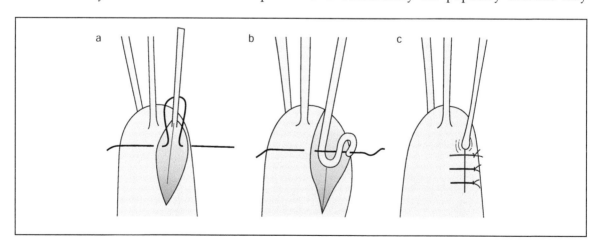

Fig. 7.6 Diagram illustrating a surgical method of shortening elongated chordae tendineae. The chorda is shortened by burying a small length within the papillary muscle. (a) A trench is created in the papillary muscle. (b) With a suture an appropriate length of the chorda is pulled and buried in the trench created in the papillary muscle. (c) After burying the chorda the trench is sutured closed.

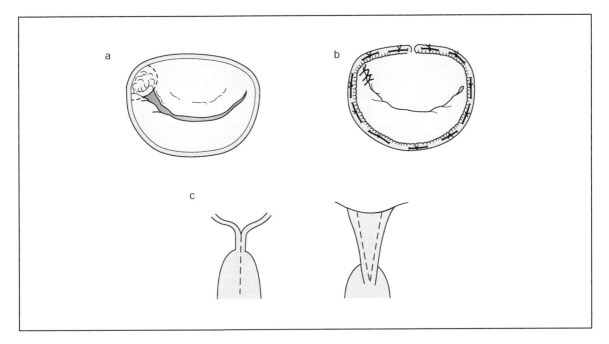

Fig. 7.7 Surgical techniques used for r epair in mitral stenosis. (a) Commissural fusion or focal ar eas of calcification may be r emoved by debridement or excision as illustrated in (b). The need for placement of a mitral annular ring is somewhat contr oversial although it pr ovides suppor t to the valve after the r epair. When chordae are thickened and fused, ar eas of thickening can be trimmed or shaved or when fused can be split or debrided with a scalpel. In fusion of the centrally placed chor ds, fenestration or the r emoval of triangular wedges of tissue is per formed. In cases of subvalvular stenosis the chor ds may need to be shaved to the level of the papillar y muscles and occasionally the papillar y muscles may need to be split and divided (c) to relieve obstr uction with unr estricted valve motion.

need to be split and divided (Figure 7.7). Although not a Carpentier technique, artificial chordae have been constructed with Gore-Tex or suture material to replace existing natural chordae.[31–33]

In stenotic valves with commissural fusion, the commissural furrow is incised with a scalpel blade (Figure 7.8). The line of commissural fusion may be identified by placing vertical traction on the free edge of both leaflets with nerve hooks, or by distending the ventricle with saline. The fused commissures are incised centrally from the valve orifice along the furrow, and should divide and spare the attached chordae to a few millimeters from the annulus. The chordae exposed after the separation of the

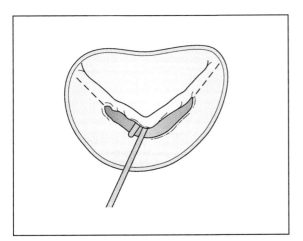

Fig. 7.8 Mitral commissur otomy. During open mitral commissur otomy, gentle traction is applied to the anterior mitral leaflet to delineate fu ther the line of fusion allowing a mor e accurate placement of the surgical incision. It is impor tant that the leaflets a e separated with chor dae intact to each r espective leaflet producing the best r esults.

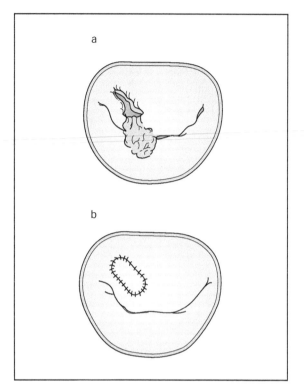

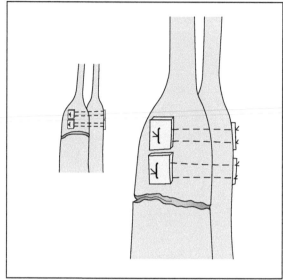

Fig. 7.10 Diagram illustrating the r eattachment of a ruptured papillar y muscle. In selected cases of partial or complete r upture the papillar y muscle can be reattached sur gically, par ticularly when ther e is good tissue to suppor t the sutur es used in the re-anastomosis.

Fig. 7.9 Diagram illustrating sur gical repair methods utilized in infective endocar ditis. In selected cases, valvular vegetations (a) can be sur gically excised as long as the underlying tissue has not been destr oyed. When per forations develop as a result of endocar ditis, the infected tissue may be debrided and a pericar dial patch (b) may be utilized to close the r emaining small hole.

commissures are repaired in the manner previously described.

Cleft or perforated leaflets can be repaired by simple closing stitches or by patches made from the patient's own glutaraldehyde-treated pericardium (Figure 7.9).[34] Complete or partial papillary muscle rupture is repaired by sewing the papillary muscle back in place, which works surprisingly well (Figure 7.10). In cases of restricted motion due to ischemic papillary muscle dysfunction, the papillary muscles may be removed at their base, repositioned, and re-implanted in the ventricle, usually in a more superior position. In the purest form of Carpentier's techniques, pledgets are not used for the repair. Instead, a larger suture

specifically designed for reconstruction is used. Pledgets are small pieces of Teflon used to reinforce suture material, and are widely used in North American cardiac surgery. Pledgets are thought to make the repair bulky, limiting mobility, and promoting thrombus formation and potential infection. Although pledgets should be avoided, papillary muscle surgery may require reinforcement with pledget material.

Mitral valve repair has also been extremely successful in acute and chronic cases of bacterial endocarditis, with a low operative morbidity and mortality, and with the same durability for the mitral reconstruction.[35–37] Mitral valve repair is done with the usual techniques, including debridement of all infected tissue and placement of an annuloplasty ring. With mitral valve replacement in the setting of bacterial endocarditis there is a 10–15% risk of subsequent endocarditis in five years, with the greatest risk occurring in the first six months postoperatively. It appears that as long as the patient has been pretreated with adequate antibiotics and all of the infected tissue is removed, mitral valve repair is associated with a lower re-infection rate than mitral valve replacement (operative mortality 7.4%; by actuarial methods 61±6% of patients are alive at ten years and have no recurrence of endocarditis). Mitral valve repairs associated with a paravalvular abscess carry the highest risk of reinfection. d'Udekem and colleagues,[38] have reported on 122 consecutive patients with active infective endocarditis and paravalvular abscess, treated with the usual reparative techniques plus wide excision of the abscess and reconstruction of the heart with glutaraldehyde-fixed bovine pericardium. There were nine operative deaths (7.4%) and only one patient had persistent infection that required re-operation. Freedom from recurrent endocarditis was 79±9% at ten years.

Mitral annular calcification (MAC) has been described in association with most of the disease processes that cause mitral disease.[39] Mitral valve replacement with extensive MAC is associated with an increased risk of ventricular rupture (18%), which has not been reported with mitral repair. Extensive annular calcification may occur, which can distort the orifice and can influence mitral repair results unfavorably. When significant MAC is present, it is removed by dissection and debridement of the affected areas of the annulus (Figure 7.11). When calcification predominantly occurs in the posterior region, exposure of the posterior annulus is accomplished by detaching the posterior leaflet from the annulus. The ventricular endothelium is then incised around the borders of the area of calcification. The bar of calcium is then removed in one piece if possible, with fine dissection using scissors, creating a trench in the annulus. Careful attention must be paid not to expose the circumflex artery or weaken the annulus by going too far into the atrioventricular groove or the ventricular myocardium. When calcium extends to the posterior leaflet, it is removed from the leaflet by shaving with a scalpel or debriding with a rongeur. Following the removal of calcium, the trench is sutured closed, and the posterior leaflet is reattached.

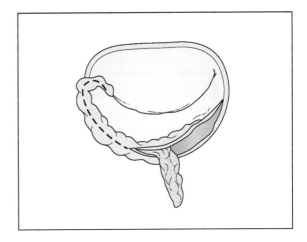

Fig. 7.11 Excision of mitral annular calcification When calcification p edominately occurs in the posterior region of the annulus, exposur e of the posterior annulus is accomplished by initially detaching the posterior leaflet f om the annulus. The ventricular endothelium is then incised ar ound the borders of the ar ea of calcification. The bar o calcium is then r emoved in one piece if possible to avoid fragmentation and embolization. Following the removal of calcium, the tr ench is sutur ed closed and the posterior leaflet is e-attached.

Whether there is associated annular dilatation or not, the surgical repair is completed with the placement of an annuloplasty ring (Figure 7.12). In cases of type I and especially type III motion, an annuloplasty ring is usually all that is required for a successful repair. The annuloplasty ring promotes remodeling of the mitral annulus, provides support for the chordal and leaflet repairs, and promotes coaptation of the anterior and posterior leaflets. The annuloplasty ring also promotes remodeling by providing a measured plication of the posterior annulus and a decrease in the anterior–posterior dimension. In this manner, the annulus is returned to its normal physiological size and shape, and should not be restrictive to the inflow tract. Care should be exercised in the choice of ring size – mitral rings will not allow for dilatation during diastole, and an undersized annuloplasty ring may result in a stenotic valve. Stenosis produced by an annuloplasty ring is unacceptable, producing obstruction to inflow, and promoting

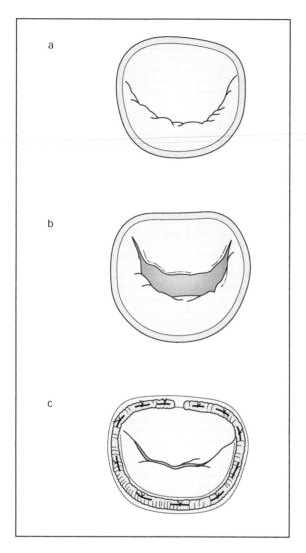

Fig. 7.12 Mitral valve drawing illustrating annular dilatation. (a) Normal mitral valve as viewed *en face*. Note the normal dimensions and shape of the mitral valve and annulus. The width of the anterior leaflet i greater than the posterior leaflet, which p oduces a line of closure towards the posterior aspect of the annulus. The normal annulus dimensions ar e described by a smaller height (anterior–posterior diameter) in comparison to the width (transverse diameter) with a 3:4 ratio, r espectively. (b) With annular dilatation the height of the annulus enlar ges becoming greater than the transverse diameter . The length and width of the posterior leaflet inc ease, which shifts the line of closur e of the mitral valve to the center of the annulus. Annular dilatation may occur as a consequence of the disease pr ocess, as in acute r heumatic mitral r egurgitation, or as a r esult of secondar y ventricular enlar gement. Dilatation occurs predominantly in the posterior aspect of the mitral annulus due to the makeup of the annular tissue. (c) Sur gical placement of a mitral annular ring returns the normal shape and dimensions to the mitral valve.

systolic anterior motion of the mitral valve and thromboembolic complications.

When measuring for ring size it is usually best to select a larger ring size for type I and II motion, and a smaller ring size for type III motion. Ring size is measured using a sizing device supplied by the manufacturer of the ring. The ring size is determined by the distance measured between the two commissures and the height of the anterior leaflet in its midportion (Figure 7.13). On average, in adults a 32–34 mm ring is used for men and a 30–32 mm ring for women. A properly positioned annular ring provides the normal apposition of the leaflets and avoids obstruction. To ensure proper alignment and geometric positioning without distortion, the natural mitral commissures must be correctly identified, and the commissure markings on the ring must be anchored appropriately at each commissure. The midpoints of the anterior and posterior leaflets should be oriented so that they are directly opposite each other, making sure that the leaflets' line of closure is parallel to the annulus of the posterior leaflet. After placement of the ring, visual inspection yields good symmetrical geometry of the line of closure ("smile") for the mitral valve leaflets with respect to the annulus.

Two types of annuloplasty ring are currently available, a fixed ring and flexible ring (Figure

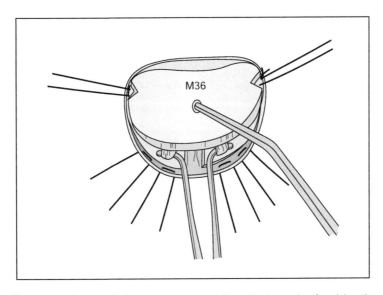

Fig. 7.13   Diagram illustrating the sur gical measur ement of the mitral annulus for sizing the mitral annular ring. The ring size is based on the size and ar   ea of the anterior mitral leaflet. Markings or g   ooves on the sizer correspond to points for matching up to the commissur   es. On average 32–34 mm rings ar e used in males and 30–32 mm rings ar e used in females. Accor ding to sur geon preference downsizing the dimension of the mitral annular ring may be per formed in patients with left ventricular enlar gement. Since mitral rings will not allow for dilatation during diastole caution must be exer   cised so as not to cause stenosis and a significant transvalvula gradient following the r epair.

7.14).[40,41] There are two Carpentier rings – the fixed "classic" ring and the semi-flexible "physiological ring". Both rings have a "D" shape which promotes remodeling of the distorted annulus to the typical systolic shape, allowing proper closure and approximation of the leaflets. With the fixed ring, the width of the annulus is preserved and the mitral annulus maintains its size and shape during the entire cardiac cycle. The flexible Carpentier ring follows the same principle, in that the anterior aspect of the ring is fixed and the posterior aspect is flexible. The anterior leaflet height dictates the use of one ring over another. If the length is larger (excessive tissue) than the sizer, then a "classic" fixed ring should be used; otherwise ring choice should probably favor the semi-flexible "physiological ring". The Duran ring is completely flexible, theoretically allowing for a normal elliptical annular shape during systole and a circular shape without obstruction during diastole, and does not produce left ventricular outflow obstruction during systole. The type of annuloplasty ring used depends on the type of repair, valvular anatomy, or preference of the surgeon.

After placement of the annular ring and before the sutures are tied in place, the competency of the valve is tested. Saline is injected into the left ventricular cavity. When the cavity is filled, the mitral leaflets expand and assume their normal position. Occasionally the anterior leaflet may require slight unfurling by manipulation with a nerve hook to expand fully. Areas of prolapse and mitral regurgitation may be visualized in this manner (Figure 7.15).

After mitral valve repair, patients receive anticoagulation for two months to promote good healing and fibrosis between the repaired tissue and the exposed cloth and sutures of the annular ring.

INTRAOPERATIVE ECHOCARDIOGRAPHIC EVALUATION OF THE MITRAL V ALVE AFTER REPAIR

After surgical repair of the mitral valve, echocardiographic analysis is done intraoperatively,

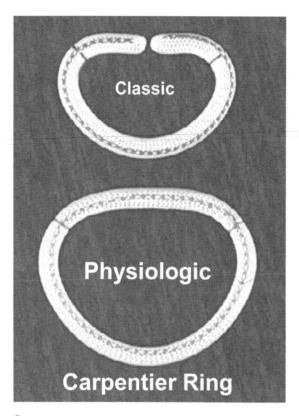

Classic

Physiologic

Carpentier Ring

a

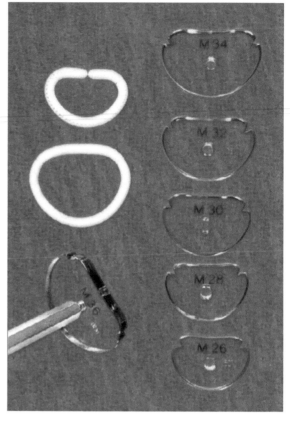

c

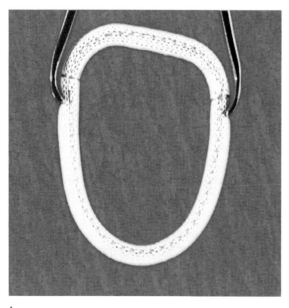

b

Fig. 7.14 Mitral valve annuloplasty rings. (a) Carpentier-Edwards classic (fixed) and physiologica (semi-flexible) rings. Both rings are D-shaped, imitating the normal shape of the mitral annulus which allows for proper closure and approximation of the leaflets during systole though remodeling of the distorted mitral annulus. To avoid annular distortion from improper alignment of the valve ring, markings indicate the fixation points for the commissues. The fixed ring preserves the width of the annulus and will maintain annular size and shape during both diastole and systole. Some flexibility is p ovided by the split of the ring anteriorly. (b) The Carpentier-Edwards physiological ring follows the same principle as the fixed ring in preserving the anterior aspect of the annulus. However, the posterior portion allows for more flexibilit, allowing the annulus to change shape during the cardiac cycle. (c) Mitral ring sizers are specifically designed for measurement of the proper ring size used during mitral valve repair surgery. The ring size is based on the size and area of the anterior mitral leaflet.

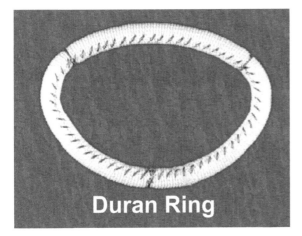

d

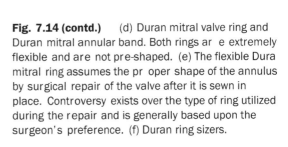

e

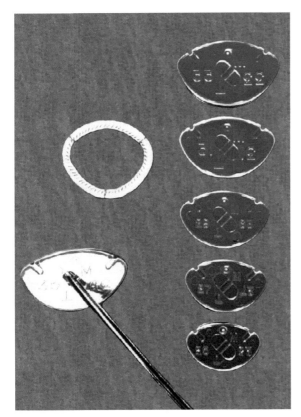

f

Fig. 7.14 (contd.) (d) Duran mitral valve ring and Duran mitral annular band. Both rings ar e extremely flexible and are not pre-shaped. (e) The flexible Dura mitral ring assumes the pr oper shape of the annulus by surgical repair of the valve after it is sewn in place. Controversy exists over the type of ring utilized during the repair and is generally based upon the surgeon's preference. (f) Duran ring sizers.

immediately after weaning from cardio-pulmonary bypass, to evaluate the success of the repair. Immediate echocardiographic evalu-ation is important since the conventional surgi-cal assessment of mitral regurgitation (filling the arrested ventricle with saline to look for a leak) is a cursory technique at best, and has not been proven reliable compared with intra-operative echocardiography. Immediate intra-operative transesophageal echocardiographic

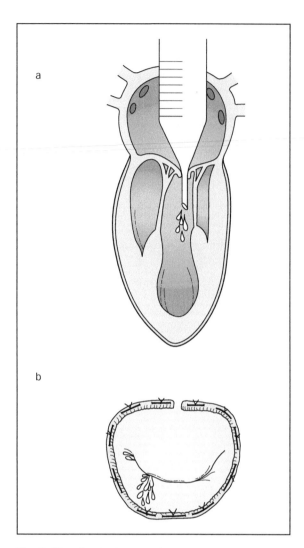

Fig. 7.15 Surgical testing for r esidual mitral regurgitation. (a) Competence of the mitral valve is tested by inser ting a syringe or catheter thr ough the valve and injecting fluid, filling the left ventricle (b) Valve leaks cor responding to mitral r egurgitation are detected when the leaflets coapt with ventricula filling

Table 7.3   Echocardiographic f ndings needing a second pump r un
Residual mitral regurgitation ≥ 2+ No change or worsening MR Color flow maximum jet a ea > 4 cm² PVF blunted systolic for ward flo PVF systolic flow eversal
Mitral inf ow obstruction Increased peak gradient acr oss mitral valve
Left ventricular outf ow tract obstr uction SAM Increased peak gradient in L VOT
Flail leaf et
Suture dehiscence
Ring dehiscence
Incomplete repair

evaluation of the repair to assess the degree of residual mitral regurgitation accurately predicts the results of mitral valve repair compared with postoperative angiographic evaluation, and does not change significantly on postoperative follow-up (Table 7.3).

The mitral leaflet motion is evaluated in the same manner postoperatively to determine the resolution of defects and to monitor the development of any new abnormalities occurring as a result of the repair. Before visualization of the heart, it is extremely helpful to compare the preoperative echocardiographic assessment with the surgical findings, and to know what techniques were used in the mitral valve reconstruction. In this manner, a quicker and more thorough echocardiographic evaluation of the leaflets and subvalvular apparatus can be made immediately after the cessation of cardiopulmonary bypass and before decannulation. Findings that require the reinstitution of cardiopulmonary bypass and repeat of a repair are very subjective (Table 7.4).[42] Careful consideration and discussion with the surgeon and anesthesiologist must be made before the initial repair is judged inadequate. Although there is a learning curve for the surgeon for valve reconstruction, a considerable degree of experience is required by the echocardiographer as well. Some findings are obvious, and need further surgery, especially if the patient develops poor hemodynamics and the regurgitation or stenosis is worse or unchanged compared to preop. Less clear are cases in which, for example, the mitral regurgitation is severe preoperatively

Table 7.4 Post pump intraoperative echocardiography at the Cleveland clinic	
Lesion (n = 611)	Number (%)
Successful repair	557 (91.2)
Failed repairs	54 (8.8)
LVOT obstruction	14 (2.2)
Persistent MS	1 (0.2)
Persistent flai	2 (0.4)
Persistent MR	33 (5.4)
Other	4 (0.6)

and moderate after the repair. Depending on many factors – including the age of the patient, the time already spent on bypass and cross-clamp time, the severity of pathology, the improvement in hemodynamics, and the experience of the echocardiographer and the surgeon – residual moderate regurgitation may be acceptable. Other questions, such as whether to perform a second repair or valve replacement, require the consideration of many of the same factors (Table 7.5).[43]

Table 7.5 Reoperations in mitral valve repair	
Causes of reoperation	Number
Early reoperation (<2 yr)	**10**
Ring dehiscence	1
Recurrent annular distension (no ring was used)	2
Triangular resection	3
Residual prolapse	4
Late reoperation (>2 yr)	**13**
Recurrent prolapse	4
Leaflet retraction	6
Valve stenosis	3

The mitral apparatus should be scanned in multiple planes to assess the continuity of the papillary muscles, chordae, and leaflets. Occasionally, small remnants of removed chordae may be seen fluttering in close proximation to the papillary muscles, but there should not be any chordae of significant length with large chaotic motion. If chordae were shortened too much the leaflets should show restricted motion. If the chordae remain elongated, there will be prolapse of the leaflets. Visualization of the posterior leaflet is limited due to the presence of the annular ring after leaflet resection. In most cases, the posterior leaflet should appear immobile and fixed in its diastolic position. The posterior leaflet usually regains its motion within 1–6 months. There should be no obvious prolapse of the leaflet margins in line of approximation in long axis views, and depending on the adequacy of repair the leaflets should show their normal height ratio (2:1 anterior to posterior). If the line of closure is visualized in the short axis plane, it should be placed posteriorly in the ventricle and follow the line of the posterior annulus. Small suture ends may be seen around the annular ring in long axis or short axis views. Suture dehiscence is characterized by long sutures that show obvious chaotic motion throughout the cardiac cycle. Use of the zoom feature or decreasing the echocardiographic field depth may help resolve the normality or abnormality of these findings.

Usually a remodeling annuloplasty ring may be visualized in the region of the mitral annulus, in the short axis proximal transgastric view at $0°–30°$, represented by increased echogenicity, hyper-reflectivity, and shadowing similar to a prosthetic valve, with the shape of ring and the annulus approximating its normal D-shape. A small decrease in the mitral valve area will be observed by the Doppler pressure half-time method, for both the Carpentier rings or flexible Duran ring.[41] There should not be a significant increase for any of the ring types, however, in the peak transmitral diastolic velocity, peak transmitral diastolic gradient ($8±4$ mmHg), mean transmitral diastolic gradient ($3±2$ mmHg), or the grade of mitral regurgitation, despite the reduction in valve area. Although patients with flexible rings have better left ventricular function initially after the repair, no significant difference is shown at one year after surgery. When suture dehiscence is present about the annular ring, the annular ring will have a rocking motion, back and forth throughout the cardiac cycle.

Color flow mapping is performed to determine reduction in the severity of mitral regurgitation compared with preoperative values. Residual mitral insufficiency is frequently in a different direction after the repair, but the maximum jet area or the ratio of jet area to left atrial area should be reduced in comparison to preoperative measurements. If necessary, the regurgitant orifice area may be calculated from the vena contracta or flow convergence method. Pulsed Doppler interrogation of the pulmonary veins should show improvement or increase in the systolic forward flow, normalizing the systolic:diastolic ratio, and preoperative systolic flow reversal should be eliminated.

At experienced centers, about 80% of cases of successful valve repair result in trivial or no mitral regurgitation, and an acceptable result should yield below 2+ mitral regurgitation.[27] Mild or trivial mitral regurgitation after mitral valve repair may be related to left ventricular function or persistent abnormality of the mitral apparatus. Patients with chronic heart disease and severe left ventricular failure may show residual mitral regurgitation immediately after heart activity has resumed, secondary to increased afterload. Type III or restricted leaflet motion may be observed after ischemic arrest due to transient left ventricular dysfunction. With continued monitoring during the completion of surgery, leaflet motion normalizes, coinciding with the return of left ventricular function. Occasionally, patients receiving inotropic and vasodilatory drugs who have reduced ventricular filling (as seen immediately after weaning from bypass) may develop left ventricular outflow obstruction with mild to moderate mitral regurgitation after repair. Correction of hemodynamics usually results in the disappearance of the left ventricular outflow obstruction and the mitral regurgita-

tion. Other causes of mild regurgitation not specifically related to the mitral repair may be abnormal cardiac rhythms, such as ventricular tachycardia or paced rhythms.

A mitral valvular repair should be considered a failure when there is no detectable change in the severity of mitral regurgitation from preoperative values, or there is 2+ or greater mitral insufficiency in the setting of normal left ventricular function. The prevalence of failed mitral valvular repair resulting in a second pump-run is about 8% as reported by the Cleveland Clinic, and may be slightly higher depending on the experience of the surgical team (Table 7.5).[27] Immediate failures may be the result of left ventricular outflow tract obstruction (3%), incomplete correction, and suture dehiscence of the annular ring or valve repair. Late failure after mitral repair is primarily due to progression of the underlying disease, especially with degenerative disease. Late failure may also be attributable to the degree of surgical experience and the difficulty of the techniques used during the repair. Chordal shortening techniques and repairs of the anterior leaflet with redundant excessive tissue are technically difficult since they require the proper assessment of length and elongation in the arrested and empty heart. Suturing the papillary muscle may be difficult in cases of reattachment after muscle rupture and burying chordae in the papillary muscle for chordal shortening, and may result in early or late suture dehiscence.

Left ventricular outflow tract obstruction complicates mitral valve repair in 3–5% of cases, with or without residual mitral regurgitation (Figure 7.16).[44–47] After mitral repair, resting gradients of 0–44 mmHg have been measured in the left ventricular outflow, which may significantly increase with isoproterenol stimulation. Left ventricular outflow tract obstruction is most common in degenerative posterior leaflet prolapse, and has not been reported after the repair of type I mitral regurgitation or rheumatic disease producing restrictive or prolapsed leaflets. The development of outflow tract obstruction has been eliminated largely with the second generation of Carpentier repair techniques.[48,49] In the first decade of repair,

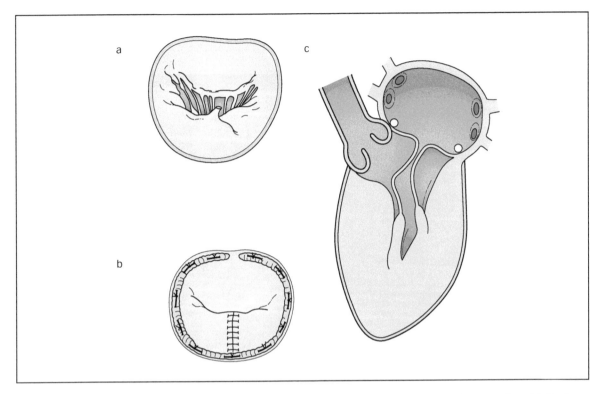

Fig. 7.16 Systolic anterior motion (SAM) following r epair. SAM of the mitral valve may be pr oduced following mitral repair due to excessive height of the posterior leaflet, which pushes the line of closu e anteriorly towards the left ventricular outflow tract. SAM may also be p oduced when too small an annuloplasty ring is utilized for the r epair, especially in hyper trophic ventricles with small cavity dimensions.

smaller rings were used more frequently, and resection of the posterior leaflet was not accompanied by shortening of the height of the leaflet. Left ventricular outflow tract obstruction has been attributed to reduction in size of the mitral annulus, secondary to the annuloplasty ring. With the placement of the annular ring, the posterior left ventricular wall and the posterior mitral leaflet are directed anteriorly towards the aorta, resulting in significant narrowing of the mitro-aortic angle to 120°–100°. Additionally, both leaflets are displaced into the left ventricular outflow tract. This distortion in ventricular geometry pushes the left ventricular inflow into the left ventricular outflow tract, with forward diastolic flow directed toward the ventricular septum instead of toward the ventricular apex. Excess tissue of the posterior leaflet (> 1 cm in height) in con-

junction with the presence of the annular ring causes the posterior leaflet to close first and pushes the anterior leaflet, and thus the line of leaflet closure, towards the left ventricular outflow tract, thereby producing systolic anterior motion (SAM). The left ventricular outflow tract and mitral valve leaflet motion should be carefully assessed in the deep transgastric view at 0°, or in the lower esophageal position between 90° and 180°, to assess for proper leaflet aspect during systole and diastole and the presence of SAM. Using these same views, color flow Doppler imaging of the inflow and outflow jets shows the direction and orientation of blood flow. Forward diastolic flow from the mitral orifice is directed anteriorly in the ventricle, while the reverse flow is deflected along the posterobasal wall and upward toward the mitral valve and aorta.

Case Studies

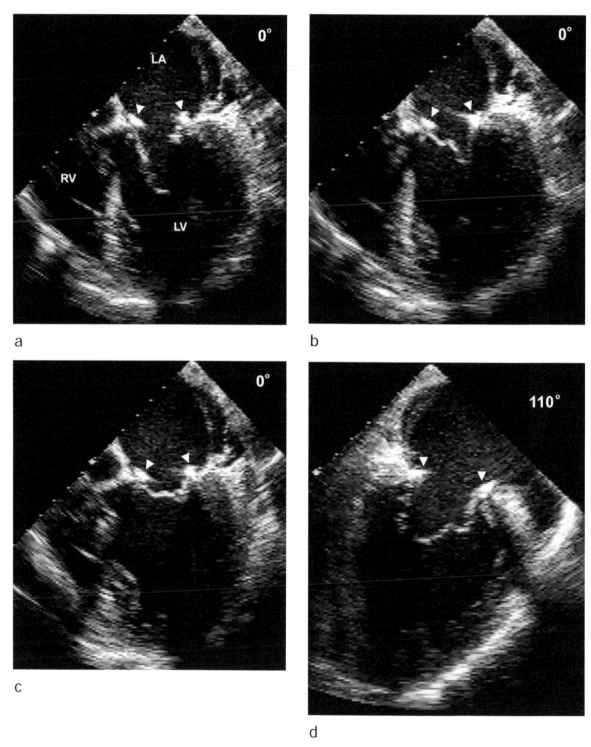

a

b

c

d

Case 7.1 Mitral valve repair. Mitral valve analysis post r epair. Lower esophageal window at 0° (a–c) and 110° (d–f) from diastole thr ough systole.

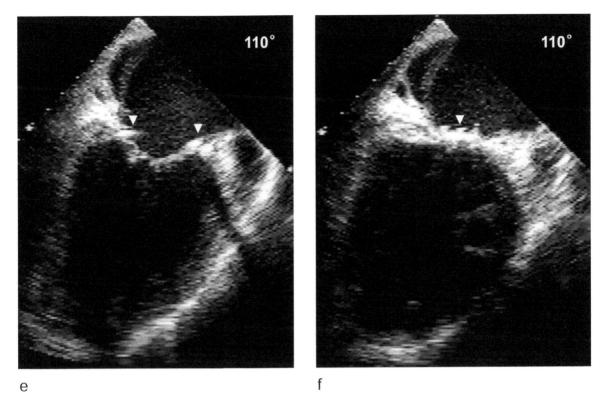

e   f

Case 7.1 (contd.)   The mitral annuloplasty ring is well visualized in cr oss-section (arrows). The anterior leafle exhibits most of the leaflet motion. The posterior leaflet often appears fixed and does not exhibit signifi motion for a period of 6–8 weeks following the r epair. There is no obvious pr olapse and leaflet motion appear normal. In addition to valve leaflet motion, left ventricular wall motion should be assessed, to ule out inferior and/or posterior wall hypokinesis or akinesis r esulting from an annular sutur e involving the cir cumflex arter y. LA, left atrium; L V, left ventricle; R V, right ventricle.

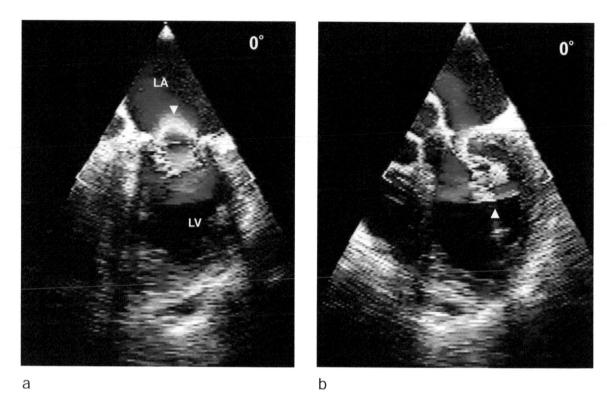

a   b

Case 7.2 Color flow Doppler following a successful mitral valve   epair. Color flow Doppler f om diastole through systole (a–d) r ecorded at 0° and corresponding views at 115° (e–h). In early diastole (a,e) flo convergence is noted above the annuloplasty ring. During mid-diastole (b,f) slightly accelerated flow velocity i noted and the inflow jet should be di ected posteriorly into the left ventricle. With closur e of the leaflets (c, g flow should diminish in the left ventricular inflow tract and sta   t to appear in the outflow tract. In systol normal velocity flow is ecorded in the outflow tract and mitral   egurgitation should not be detected. Pulsed and continuous wave Doppler may be guided by color flow to   ule out the pr esence of a significant gradient ac oss the annuloplasty ring or in the outflow tract that would suggest either   estriction of the mitral orifice o obstruction to the outflow tract esulting in SAM. LA, left atrium; L V, left ventricle.

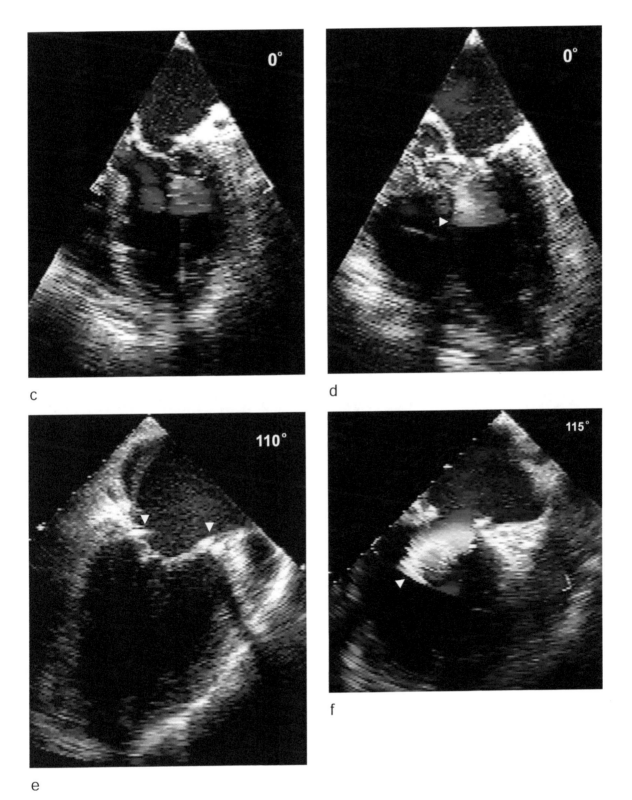

c

d

e

f

Case 7.2 (contd.)

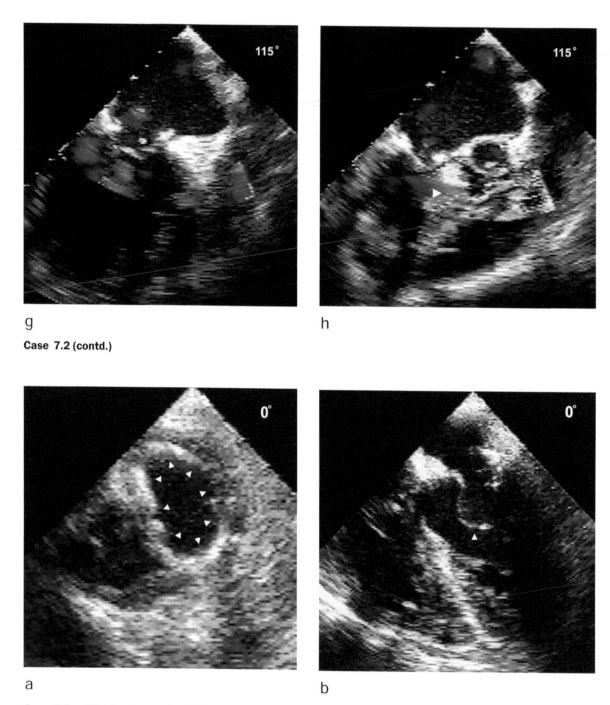

g

h

Case 7.2 (contd.)

a

b

Case 7.3 Mitral valve repair. (a) Shor t-axis echocardiographic image illustrating the full extent of the mitral annuloplasty ring. (b–d) Serial echocar diographic images obtained fr om the lower esophageal window at 0° with mild anteflexion of the p obe, demonstrating chor dal analysis following the r epair. Redundant chor dae to the anterior leaflet a e noted, visualized as an undulating motion fr om diastole to systole. This was the only obvious abnormality visualized and indicates an unsuccessful r epair. Echogenicity of the annuloplasty ring leaflet may deter analysis of leaflet motion following the epair, making it impor tant to per form a complete analysis from multiple views of the mitral leaflets and subvalvular apparatus

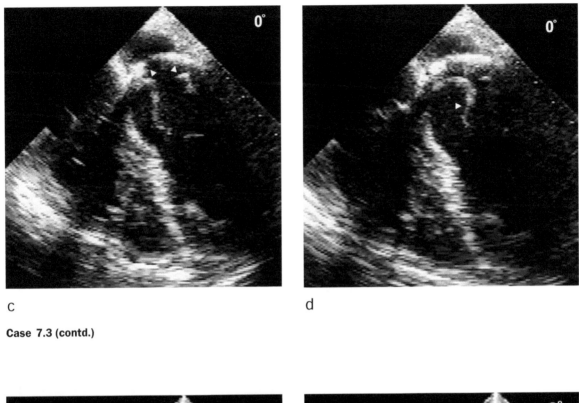

c

d

Case 7.3 (contd.)

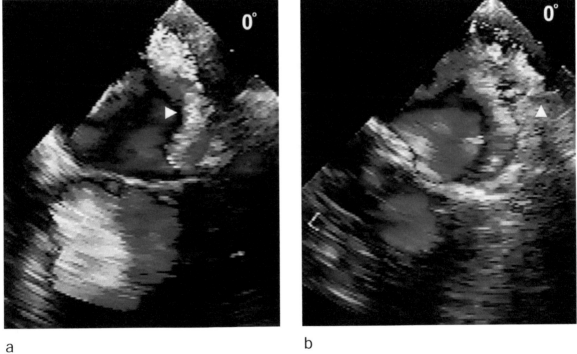

a

b

Case 7.4 Successful mitral repair of mitral valve prolapse and annular dilatation. (a–c) Color flow Dopple illustrating significant mitral regurgitation before mitral repair.

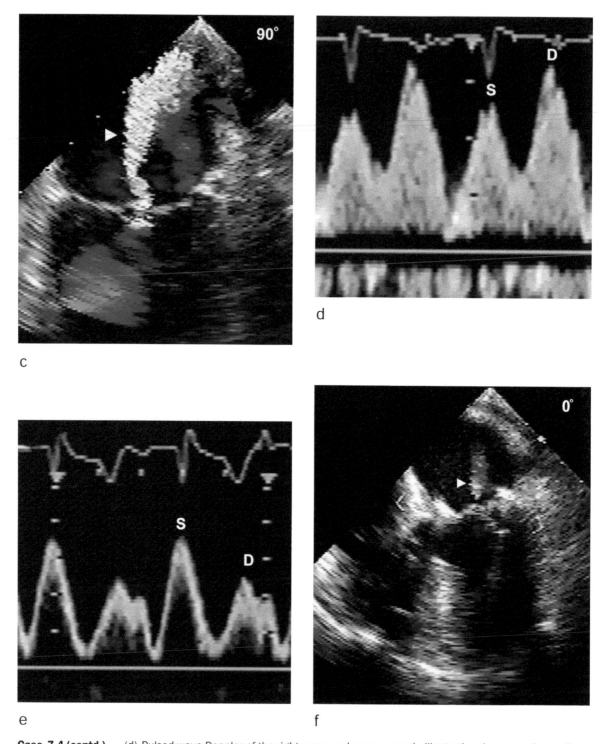

c

d

e

f

Case 7.4 (contd.) (d) Pulsed wave Doppler of the right upper pulmonar y vein illustrating decr eased systolic flow in comparison to diastolic flo . Following successful mitral valve r epair (e) systolic flow has no malized in relationship to diastolic flow as epresented by absence of significant mitral egurgitation (f). S, systolic flow D, diastolic flo .

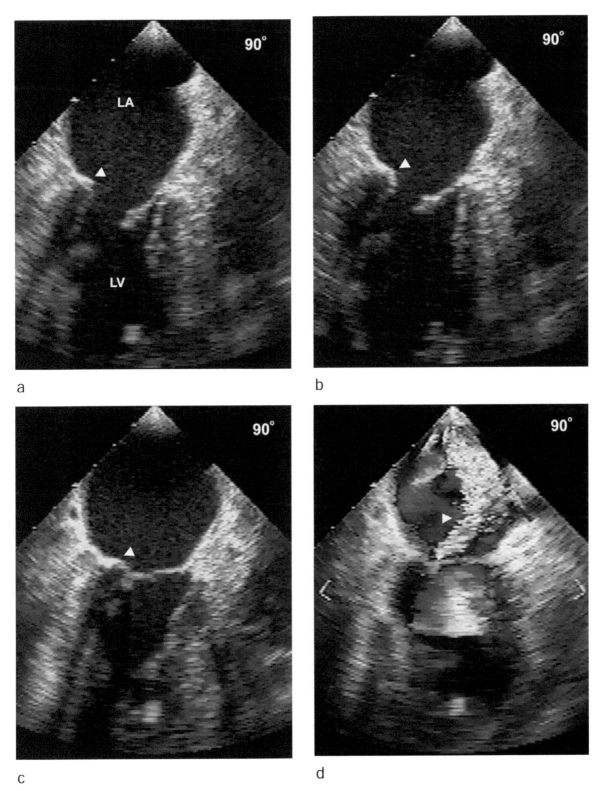

a

b

c

d

Case 7.5 Unsuccessful mitral repair of type III restrictive mitral regurgitation. (a–c) Diastolic through systolic frames demonstrating an immobile posterior leaflet. In addition there was a small posterior wall aneurysm. (d) Color flow Doppler demonstrating significant mitral regurgitation.

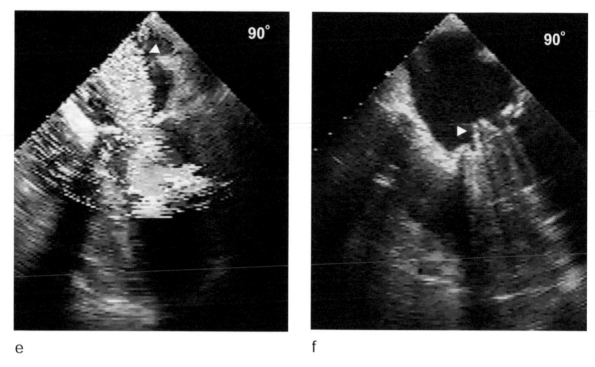

e   f

Case 7.5 (contd.)   (e) Immediately following the r epair severe mitral regurgitation is noted almost entir ely filling the left atrium. (f) St. Jude pr osthesis replacing the repair. LA, left atrium; L V, left ventricle.

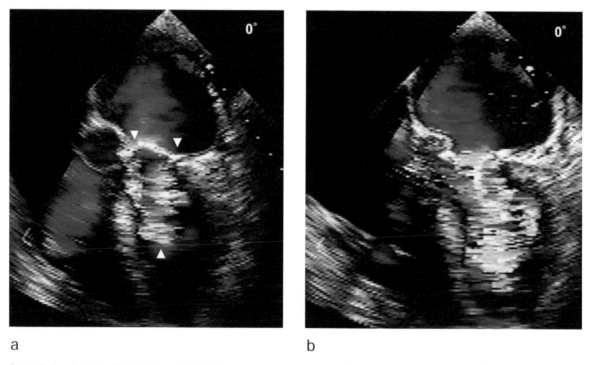

a   b

Case 7.6   Doppler illustration of SAM following mitral r epair. (a) End-systolic frame obtained fr om the lower esophageal window at 0°. Note the tilt of the mitral annuloplasty ring (ar rows) in relation to the aor tic valve. This finding co responds to a decr eased aorto-mitral angle. Ther e is high velocity flow demonstrated in the lef ventricular outflow tract by color Dopple . (b) Subsequent diastolic frame demonstrating left ventricular inflo color flow jet di ected anteriorly towar ds the left ventricular outflow tract

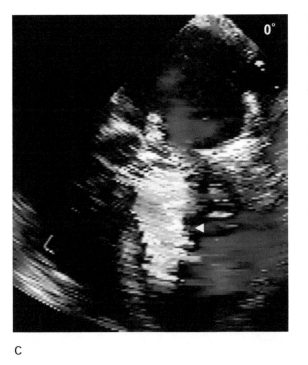

c

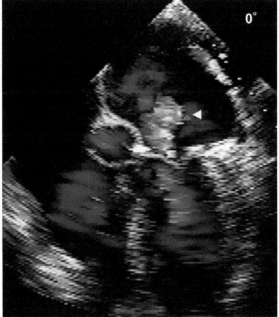

d

e

Case 7.6 (contd.) (c) Early systolic frame demonstrating high velocity flow in the left ventricula outflow tract. (d) End-systolic frame demonstrating mitral regurgitation. (e) A 5 m/sec high-velocity jet recorded with continuous wave Doppler of the left ventricular outflow tract suggesting significant S and failed repair.

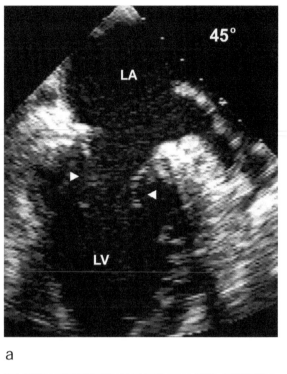

a

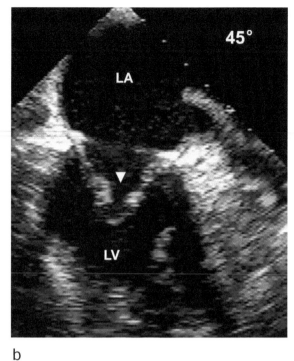

b

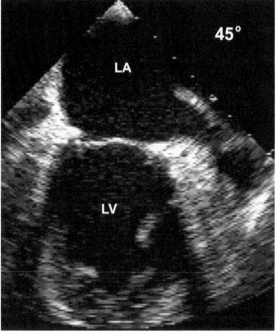

c

Case 7.7 Left ventricular inflow obst uction secondar y to a small mitral annuloplasty ring. (a) Diastolic frame obtained fr om the lower esophageal window at 90° exhibiting restricted anterior mitral valve motion following r epair. Note the annular diameter, which appears significantly smalle or "pinched" in r eference to the left atrium and left ventricle at that level. (b) Thickened anterior and posterior leaflets during mid-diastole. The posterio leaflet exhibits much mor e motion than usual following mitral r epair, which is consistent with excessive remaining tissue. (c) Systolic frame suggesting normal leaflet closu e.

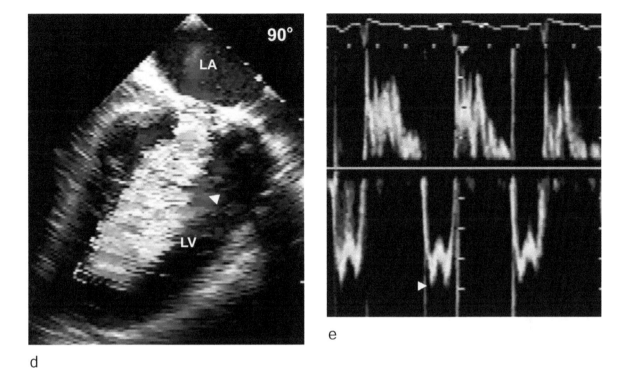

d

e

Case 7.7 (contd.)   (d) Color flow Doppler demonstrating high velocity flow during diastole in the le
ventricular inflow tract. (e) Pulse wave Doppler during diastole. The flow a   oss demonstrates a 1.75 m/sec
flow jet and a 12 mmHg gradient acr   oss the mitral valve.

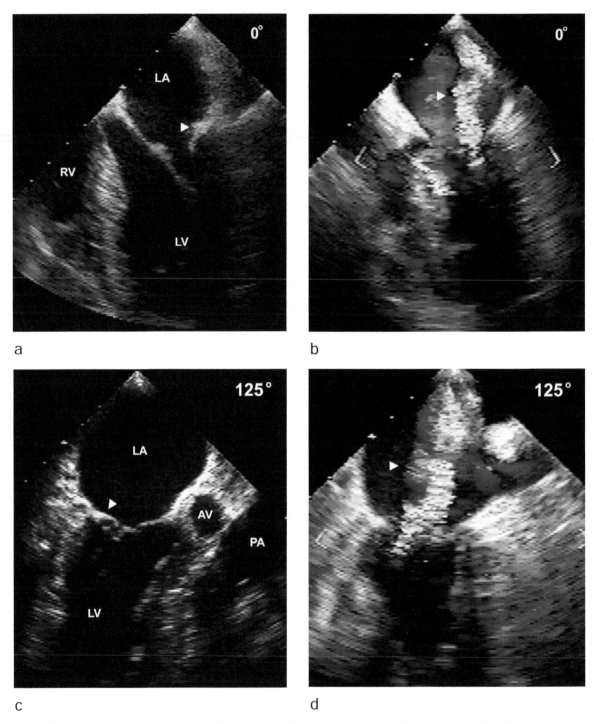

Case 7.8 Failed mitral valve r epair. (a) Mitral r egurgitation secondar y to mitral annular calcification (a row) and prolapse of the posterior leaflet seconda y to excessive leaflet tissue, ecorded from the lower esophageal window at 0° and at 125° (c). (b) Cor responding color flow Doppler image demonstrating a mitral egurgitant jet (arrow) at 0° and 125° (d). Image following r epair involving a triangular r esection of the posterior leaflet withou removal of the mitral annular calcification.

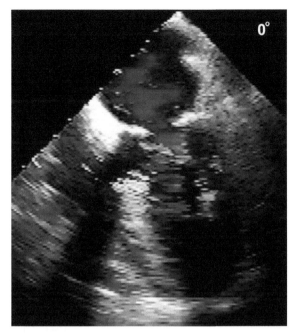

e

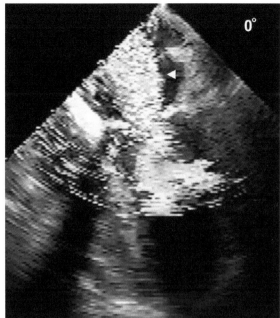

f

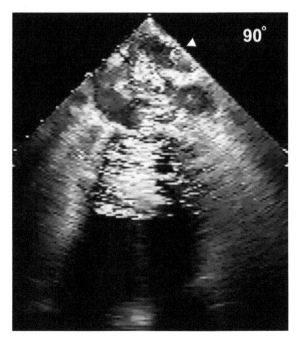

g

Case 7.8 (contd.) (e) The mitral annuloplasty ring is readily apparent and appears small in r elation to the mitral annulus, although color flow Doppler doe not demonstrate significant flow obs uction during diastole. (f) Sever e mitral r egurgitation (arrow) demonstrated in diastole at 0° and with r eversal of flow in the pulmonar y veins at 90° (g). LA, left atrium; LV, left ventricle; R V, right ventricle; A V, aortic valve; PA, pulmonar y artery.

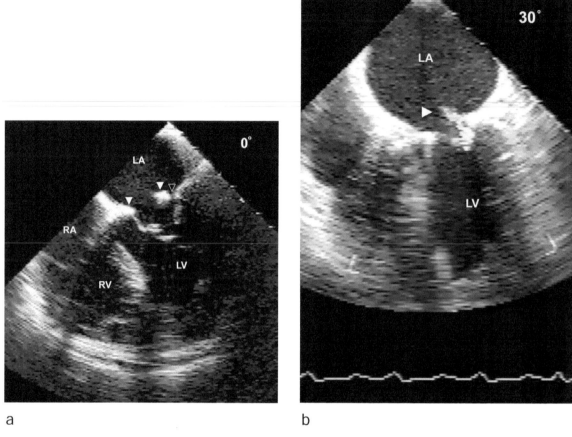

a
b

Case 7.9   Mitral valve repair. Immediately following weaning fr om cardiopulmonar y bypass a fairly lar ge mitral regurgitant jet (a) is suggested with ventricular pacing. With r esumption of sinus r hythm (b) the mitral regurgitant jet is dramatically r educed and represents the tr ue result of the mitral r epair.

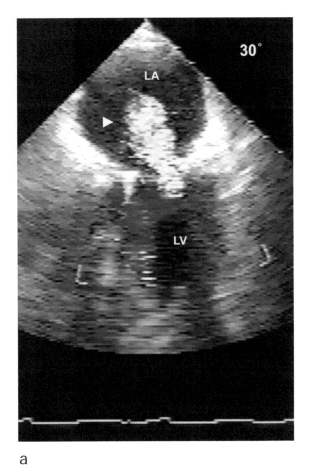

a

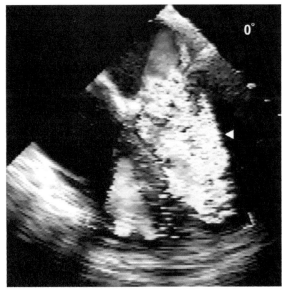

b

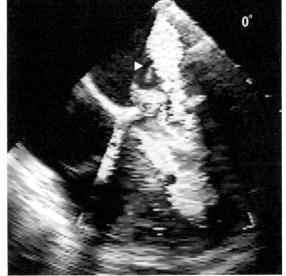

c

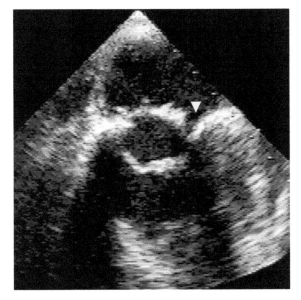

d

Case 7.10 Ring dehiscence post mitral r epair.
(a) Mid-diastolic frame obtained fr om the lower
esophageal window at 0°. Ther e is an echo-fr ee
space between the mitral annuloplasty ring and the
valve annulus. Color flow Doppler during systole (b
and diastole (c) demonstrating abnor mal flow in th
region of the space and a significant mitra
regurgitant jet originating between the mitral
annuloplasty ring and the mitral annulus. (d) With
anteflexion of the pr obe at 75° the annuloplasty ring
is demonstrated again with an echo-fr ee space
suggesting ring dehiscence.

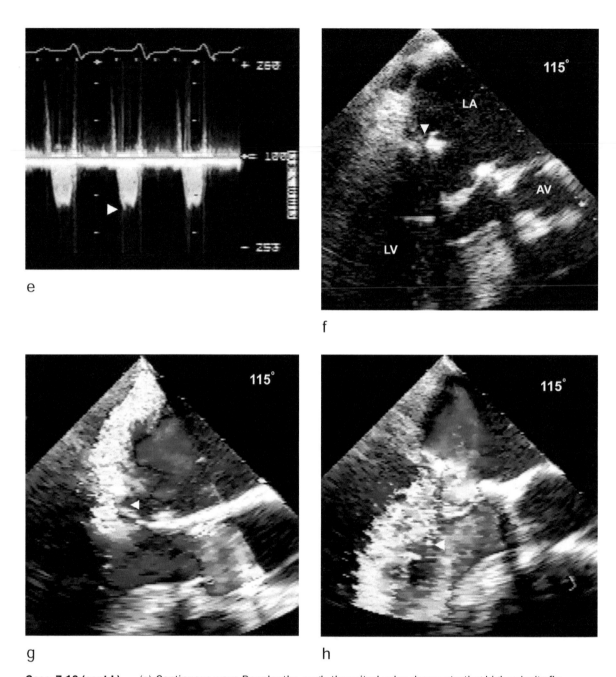

Case 7.10 (contd.) (e) Continuous wave Doppler thr ough the mitral valve demonstrating high velocity flo during diastole in the range of 1.3 m/sec. (f) Echo-fr ee space demonstrated between the annuloplasty ring and the annulus at 115°, with color flow Doppler again demonstrating significant mitral egurgitation (g) and high velocity flow during systole (h). During the second ca diopulmonar y bypass r un, the mitral annuloplasty ring was deter mined to be too small and had separated fr om the annulus. LA, left atrium; L V, left ventricle; RA, right atrium; R V, right ventricle; A V, aor tic valve.

REFERENCES

1. Carpentier A, Deloche A, Dauptain J, et al. A new reconstructive operation for correction of mitral and tricuspid insufficiency. J Thorac Cardiovasc Surg 1971;61:1–13.

2. Carpentier A. Cardiac valve surgery-the "French correction". J Thorac Cardiovasc Surg 1983;86:323–337.

3. Cohn LH. Surgery for mitral regurgitation. JAMA 1988;260:2883.

4. Cooley DA. Technical problems in mitral valve repair and replacement. Ann Thorac Surg 1989;48:S91–2.

5. Lessana A, Carbone C, Romano M, et al. Mitral valve repair: results and the decision-making process in reconstruction. Report of 275 cases. J Thorac Cardiovasc Surg 1990;99:622.

6. Cooper GJ, Wright EM, Smith GH. Mitral valve repair: a valuable procedure with good long-term results even when performed infrequently. Br Heart J 1991;66:156–160.

7. Krause AH, Okies JE, Bigelow JC, et al. Early experience with mitral valve reconstruction for mitral insufficiency. Am J Surg 1991;161:563–566.

8. Loop FD, Cosgrove DM, Stewart WJ. Mitral valve repair for mitral insufficiency. Eur Heart J 1991;12(suppl B):30–33.

9. Cohn LH. Reparative mitral valve surgery. Choices in Cardiology 1992;7:7–9.

10. Odell JA, Hartzell VS, Orszulak TA. Early results of a simplified method of mitral valve annuloplasty. Circulation 1995;92:II-150.

11. Rao V, Christakis GT, Weisel RD, et al. Changing pattern of valve surgery. Circulation 1996; 94:II113–119.

12. Michel PL, Lung B, Blanchard B, et al. Long-term results of mitral valve repair for non-ischaemic mitral regurgitation. Eur Heart J 1991;12(suppl B):39–43.

13. Grossi EA, Galloway AC, LeBoutillier M, et al. Anterior leaflet procedures during mitral valve repair do not adversely influence long-term outcome. J Am Coll Cardiol 1995;25:134–136.

14. Cohn LH, DiSesa VJ, Couper GS, et al. Mitral valve repair for myxomatous degeneration and prolapse of the mitral valve. J Thorac Cardiovasc Surg 1989;98:987–993.

15. Cosgrove DM. Surgery for degenerative mitral valve disease. Sem Thorac Cardiovasc Surg 1989;1:183–193.

16. Loop FD. Long-term results of mitral valve repair. Sem Thorac Cardiovasc Surg 1989;1:203–210.

17. Hendren WG, Nemec JJ, Lytle BW, et al. Mitral valve repair for ischemic mitral insufficiency. Ann Thorac Surg 1991;52:1246–1252.

18. Kay GL, Kay JH, Zubiate P, et al. Mitral valve repair for mitral regurgitation secondary to coronary artery disease. Circulation 1986;74:I–88.

19. Rankin JS, Feneley MP, Hickey M, et al. A clinical comparison of mitral valve repair versus valve replacement in ischemic mitral regurgitation. J Thorac Cardiovasc Surg 1988;95:165–177.

20. Craver JM, Cohen C, Weintraub WS. Case-matched comparison of mitral valve replacement and repair. Ann Thorac Surg 1990;49:964.

21. Yun KL, Miller DC. Mitral valve repair versus replacement. Cardiol Clin 1991;9:315.

22. Cohn LH, Kowalker W, Bhatia S, et al. Comparative morbidity of mitral valve repair versus replacement for mitral regurgitation with and without coronary artery disease. Ann Thorac Surg 1988;45:284.

23. Rankin JS, Livesey SA, Smith LR, et al. Trends in the surgical treatment of ischemic mitral regurgitation: effects of mitral valve repair on hospital mortality. Sem Thorac Cardiovasc Surg 1989;1:149–163.

24. Acar J, Michel PL, Luxereau P, et al. Indications for surgery in mitral regurgitation. Eur Heart J 1991;12(suppl B):52–54.

25. Lessana AL, Romano M, Lutfalla G, et al. Treatment of ruptured or elongated anterior mitral valve chordae by partial transposition of the posterior leaflet: experience with 29 patients. Ann Thorac Surg 1988;45:404.

26. Deloche A, Jebara VA, Relland JY, et al. Valve repair with Carpentier techniques: the second decade. J Thorac Cardiovasc Surg 1990;99:990–1002.

27. Cosgrove DM, Stewart WJ. Current problems in cardiology: mitral valvuloplasty. Curr Probl Cardiol 1989; 14(7):353–416.

28. Antunes MJ, Magalhaes MP, Colsen PR, et al. Valvuloplasty for rheumatic mitral valve disease. A surgical challenge. J Thorac Cardiovasc Surg 1987;94:44–56.

29. Antunes MJ. Mitral valvuloplasty for rheumatic heart disease. Sem Thorac Cardiovasc Surg 1989;1:164.

30. Duran CMG, Gometza B, DeVol EB. Valve repair in rheumatic mitral disease. Circulation 1991; 84:III–125.

31. Frater RWM, Vetter HO, Zussa C, Dahm M. Chordal replacement in mitral valve repair. Circulation 1990;82:IV–125.

32. Kobayashi Y, Seiki N, Ohmori F, et al. Mitral valve dysfunction resulting from thickening and stiffening of artificial mitral valve chordae. Circulation 1996;94:II129–32.

33. David TE, Bos J, Rakowski H. Mitral valve repair by replacement of chordae tendineae with polytetrafluoroethylene sutures. J Thorac Cardiovasc Surg 1991;101:495–501.

34. Chauvaud S, Jebara V, Chachques J-C, et al. Valve extension with glutaraldehyde-preserved autologous pericardium. Results in mitral valve repair. J Thorac Cardiovasc Surg 1991;102:171–178.

35. Hendren WG, Morris AS, Rosenkranz ER, et al. Mitral valve repair for bacterial endocarditis. J Thorac Cardiovasc Surg 1992;103:124–129.

36. Aranki SF, Adams DH, Rizzo RJ, et al. Determinants of early mortality and late survival in mitral valve endocarditis. Circulation 1995;92:II143–49.

37. Pagani FD, Monaghan HL, Deeb GM, Bolling SF. Mitral valve reconstruction for active and healed endocarditis. Circulation 1996;94:II–133.

38. d'Udekem Y, David TE, Feinder CM et al. Long term results of surgery for active infective endocarditis. Euro J Cardiothorac S 1997;11(1):46–52.

39. Asmar BE, Acker M, Couetil JP, et al. Mitral valve repair in the extensively calcified mitral valve annulus. Ann Thorac Surg 1991;52:66–69.

40. David TE, Komeda M, Pollick C, Burns RJ. Mitral valve annuloplasty: the effect of the type on left ventricular function. Ann Thorac Surg 1989;47:524–528.

41. Unger-Graeber B, Lee RT, St. John Sutton M, et al. Doppler echocardiographic comparison of the Carpentier and Duran annuloplasty rings versus no ring after mitral valve repair for mitral regurgitation. Am J Cardiol 1991;67:517–519.

42. Stewart WJ, Salcedo EE, Cosgrove DM. The value of echocardiography in mitral valve repair. Cleveland Clin J Med 1991;58(2):177–183.

43. Deloche A, Jebara VA, Relland JYM, et al. Valve repair with Carpentier techniques. The second decade. J Thorac Cardiovasc Surg 1990; 99:990–1001.

44. Galler M, Kronzon I, Slater J, et al. Long-term follow-up after mitral valve reconstruction: incidence of postoperative left ventricular outflow obstruction. Circulation 1986;74:I99–103.

45. Kronzon I, Cohen ML, Winer HE, Colvin SB. Left ventricular outflow obstruction: a complication of mitral valvuloplasty. J Am Coll Cardiol 1984;4:825–828.

46. Freeman WK, Schaff HV, Khandheria BK, et al. Intraoperative evaluation of mitral valve regurgitation and repair by transesophageal echocardiography: incidence and significance of systolic anterior motion. J Am Coll Cardiol 1992;20:599–609.

47. Kreindel MS, Schiavone WA, Lever HM, Cosgrove D. Systolic anterior motion of the mitral valve after Carpentier ring valvuloplasty for mitral valve prolapse. Am J Cardiol 1986;57:408–412.

48. Assoun B, Diebold B, Abergel E, et al. Morphology-function relationship after mitral valve repair (abstr). Circulation 1992;86(suppl I):I–724.

49. Mihaileanu S, Marino JP, Chauvaud S, et al. Left ventricular outflow obstruction after mitral valve repair (Carpentier's Technique): Proposed mechanisms of disease. Circulation 1988;78(suppl I):I–78–84.

8

Mitral Valve Prostheses

Types of prosthetic heart valves • Prosthetic valve endocarditis • Prosthetic valve thrombosis

The prosthetic heart valve has played a large role in clinical cardiology over the past thirty years. In many instances prosthetic heart valve replacement represents the last stage of the natural history for cardiac valvular heart disease, and has dramatically improved the lives of many patients. Unfortunately, prosthetic valves are far from perfect, have a limited lifespan and may introduce a different set of problems for the cardiac patient, by substituting one disease process for another.

The ideal artificial heart valve should permit the unimpeded flow of blood from cardiac chamber to chamber, restore near normal hemodynamics, and offer the best chance for regression or remodeling from the effects of the primary valvular disease. In addition, the ideal prosthetic valve should be durable and non-thrombogenic. Since the 1950s many prosthetic valves have been introduced in order to overcome the inadequacies of previous models.[1,2] Flaws in performance or in structural integrity have eliminated many valve designs and new models have been introduced that include refinements to some previously successful valves.[3] Trends in surgical management have also moved from routine replacement to valve repair. Prosthetic heart valves require routine evaluation of the physiological function and detection of structural malfunction.

In the past, the non-invasive evaluation of prosthetic valves has included phonocardiography, cinefluoroscopy, and ultrasound. Transthoracic echocardiography has been the routine evaluation of prosthetic heart valves, despite the limitations due to their non-biological components.[4–6] Multiplane transesophageal echocardiography, with its improved resolution and ability to provide multiple imaging planes, has greatly enhanced the evaluation of prosthetic heart valves.[7–10] However the transesophageal echocardiographic evaluation of prosthetic valves is often a challenging task. In most instances transesophageal echocardiography is performed when the transthoracic study is inconclusive and/or malfunction of the prosthesis is suspected. An accurate diagnosis is important because prosthetic valve malfunction can be catastrophic, and re-operation has a significantly higher mortality and morbidity than the initial valve surgery.

To simplify the transesophageal echocardiographic examination it is helpful for the echocardiographer to have a working knowledge of the different prosthetic valve types and their echocardiographic appearances. Prior to performing the transesophageal examination it is important to know the type of prosthetic valve, date of implant, model number (if available) and anticoagulation status.[11] Most prosthetic valves have specific echocardiographic and structural characteristics. In our experience, due to the inherent problems unique to individual types and models of each prosthetic valve, the length of the transesophageal echocardiographic examination is dramatically shortened and the interpretation process is simplified when all of this information is available prior to performing the study.

TYPES OF PROSTHETIC HEAR T VALVES

There are two basic categories of prosthetic valve design. Mechanical prosthetic valves have been engineered to promote structural integrity over long periods. Bioprosthetic valves have been made to simulate native-valve hemodynamics which promote less thrombogenicity.

Mechanical prostheses

Mechanical prosthetic heart valves may be classified by their supporting structure (strut or cage) and type of occluder mechanism (Table 8.1). Mechanical valves comprise the central occluder ball-cage valve, central occluder disk-cage valve, eccentric tilting-monocuspid disk valve, and tilting bileaflet disk valve.

Due to their structural composition, mechanical prosthetic valves inherently produce obstruction and turbulent blood flow. The first mechanical valves were constructed with a cage mounted in a sewing ring with a ball-shaped poppet. In the mitral position the cage is oriented such that it protruded into the valvular outflow tract (Figure 8.1). When the valve was in the open position with the ball at the top of the cage, turbulence occurred. Since the metallic cage had to be mounted in a stiff sewing ring for support, the result was a somewhat bulky valve with a small effective orifice area relative to the ring circumference. In addition, mechanical valves are thrombogenic due to turbulence associated with their non-biological components. Advances and modifications in mechanical valve technology have largely sought to address problems of thrombogenicity and valve obstruction (Figure 8.2). Increased valve orifice

Table 8.1 Mechanical prosthetic valves
Central ball occluder
Starr-Edwards
Smelof f-Cutter (Smelof f-Sutter)
Braunwald-Cutter
Magover n-Cromie
Harken
DeBakey-Sur gitool
Hufnagel
Central disk occluder
Beall-Sur gitool
Starr-Edwards disk
Cooley-Cutter
Kay-Shiley
Kay-Suzuki
Cross-Jones
Starr-Edwards (models 6500, 6520)
Eccentric monocuspid disk
Bjork-Shiley (standar d, convexo-concave, monostr ut)
Lillehei-Kaster
Kaster-Hall (Medtronic-Hall)
Wada-Cutter
Omniscience I and II
Bileaf et bicuspid disks
St. Jude
Duromedics
Carbomedics
On-X

areas have reduced turbulence and improved materials have increased durability. In addition, efforts have centered on decreasing the profile of the valve by incorporating tilting disks (Figures 8.3 and 8.4) instead of central occluders, and changing from cages to shorter struts and finally to leaflet disks with only hinge supports (Figures 8.5–8.7). In comparison to tissue valves, mechanical valves are extremely durable and enjoy a long life expectancy.

Bioprosthetic valves

The development of tissue or bioprosthetic cardiac valves was an attempt to manufacture a

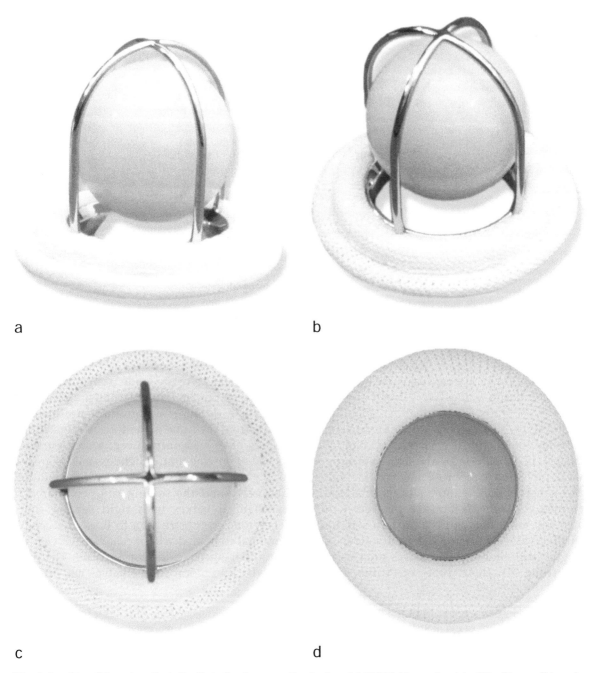

a

b

c

d

Fig. 8.1 Starr-Edwards mitral silastic ball valve pr osthesis (model 6120). The major risk of the Star r-Edwards prosthesis is for thr omboembolic complications, similar to the other cur rently available mechanical valves. There is a r eported low rate of thr ombotic occlusion, mechanical sticking and encasement. The high valve profile and hemodynamic characteristics distinguish the Star r-Edwards valve from the other available mechanical valves. Satisfactor y hemodynamics ar e usually pr oduced with prostheses in the mitral position.

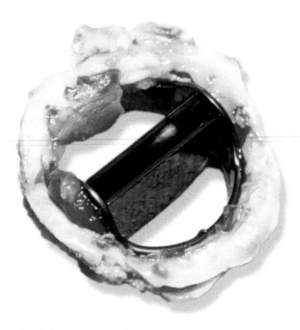

Fig. 8.2 Explanted St. Jude bileaflet valve wit pannus formation and thrombus which interfered with leaflet opening and closu e with protrusion to the orifice of the sewing ring

Table 8.2	Bioprosthetic tissue valves

Heterograft
- Porcine aortic leafle
  Hancock
  Carpentier-Edwards
  St. Jude BioImplant (Liotta)
  Medtronic Intact
  Tascon
  Angell-Shiley
- Bovine pericardium
  Hancock Pericardial
  Carpentier-Edwards Pericardial
  Ionescu-Shiley
  Mitro-flow (Mitral Medical)

Homograft
- Preserved human aortic valve Cryolife
- Dura mater

Autograft
- Fascia lata

Stentless

facsimile of the native cardiac valve (Table 8.2). The first tissue valves were fresh cadaveric aortic homografts. Due to the unavailability of fresh valves, bioprosthetic valves or valves constructed of chemically stabilized biological tissue with metallic or plastic structural support were developed. Bioprosthetic cardiac valves are constructed of human or animal tissue formed as valve leaflets suspended within struts in an orientation typical to a semilunar cardiac valve and mounted in a sewing ring (Figure 8.8). Bioprosthetic valves are classified according to their type of valve tissue.

Heterograft valves are made from animal tissue (bovine or porcine), homografts are composed of human tissue, and autografts are made of tissue from the same patient. Recently, stentless valves have been introduced, which are composed of porcine tissue. Stentless valves are less bulky, and there is some degree of flexibility to the valve and the sewing ring, compared to mechanical valves with rigid sewing rings. Therefore, the obstruction to flow produced is minimal compared with mechanical valves, and thrombogenicity is less of an issue. The main drawback to bioprosthetic valves has been the

Fig. 8.3 Björk-Shiley mitral valve. The Bjö rk-Shiley valve is a low pr ofile, tilting-disk valve and was intr oduced in 1969. Thr ee types of Bjö rk-Shiley valves wer e manufactured: the standar d, spherical disk valve (R/S), and the 60° and 70° degree convexo-concave disk valves (CC). The Bjö rk-Shiley convexo-concave (C/C) valve replaced the R/S valve ar ound 1976 and for the next ten years was one of the most popular pr osthotic valves in the world. The C/C valve was initially manufactur ed with a 60° opening angle. The later model with a 70° opening was never available in the United States. With the 60° C/C disk valve the pivot point was moved 2.5 mm downstr eam to reduce obstr uction by cr eating a lar ger minor orifice and a 12 larger opening angle. The C/C valve, despite impr oved hemodynamics, was plagued with design fatigue of the outlet str ut, due to the unique motion of the convexo-concave disk, r esulting in str ut fracture and hemodynamic catastr ophe due to expulsion of the occluder disk. Repeated modification in the welding technique and later imp oved design of the outlet str ut remedied the pr oblem, but the valve was still r emoved from the market. ▶

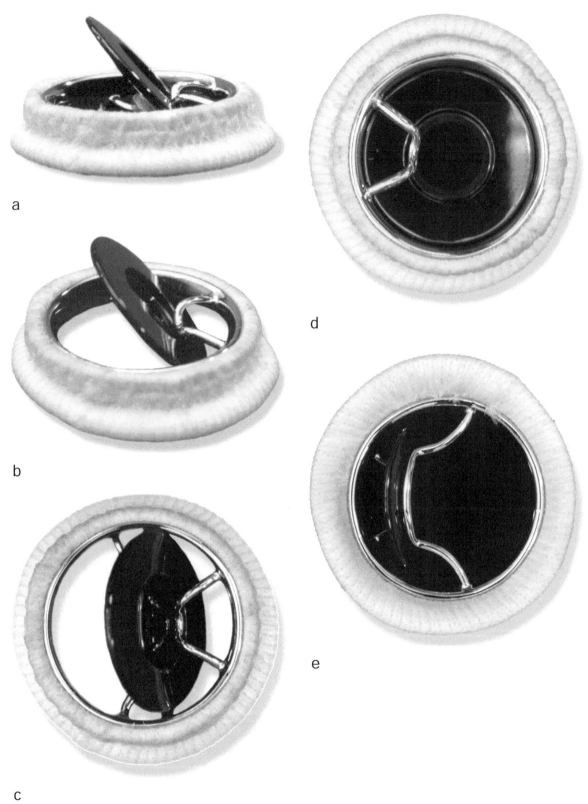

a

b

c

d

e

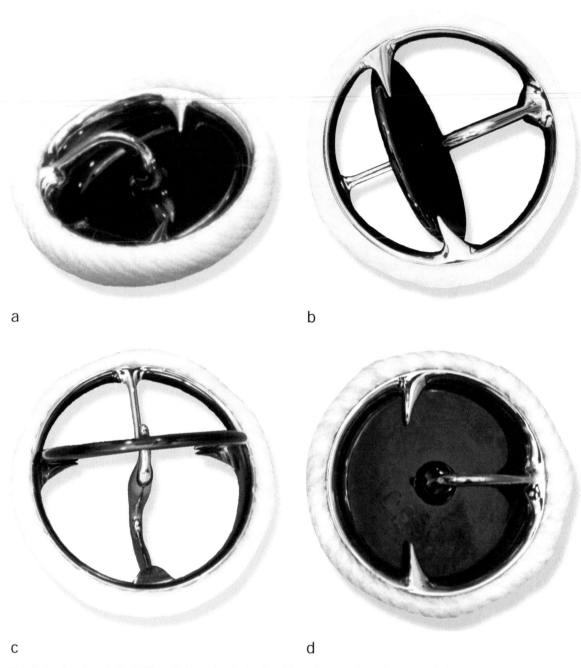

a

b

c

d

Fig. 8.4   Medtronic-Hall tilting disk mechanical valve. The valve consists of a pyr   olytic carbon-covered disk that is suspended in a titanium cage and suppor   ted with an S-shaped central str ut without welds, mounted to a Teflon sewing ring. The disk is guided during opening and closing by a r   od guide str ut projecting through a central disk per foration. The disk opens to a maximum of 75°. The valve can be r   otated to allow for a disk parallel to flow orientation to p   oduce an eccentric flow p   ofile and provide good hemodynamics.

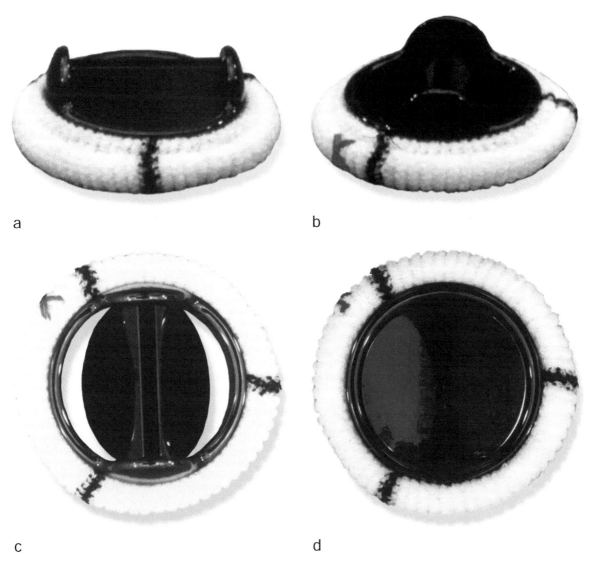

a   b

c   d

Fig. 8.5 St. Jude bileaflet mitral p osthesis. The St. Jude valve was the first comme cially available, low profile bileaflet p osthesis and was intr oduced in 1977. The St. Jude Standar d bileaflet valve comprises pyrolytic carbon-coated graphite frame, two pyr olytic carbon leaflets imp egnated with tungsten to make them radiopaque, and a Dacr on sewing ring. The leaflets open f om an angle of 30° to a maximum of 85° from a central hinge point, which pr ovides two lar ge lateral orifices and one smaller central orifice, with rapid openi which is not position-sensitive.

durability of the tissue used to produce the valves.

Due to the inflammatory response, a form of rejection to the leaflet tissue occurs and bioprosthetic leaflets tend to degenerate and calcify, which may greatly shorten the durability of these valves. The first bioprosthetic tissue valves were made from animal valve leaflets. These were later replaced by animal pericardium which produced better valve flow dynamics and increased strength with less tendency to calcify, degenerate and subsequently tear or rupture. Modifications of the preservation process, with the use of glutaraldehyde fixation of the valve tissue, have served to strengthen the tissue and reduce the degenerative response.[12] This

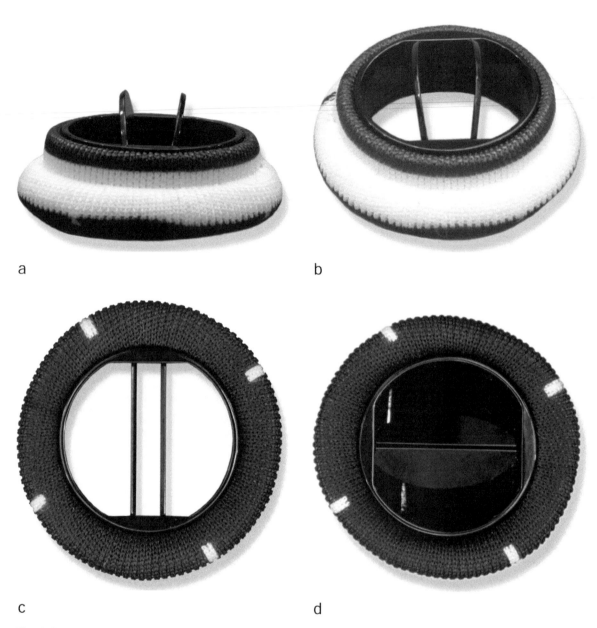

Fig. 8.6 CPHV standard mitral valve. The Carbomedics pr osthetic heart valve is a bileaflet mechanical valve first introduced in 1986 and manufactur ed by Sulzer Carbomedics, Inc. The CPHV standar d series has pyr olytic carbon leaflets designed for an intra-annular position and otatable for optimum orientation. The valve design includes a recessed pivot mechanism, which pr omotes 'washing' of the mechanism as blood flows th ough the valve orifice. The sewing cu f is made of knitted polyester and is contour ed, which aids seating the valve during implantation. A few models have sewing rings coated with Biolite Carbon to r educe pannus gr owth. The Orbis Universal model, as its name implies, incorporates a sewing ring that may be implanted in either the aortic or mitral position.

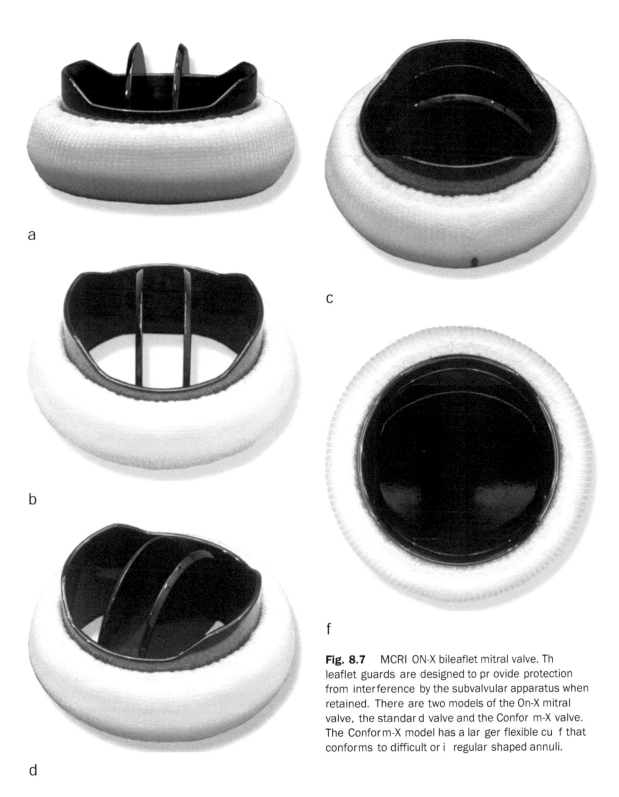

a

b

c

d

f

Fig. 8.7 MCRI ON-X bileaflet mitral valve. Th
leaflet guards are designed to pr ovide protection
from interference by the subvalvular apparatus when
retained. There are two models of the On-X mitral
valve, the standar d valve and the Confor m-X valve.
The Confor m-X model has a lar ger flexible cu f that
conforms to difficult or i regular shaped annuli.

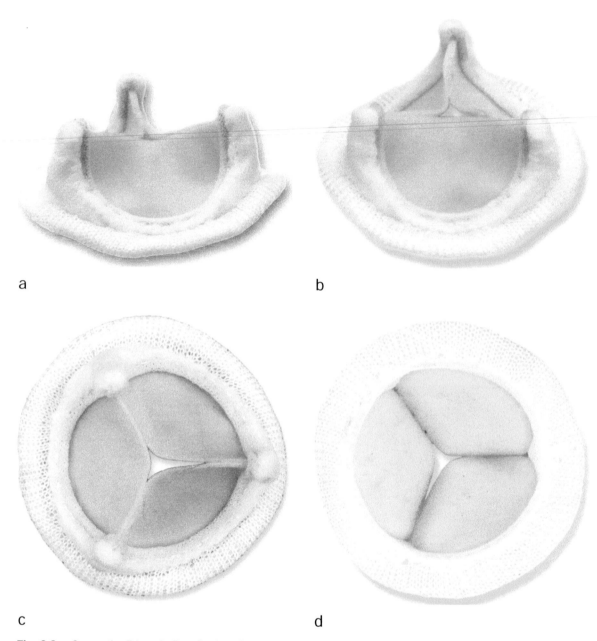

a

b

c

d

Fig. 8.8 Carpentier-Edwards Duraflex Low P essure Porcine Mitral biopr osthesis. The valve is constr ucted with a XenoLogiX tr eatment which is thought to r educe phospholipid content and pr event calcification. Th mitral valve receives a low pr essure fixation to dec ease the str ess of the valve. The mitral model has an extended sewing ring to pr ovide a lar ger sur face area for attaching to the native annulus.

degenerative and calcification process is accelerated in younger patients, limiting the use of bioprosthetic valves in children.

A major problem with porcine valves is the septal shelf or muscular bar that is naturally associated with the right coronary cusp in the pig. When a porcine valve is removed and prepared, the right coronary cusp cannot be removed without a significant portion of septal muscle which, when mounted in a sewing ring, tends to reduce the valve orifice, which impedes blood flow.

Improvements in bioprosthesis technology have addressed the issues of premature degeneration by varying tissue type and fixation methods. Porcine valves have many configurations and sizes closely resembling human valves. The treated valves are nonviable and become stiffer than normal valves. Thrombogenicity is low since flow through the triangular central orifice is less turbulent.[13] In smaller valves, the orifice opening may be asymmetrical at low flow rates, and can produce obstruction to forward flow.[14]

Porcine valves have less regurgitation than mechanical valves, with regurgitation occurring in only approximately 10% of valves.[15–17] Dysfunction is usually associated with progressive leaflet thickening and calcification. As the process progresses, the leaflets become more rigid and tears or progressive stenosis result. Tears most commonly occur in the mitral position due to back-pressure and occur along the site of attachment to the strut.

Echocardiographic examination of prosthetic heart valves

Prosthetic heart valves require serial examinations on a routine basis, due to the inherent problem of valve malfunction that occurs over the lifetime of the valve. Echocardiographic examinations are routinely performed at six-to-twelve-month intervals depending on various clinical variables. In many hospitals, transesophageal echocardiography is routinely performed during the surgical implantation of the prosthetic valve to establish the initial valve function which serves as the baseline for subsequent evaluations. Performing transesophageal echocardiography during surgery has had a major impact on reducing both early valve malfunctions and perioperative mortality and morbidity.[18] Transthoracic evaluations are usually sufficient for routine follow-up examinations, with transesophageal echocardiography performed only when questions arise from the transthoracic imaging. In patients with hemodynamic compromise and suspected prosthetic

Table 8.3	Prosthetic valve malfunction
1.	Pannus formation, fib ous tissue in growth – obstructive
2.	Paravalvular regurgitation
3.	Endocarditis
4.	Poppet variance, abnormal motion or sticking
5.	Disk wear
6.	Sewing ring dehiscence
7.	Valve outflow turbulence, obst uction
8.	Strut fracture
9.	Leaflet tear or rupture
10.	Annulus abnormality, pseudoaneurysm
11.	Thrombogenicity, systemic embolism

valve malfunction, however, transesophageal echocardiography is increasingly the diagnostic method of choice (Table 8.3).[19] In order to adequately describe echocardiographic findings for prosthetic heart valves it is helpful to fully understand and know the specific terminology. Table 8.4 summarizes some of the most common terms used with prosthetic valves.

Transesophageal echocardiographic examinations are frequently requested and may provide vital information in patients with thromboembolic events, suspected endocarditis, or certain prosthetic valves that are nearing the end of their working lives. As a result, 16% of all transesophageal echocardiographic examinations are performed in our laboratory for prosthetic valve evaluations.

Echocardiographic artifacts such as reverberations and shadowing or ghosting are frequently produced by the non-biological components of the prosthesis. These artifacts prevent the visualization of anatomic structures and prosthetic valve components and frequently attenuate color and conventional Doppler flows that lie posterior to or behind the valve in the far field of the image sector. The depth of these structures in the imaging sector, and the

---

Table 8.4 Prosthetic valve def nitions

Ball swelling – enlar gement of the occluder ball (silicon r ubber) due to absorption of materials, i.e. lipids etc.

Cloth wear – disintegration of the cloth material used to cover the sewing ring and/or str uts due to wear and tear.

Disk embolization – dislodgment of the occluder device fr om the valve suppor ting apparatus due to mechanical failure, usually lethal.

Disk notching – defor mity of the occluder disk due to wear and tear .

Effective valve orifice – the t ue orifice a ea of the valve. Due to the geometr y of the pr osthetic valve and leaflets that ar e inside the sewing ring the tr ue valve opening is smaller than the inter nal diameter of the sewing ring.

Fatigue failure – mechanical failur e due to wear and tear over time.

Flange – metallic ring which r etains the occluder disk or ball.

Occluder – portion of the mechanical valve that simulates the valve leaflet

Pannus formation – migration of excessive fib ous tissue to the pr osthetic valve str uctures from the native annulus as par t of the nor mal endothelialization pr ocess.

Paravalvular regurgitation – regurgitation occurring in between the valve sewing ring and the native valve annulus, due to par tial or complete dehiscence.

Physiological regurgitation – backflow leakage due to the eversal of blood flow pushed backwa ds as the leaflets close, or nor mal leak when the valve is closed due to the mechanics of the valve.

Primary tissue failur e – leaflet calcification or olapse in a biopr osthesis secondar y to tissue degeneration resulting from inflammation, infection or tissue ejection.

Primary valve orifice – inte nal diameter of the sewing ring.

Ring abscess – spr ead of infection in between the sewing ring and the native annulus to the soft tissues of the fib ous skeleton and contiguous car diac str uctures.

Ring or valve dehiscence – displacement or excessive motion of the pr osthetic sewing ring in r elation to the native annulus due to br oken sutures or abscess, etc.

Stent – mechanical suppor ting str ucture for the tissue leaflets in a biop osthesis.

Stent creep – the inward migration of the stents towar ds the valve opening of a pr osthetic valve due to tension on the stents pr oduced by thickened and/or r estricted leaflets

Strut – occluder suppor ting structures projecting from the ring str ucture.

Strut fracture – mechanical separation of the str ut from the valve ring due to material fatigue or a br oken weld.

Transvalvular regurgitation – pathological r egurgitation through the valve leaflets as a esult of valve malfunction.

Valve profile – height of valve fr om the sewing ring to the top of the valve.

Variance – abnormal occluder motion pr oduced by defor mity of the occluder due to wear and tear .

---

position of the prosthetic valve between the posterior structures of the heart and the transducer, also limits transthoracic echocardiographic examinations. Spatial distortion, due to the high acoustic impedance of artificial material, affects both transthoracic and transesophageal echocardiography. To some degree these limitations may be overcome with multiplane transesophageal imaging at higher transducer frequencies, with the better echo windows produced in multiple planes. Optimized planes obtained with rotation of the multiplane transducer improve spatial understanding of both morphological and color Doppler findings, thereby producing a more complete examination. One drawback of transesophageal echocardiography is the inability to provide imaging planes with adequate parallel alignment of cardiac blood flow for conventional Doppler analysis in all patients. Doppler examinations may often be better performed with transthoracic imaging. For total echocardiographic analysis of a prosthetic valve in our laboratories, transesophageal and transthoracic imaging are frequently complementary.

The transesophageal echocardiographic evaluation of prosthetic heart valves is similar to a transthoracic evaluation. To assure a complete assessment, the echocardiographer should apply a systematic approach to evaluating the prosthetic valve, as outlined in Table 8.5. When interpreting prosthetic valve echocardiographic studies it is important to know the specific type of valve being visualized including the model number, the size of the valve, the date it was implanted and also the results of previous echocardiographic analyses. The anticoagulation status of the valve is also important, especially if there have been abrupt alterations in the anticoagulation state. Although prosthetic valves are usually easily identifiable on echocardiography, it may be difficult to establish the exact type of prosthesis, other than mechanical versus bioprosthetic, if the type of valve is not known. Each type of prosthetic valve has specific characteristics that require individual attention before excluding a diagnosis of malfunction.

Certain pathologies affect all prosthetic valves, whereas a few structural conditions are more specific to mechanical or bioprosthetic valves. In general, prosthetic valves must be evaluated for obstruction or stenosis, valve regurgitation, endocarditis, and mechanical or structural failure. A complete echocardiographic evaluation often requires two-dimensional and M-mode imaging, together with conventional color flow Doppler, to rule out these pathologies.

Transthoracic echocardiographic examination of prosthetic valves has been adequately described in many echocardiographic textbooks, and the physician performing transesophageal echocardiography should be well versed in these techniques, as the principles are identical in transesophageal studies.[20–23]

The multiplane transesophageal echocardiographic examination should include a full evaluation of the heart and particularly the prosthetic valves. It is important to identify the appropriate window for visualizing the prosthetic valve. Once identified, the valve should be centered in the field of view and the transducer should be rotated slowly through a full 180 degrees to allow close inspection of the valve. Rotation of the transducer invariably provides an imaging plane that is perpendicular to leaflet motion, allowing direct visualization of the leaflet opening and closing within the sewing ring. The depth of field of the

---

Table 8.5　Evaluation of prosthetic valves

1. Two-dimensional evaluation of valve structural integrity

2. Opening and closing ability

3. Fixation of the sewing ring

4. Measure gradient

5. Evaluate physiological regurgitation, transvalvular regurgitation, or paravalvular regurgitation

6. Individual valve idiosyncrasies

echocardiographic sector should be adjusted to allow full evaluation of the valve, using the zoom feature when necessary. It is frequently helpful to use less gain when visualizing the prosthesis to help reduce echocardiographic artifact, which may be more pronounced with transesophageal echocardiography. After evaluating the valve structure, it is necessary to perform a continuous wave and color Doppler evaluation to correlate abnormal hemodynamics with suspected structural abnormalities.

When visualizing the prosthesis, the appearance of the valve ring should be noted to determine whether the valve is intact and seated properly, orientated normally with the valve annulus. Excessive movement or abnormal rocking of the valve ring demonstrates valvular dehiscence. The location and extent of dehiscence should be noted along with associated abnormal flows detected by color Doppler. In magnified views, suture material or remnants of the native valve may be visible and

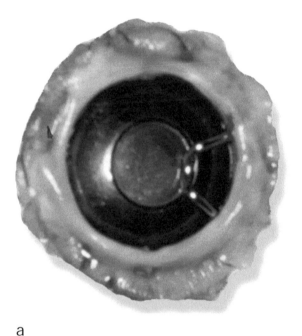

a

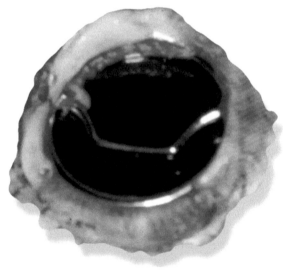

b

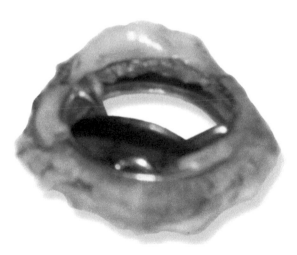

c

Fig. 8.9 Explanted Björk-Shiley valve with pannus formation which covered the sewing ring, encroached on the valve orifice, and interfered with leaflet motion. Sticking occurred on opening, and was visualized with echocardiography by demonstrating the characteristic motion on m-mode.

associated with malfunction. Large thrombi, and vegetations or pannus tissue, which may interfere with occluder (disk, ball or leaflet) motion velocity and valve opening or closing, should be excluded (Figure 8.9). With bioprosthetic valves, excessive chaotic motion or prolapse suggests flail leaflets. Abnormal or chaotic occluder motion may be better demonstrated with m-mode echocardiography when performing a transesophageal examination. In addition to observing the prosthesis it is important to note cardiac chamber dimensions and function, as this may be the source of hemodynamic dysfunction, rather than malfunction of the cardiac prosthesis. With multiplane transesophageal echocardiography, multiple windows permit examination of the cardiac chambers that are obscured by prosthetic valve artifact during transthoracic echocardiographic examinations.

TEE imaging mitral valve prosthesis
Multiplane transesophageal echocardiography is superior to transthoracic echocardiography for the evaluation of the mitral valve prosthesis when malfunction is suspected. For routine evaluations, transthoracic echocardiography may be sufficient as long as there are no abnormalities detected and no clinical suspicion for malfunction.

The mitral valve prosthesis is visualized in long axis from the mid-esophagus in views similar to the standard transthoracic four- and two-chamber apical views, except that with transesophageal echocardiography the prosthetic artifacts are projected towards the left ventricle allowing examination of the left atrium and the atrial surface of the valve. Starting with the transducer at 0° and rotating the transducer through 180°, the mitral prosthesis, especially the sewing ring, may be examined in detail. The mitral valve leaflets or poppets open toward the ventricular apex, allowing rapid identification of the type of valve and assessment of the opening and closing motion. The maximum opening excursion may therefore be directly assessed in this view. The orientation of the sewing ring to the annulus is easily demonstrated throughout its circumference. Excessive motion of the sewing ring is visible, as are gaps between the ring and the native annulus. The sewing ring should appear firmly attached to the native mitral annulus and should not move during the cardiac cycle. Note that when the posterior leaflet of the mitral valve is preserved, the sewing ring appears to have more motion postoperatively than when the mitral prosthesis is sewn directly to the annulus. Paraprosthetic mitral valve leaks due to lack of approximation of the sewing ring to the annulus are commonly visualized with transesophageal echocardiography. Surgical debridement of the annulus (similar to debridement in mitral repair) allows better seating of the sewing ring. Despite these techniques, small mitral prosthesis paravalvular leaks are most frequently seen in the central portion of the posterior annulus, which is the area most prone to distortion (see Chapter 2). Many newer valves are being developed with deformable sewing rings to address this issue. The mid-esophageal long axis views of the mitral prosthesis enable optimal visualization of masses that may be present with normal prostheses or with prosthetic malfunction, such as thrombi or vegetations attached to the prosthetic valve components, or clots in the left atrium and the left atrial appendage.

Color and conventional Doppler is performed in these views since parallel alignment to the antegrade and retrograde flow through the valve is easily obtained. Color flow Doppler determines the direction and orientation of normal and abnormal flows to assist in directing pulsed and continuous lines of interrogation for determining maximum velocities, for peak and mean gradients, deceleration and pressure half-time measurements, and effective valve orifice areas. Posterior orientation of the transesophageal probe ensures that regurgitant jets are rarely missed. Continuous wave Doppler may also be used in the continuity formula or PISA method for determining valve areas and valve obstruction.

The mitral prosthesis is also visualized in the short axis view at 0° and in longitudinal views at 90° from the gastric windows, similar to the transthoracic parasternal long and short axis views. The short axis views at 0–15° are ideal for evaluating mitral bioprostheses, but not satisfactory for evaluating mechanical prostheses. As with the mid-esophageal views, the mitral prosthesis type, leaflet or poppet motion, sewing ring stability, and approximation to the annulus may be assessed. Thrombi, vegetation and prosthetic valve material degeneration are often demonstrated in these views. Excessive bioprosthesis leaflet motion, suggesting torn or flail leaflet segments as well as limited amplitude excursion, may be recognized in the longitudinal views. Color Doppler should be performed in longitudinal views for determining regurgitant flow jet and vena contracta width.

The deep transgastric view from 10° to 30° provides the optimal images, free of prosthetic valve artifacts, for evaluating the ventricular surface of a mitral valve prosthesis.

Doppler interrogation: gradients and prosthetic stenosis

The assessment of blood flow through a prosthetic valve can be measured with transesophageal echocardiography with pulsed wave and continuous wave Doppler techniques with similar accuracy to transthoracic imaging, provided that imaging planes parallel to the prosthetic valve flows are obtained.[24–29] All prosthetic valves are inherently obstructive since their effective valve orifice area is less than the normal native valve area. It is important to take into consideration the specific flow profile through a given prosthesis, and not to assume that Doppler interrogation should be directly perpendicular to the valve plane as suggested by the sewing ring. Alignment of the Doppler beam may be aided by observing the direction and orientation of the color flow jet.[30–33]

Using the peak instantaneous transvalvular flow velocities obtained with continuous wave Doppler, the peak and mean pressure gradients may be determined using the modified Bernoulli equation ($p = 4v^2$).[34] Excellent correlation has been obtained between gradients obtained by Doppler methods and catheterization pressure measurements of prosthetic valves, despite the possibility that the assumptions made by the Bernoulli formula may not have been fully validated for artificial valves.[35–38] Various reports[17,39–57] have defined the normal gradients obtained with individual cardiac prosthetic valves in relation to the position and size of the valve as obtained with echocardiography, cardiac catheterization and *in vitro* testing, as summarized in the Appendix.

As with normal native cardiac valves, Doppler peak instantaneous gradients across prosthetic valves may demonstrate higher velocities than are obtained by measuring peak-to-peak pressure gradients at catheterization. Mean gradients obtained with both methods should therefore be compared. In any given prosthesis, high velocities may be recorded initially as the valve opens, which may give the erroneous impression of prosthetic valve obstruction.[58,59] Since higher velocities may be temporally related to forward blood flow due to valve dynamics, the mean gradient measurement is the most reliable gradient measurement in clinical practice.

Artificially high peak gradients may be obtained due to the effect of pressure recovery related to the geometry of the prosthetic valve.[60,61] This phenomenon is principally noted with high flow velocities recorded from the central orifice of bi-leaflet mechanical valves in the aortic position, but can occur with any prosthesis. It is noteworthy that these velocities are recorded on the initial post-implant echocardiogram and remain unchanged on subsequent follow-up echocardiographic studies. In such patients, transesophageal echocardiography demonstrates normal valve structure and mechanics despite the high mean and peak transvalve gradients. However, it is important to recognize increasing gradients on serial studies, since this finding is usually related to valve stenosis and not to pressure recovery. Baumgartner and colleagues have shown that in patients who show high-localized Doppler gradients due to the pressure-recovery phenomenon, if the valve truly becomes pathologically stenotic, the high-pressure gradients tend to disappear,[62] emphasizing the importance of routine serial echocardiographic follow-up.

In addition to prosthetic valve gradients, Doppler sampling using the continuity principle or the vena contracta jet method provides an accurate assessment of effective orifice area for the prosthetic valve. Using the continuity principle, blood flow is calculated in one area of the heart and compared to the flow through the prosthetic valve, similar to quantification of native valve orifice areas. The continuity principle is valid provided that there is no significant regurgitation of the corresponding valve used for calculation of the forward flow. The pressure half-time method for measuring prosthetic valve obstruction has not been as successful as the continuity principle and therefore should not be routinely used for comparison with catheterization methods. However, the pressure-half-time method is valid for serial measurements in the same patient over time for the assessment of prosthetic valve obstruction.[30,33,62–65]

Doppler interrogation: physiological, transvalvular and paravalvular regurgitation

Due to the intrinsic design characteristics of prosthetic valves it is common to detect small regurgitant jets with transesophageal echocardiography.[66–75] This regurgitation is similar to that seen in native valves and known as physiological regurgitation. Physiological regurgitation is most prominent with mechanical valves and is produced by the backward motion of the occluder device or leaflet. Additionally when the valve is closed, there are small gaps that remain between the occluder or leaflets and the

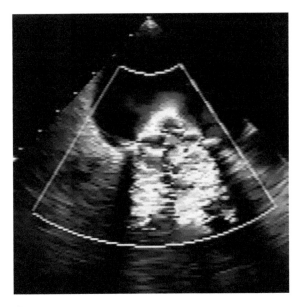

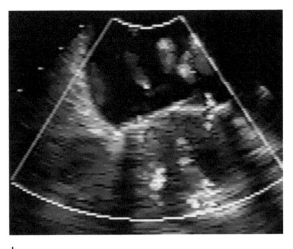

a   b

Fig. 8.10 Normal color-flow Doppler with a St. Jude bileaflet   osthesis. (a) Flow thr ough the bileaflet valv usually occurs thr ough three orifices c eated by the valve leaflet a rangement of two major orifices and on minor central orifice, and is exhibited by th   ee areas of flow conve gence on the opening sur face of the valve ring. (b) Transesophageal echocardiography provides an excellent assessment of the r   egurgitant jets to determine normal versus abnor mal flows. Typically no mal regurgitation of the St. Jude pr osthesis consists of three small jets, two fr om the lateral por tions of the leaflets and the sewing ring and one central je representing a small amount of r egurgitation during the valve' s closing phase, as demonstrated by systolic flow reversal on conventional Doppler . Color flow Doppler   eadily demonstrates abnor mal regurgitation associated with bileaflet mechanical valves. Characteristics of abno   mal transvalvular or paravalvular leaks in the mitral position ar e regurgitant jets that ar e asymmetric and cr oss the valve midline, jets of long duration (pansystolic), or jets that exhibit a mosaic or turbulent flow patte   n often along the atrial wall.

sewing rings which allow the backward flow of small amounts of blood. As each valve has an inherent forward flow dynamic velocity profile, each also has a specific profile for physiological regurgitation (Figure 8.10). The amount of regurgitant flow is usually small, depending on the specific prosthetic valve type, and may only be present during part of the cardiac cycle. Color flow Doppler imaging demonstrates that the physiological regurgitant jet appears confluent in color without significant variance, resembling a 'flame-like' jet that flickers in and out of view.

The size of the color flow jet with physiological prosthetic regurgitation is often larger than in physiological regurgitation of a native valve. An important observation is that physiological regurgitant jets usually remain the same size and appearance on serial echocardiographic studies. Physiological regurgitation with mitral prostheses yields regurgitant jet areas of less than 2 cm^2 and jet lengths of less than 2.5 cm. In the aortic prosthesis, physiological jet areas are less than 1 cm^2 and jet lengths are less than 1.5 cm.[67] Bioprosthetic valves leak less frequently than mechanical valves. Physiological regurgitation jets seen with bioprostheses are usually small and do not usually occur over the entire duration of valve closure. One of the quality control issues for pericardial bioprostheses is the *in vitro* testing and recognition of valvular regurgitation for each valve during the manufacturing process.

Pathological prosthetic regurgitation results from valve malfunction, and may occur primarily as leakage through the valve (transvalvular regurgitation) due to leaflet or occluder damage, or as a result of paravalvular regurgitation due to blood flow between the valve-sewing ring and the native valve annulus. Pathological valvular regurgitation may be underestimated and falsely labeled as physiological or mild, due to attenuation of the conventional or color Doppler signal by the prosthetic valve. Transesophageal echocardiography is extremely helpful for assessing true regurgitation either through or around the prosthesis. Color flow Doppler usually demonstrates a significant regurgitant jet with marked flow variance, producing a mosaic color display.

The echocardiographic techniques for identifying transvalvular regurgitation are identical to those for native valvular regurgitation. Transvalvular prosthetic regurgitation may appear similar to physiological regurgitation, but the transvalvular regurgitant jet is usually larger, and is associated with hemodynamic abnormalities that are readily demonstrated during the echocardiographic study. Pathological transvalvular regurgitation is usually associated with prosthetic valve malfunction, especially with mechanical-type prostheses. In distinguishing pathological from physiological transvalvular regurgitation, it is vital to use conventional as well as color flow Doppler, as the timing of regurgitant flow signals may be better described with pulsed or continuous wave techniques. Once the exact origin of the regurgitant flow jet is identified with color flow Doppler, conventional Doppler may assist in determining the severity of regurgitation. Color flow Doppler enables the jet area to be determined for mitral prostheses, provided that the jet is not eccentric and impinging on the atrial surface: areas less than 4 cm^2 are consistent with mild regurgitation; areas of 4–8 cm^2 are consistent with moderate regurgitation; and areas greater than 8 cm^2 signify severe regurgitation.

Continuous wave Doppler with a higher signal-to-noise ratio may be more accurate for detecting abnormal flows by identifying weaker flow signals. Pulsed Doppler is limited by the Nyquist limit, since many prosthetic valves intrinsically produce flow with higher signals then can be accurately recorded with this technique. If the flows are accurately detected with pulse Doppler, this technique may be most helpful in determining the timing of the abnormal flow, which helps in determining the severity of regurgitation.

Structural failure of a bioprosthetic valve due to deterioration of the valve leaflets most commonly produces transvalvular regurgitation.[75–78] Degeneration of the valve leaflets results in thickened and stiff leaflets that can produce ruptures or tears in the leaflet surface due to the wear and tear of motion during the cardiac cycle. Leaflet rupture may produce prolapse of the leaflet with significant regurgitation. In addition to leaflet rupture, the leaflet may tear completely away from the strut or sewing ring producing a flail leaflet with acute severe regurgitation. With severely abnormal leaflet deformities, banding of the Doppler spectral display has been noted as a result of the high-velocity fluttering of the flail leaflet segment.

Transesophageal echocardiography is pivotal for distinguishing transvalvular regurgitation from paraprosthetic regurgitation, especially for prostheses in the mitral position. In paraprosthetic regurgitation, the actual defect producing the leak is frequently visualized with careful observation during rotation of the transducer from 0° to 180°. The addition of color Doppler allows flow to be readily visualized emanating from the defect directed toward the left atrium. In patients with large paraprosthetic leaks, color flow Doppler may demonstrate antegrade and retrograde flow (to-and-fro flow) through the defect. Small paraprosthetic leaks are frequently detected immediately after implant, and have been reported to decrease or disappear over time. Transesophageal echocardiography plays a critical role at the time of surgical valve replacement, defining severe paraprosthetic leaks and allowing the surgeon to correct them immediately, thus reducing early morbidity and mortality.

The early development of paraprosthetic leaks not present immediately after implant are usually the result of suture and/or annulus failure and must be monitored echocardiographically for acute or progressive worsening. Late-developing paraprosthetic leaks may be the earliest signs of prosthetic valve endocarditis and coexistent annular abscess, which may result in valve dehiscence.[16,79–82] Large regurgitant jets are detected by color flow Doppler, in addition to rocking of the sewing ring during the cardiac cycle adjacent to the defect. Valve dehiscence is usually an ominous sign associated with severe regurgitation, requiring surgical correction and valve re-implantation.

PROSTHETIC VALVE ENDOCARDITIS

Insertion of any foreign material such as a prosthetic valve introduces the risk of infection at the implant site during episodes of bacteremia. The risk of infection decreases once the prosthesis has endothelialized. Mechanical and bioprosthetic valves have a similar incidence for endocarditis. When patients with valvular prostheses develop signs of systemic infection such as fever, it is imperative to rule out prosthetic valve endocarditis.

The hallmark of endocarditis echocardiographically is the detection of valvular vegetations. Traditionally, transthoracic echocardiography has been the technique of choice to visualize vegetations even though the sensitivity in prosthetic valve endocarditis is less than that for native valve endocarditis.[83–87] Echocardiographic artifacts such as reverberations and shadowing from the prosthetic valve frequently obscure vegetations. New abnormalities, such as valve instability, abnormal sewing ring motion, development of paraprosthetic regurgitation, and increased transvalvular gradient with or without abnormal motion of the valve poppet or leaflet, are suggestive of infected prosthetic valve endocarditis. Destruction of bioprosthetic leaflets with worsening hemodynamics may be detected even when vegetations are not visualized. Annular abscess is a known complication of endocarditis and may be the first evidence of infection.

Numerous studies have demonstrated that biplane and multiplane transesophageal echocardiography has a higher sensitivity than transthoracic echocardiography for detecting prosthetic valve endocarditis, and especially for detecting small vegetations.[88–103] When the transthoracic echocardiogram is negative in patients with suspected prosthetic valve endocarditis, transesophageal echocardiography should therefore be recommended. Vegetations appear echocardiographically as small irregular masses attached to some part of the valve structure, and are often indistinguishable from thrombus. Small vegetations may appear as small discrete masses without significant mobility.[89] Larger vegetations usually appear mobile with chaotic motion. Occasionally vegetations impair valve poppet or leaflet motion, and produce obstruction and/or regurgitation.

Spread of infection to the annulus ring results in paravalvular abscess, pseudoaneurysms and fistulas, and is associated with a higher complication rate and a poor clinical outcome.[93–99] Paravalvular abscess usually appears as an echo-free space adjacent to the prosthetic sewing ring, is more common in the aortic position than the mitral, and is equally likely to occur in mechanical and bioprosthetic valves. When a clear space is present within an area of thickening, an abscess is easier to diagnose, and represents rupture of the abscess and communication with the blood pool. An abscess can be missed due to the surrounding echo artifact from the prosthesis, so identification of the abscess requires a meticulous search. Occasionally the diagnosis of abscess can be made by visualizing exaggerated motion of the valve and sewing ring, with new paravalvular regurgitation and partial dehiscence of the prosthesis. The importance of serial follow-up echocardiographic studies with prosthetic valves cannot be overemphasized. We have frequently diagnosed abscesses by recognizing new abnormalities that were not present on previous studies, and valve abscess is an indication for repeat valve replacement.

Transesophageal echocardiography has greatly enhanced our ability to detect paravalvular abscesses. Daniel and colleagues obtained a sensitivity of 87% and specificity of 95% for the diagnosis of abscesses for prosthetic and native valve endocarditis with transesophageal echocardiography.[96] San Roman and colleagues studied only patients with prosthetic valve endocarditis and were able to identify 90% of paravalvular abscesses that were confirmed at the time of surgery.[98] The same group was able to identify 100% of pseudoaneurysms and fistulas with transesophageal echocardiography in the setting of prosthetic valve endocarditis.[98]

PROSTHETIC VALVE THROMBOSIS

Prosthetic heart valve thrombosis is a rare but potentially fatal complication that invariably involves mechanical prostheses.[104–107] Prosthetic valve thrombi range from small thrombi that may slightly interfere with valve function, to thrombi that totally prevent poppet or leaflet motion, leaving the valve partially open or partially closed and resulting in either significant obstruction to antegrade flow or massive regurgitation. Thrombi may occur in the setting of altered or insufficient anticoagulation, or may occur in adequately anticoagulated patients secondary to a structural abnormality associated with mechanical failure of the prosthetic valve components. Clinically, thrombosis should be suspected in any patient with a prosthetic valve who suddenly presents with florid heart failure.

Transthoracic or transesophageal echocardiography can be life-saving in establishing the diagnosis of a thrombosed valve in time to allow appropriate treatment.[104–111] Thrombus should be suspected when there is an increased echodensity within the valve structure and poppet or leaflet motion is either abnormal or undetectable. Doppler examination usually demonstrates an increased transvalvular gradient, indicating partial obstruction or new and significant regurgitation. It is important to realize that when the valve is fixed in the open position, regurgitation may exhibit low velocities so that the severity of regurgitation may be underestimated. Transesophageal echocardiography can demonstrate the presence of a mass or thrombus, the degree of hemodynamic impairment resulting from restricted poppet or leaflet motion, or an occluder fixed either in the open or closed position.[108–111]

Numerous reports have described the diagnosis of prosthetic valve thrombosis with cine-fluoroscopy and transthoracic and transesophageal echocardiographic imaging. Urgent transesophageal imaging is essential for diagnosing prosthetic malfunction in a hemodynamically unstable patient when the findings with cine-fluoroscopy or transthoracic imaging are equivocal. Transesophageal echocardiography has a clear advantage over other techniques in evaluating patients with mitral prosthesis, atrial fibrillation and systemic embolic events.[111] Prosthetic valve thrombi appear as distinct masses attached to the valve components and are visualized throughout the entire cardiac cycle. Pannus formation tends to be associated with the sewing ring, extends to the other valve structure and is more echo-dense than a thrombus. Ultrasound video intensity ratios of the mass as compared to the prosthesis have corroborated these findings. Differentiation of thrombus from pannus may still be difficult, especially since pathological studies have shown that a thrombus may be adherent to pannus formation. Barbetseas and colleagues have reported the clinical and echocardiographic parameters that may help differentiate thrombus from pannus formation in prosthetic valve obstruction.[111] Factors that are associated with thrombus are short duration from time of valve insertion to malfunction, inadequate anticoagulation, shorter duration of

symptoms, and no change in NYHA class from the time of surgery. Thrombi tend to be larger, and extend to the left atrium surface of the valves in the mitral position, and always produce abnormal valve motion, in contrast to pannus formation where abnormal motion is detected in only 60%. In addition, the documentation of a soft mass on transesophageal echocardiography and a history of inadequate anticoagulation is similar to ultrasound video intensity alone in differentiating thrombus from pannus formation.

Recent reports have described the role of transesophageal echocardiography in monitoring thrombolytic therapy in the treatment of thrombosed valves.[112–121]

Case Studies

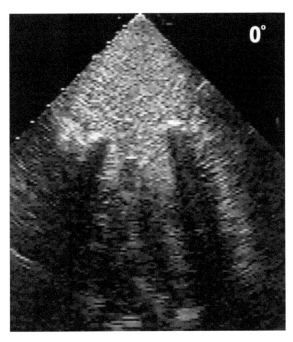

a

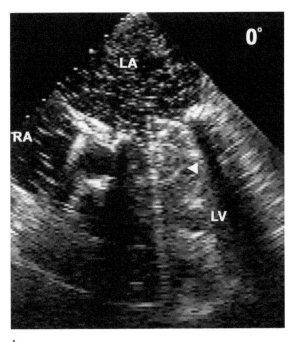

b

Case 8.1 Transesophageal echocardiography plays a major role in determining the success of valve replacement. (a) Four-chamber view from the lower esophageal window immediately after closure of the left atrium and at the start of weaning from bypass. Contrast fills the left atrium demonstrating sluggish flow with the left atrium with the start of valve motion. (b,c) With continuous observation the echocardiographic contrast clears with resumption of cardiac function. The two leaflets of the St. Jude mitral prosthesis can be seen opening and closing during the cardiac cycle.

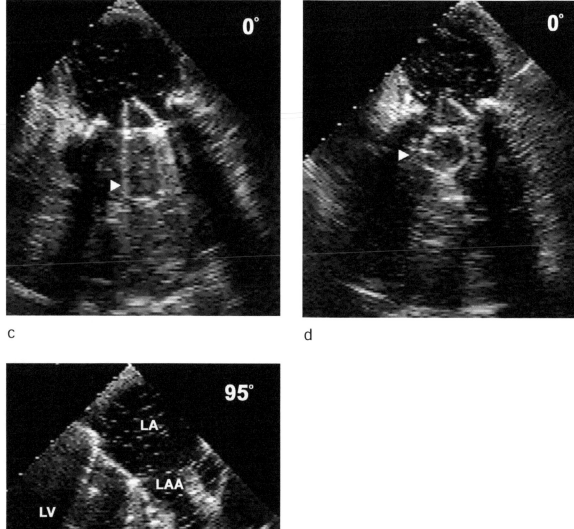

c

d

e

Case 8.1 (contd.) (d) During the weaning pr ocess a left ventricular vent balloon catheter (ar row) is visualized across the mitral pr osthesis which promotes the evacuation of r etained air from the left ventricle and left atrium. (e,f) Two-chamber view demonstrating the St. Jude mitral pr osthesis in a plane 90° to the pr evious views. Only one leaflet i seen opening during the systolic frame (e) and closing during the diastolic frame.

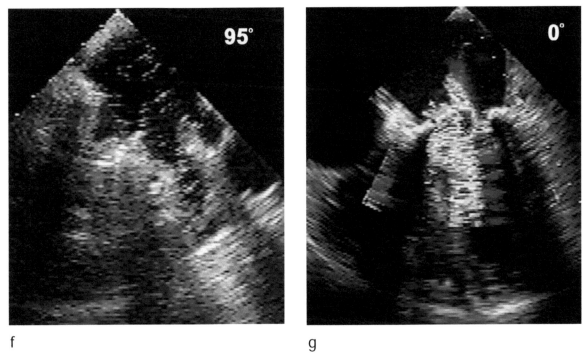

f   g

Case 8.1 (contd.)   (f) secondary to the vent crossing the valve. (g) Color flow Doppler of the four-chambe
view demonstrating diastolic flow acoss the valve before removal of the left ventricular vent catheter. LA, left
atrium; LV, left ventricle; LAA, left atrial appendage; RA, right atrium.

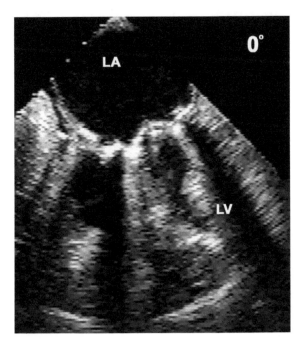

a

Case 8.2   Post-operative evaluation of a St. Jude
bileaflet mitral prosthesis. (a) Four-chamber view
demonstrating the normal leaflet closue
configuration following weaning from bypass. The
valve leaflets, sewing ring and native annulus ae
easily visualized with transesophageal
echocardiography in this view.

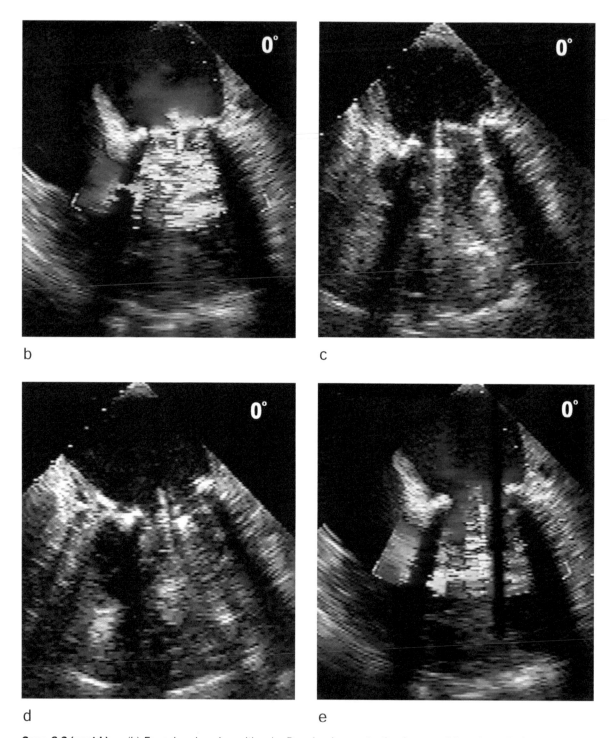

b

c

d

e

Case 8.2 (contd.)   (b) Four-chamber view with color Doppler demonstrating for ward flow th ough the pr osthetic orifices. Forward flow demonstrates a mosaic patte n as flow mixes in the left ventricle. Flow conve   gence is noted on the left atrial side of the valve demonstrating the thr   ee orifices of the bileaflet valve. (c,d) Only o leaflet is opening and closing nor mally with the other leaflet demonstrating delayed motion in   eference to the normally moving leaflet. This is a f   equent finding immediately following weaning which is due to low atria pressur e upon weaning of car diopulmonar y bypass. (e) Color flow Doppler th   ough the mitral pr osthesis with only one leaflet opening demonstrating most of the flow t   ough the side of the nor mally moving leaflet.

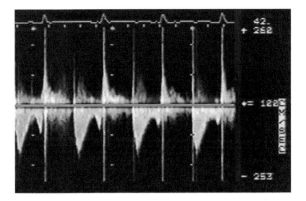

f

Case 8.2 (contd.) (f) Continuous wave Doppler interrogation in the same view. Note the r egurgitant jet with lower-than-expected for ward flow velocit recorded through the valve orifice. LA, left atrium; LV, left ventricle.

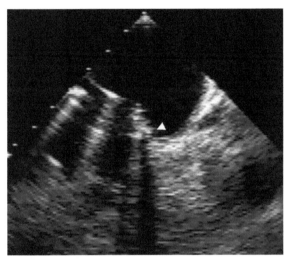

a

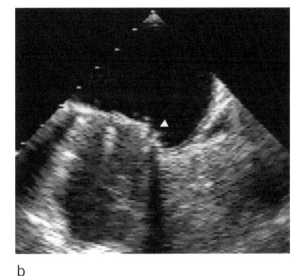

b

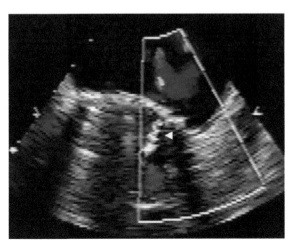

c

Case 8.3 St. Jude peripr osthetic leak. Small periprosthetic leaks between the native annulus and the outer sur face of the pr osthetic valve sewing ring are frequently detected post-operatively. Many of these leaks disappear during the endothelialization process that occurs with the valve ring. In mitral valve replacements periprosthetic leaks fr equently occur in the posterior por tion of the annulus, and this is fr equently associated with the loss of the normal oval orifice caused by annular calcification. distor ted annulus due to calcification may p esent a problem technically in appr oximating the sewing ring and may promote stress and br eakage of the sutur e ring. (a) Nor mal opening of a bileaflet valve. (b Normal closure of the valve. Note the ar ea of separation (dehiscence) between the sewing ring and the native annulus. (c) Color flow Dopple demonstrates the defect as a r eal communication between the left atrium and ventricle.

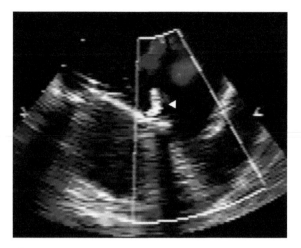

d

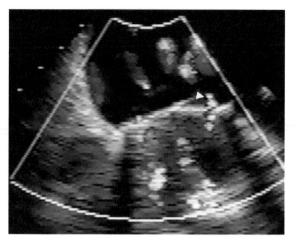

e

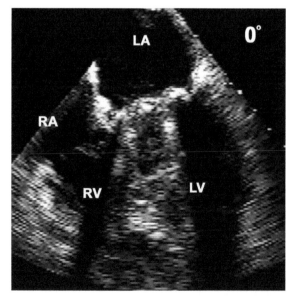

f

Case 8.3 (contd.) (d,e) Color flow Dopple
demonstrating regurgitant flow f om the defect which
is distinct fr om the physiological r egurgitation
expected with a bileaflet valve in two planes 90
apar t. Small color Doppler flow disturbances a e
seen on both leaflet su faces of the bileaflet valv
ring. Note the small transvalvular jets in the left
atrium originating fr om each orifice of the bileafl
valve in distinction to the paravalvular leak.
(f) Continuous wave Doppler thr ough the defect
demonstrating a small paravalvular leak in the firs
and last beats.

a

Case 8.4 St. Jude mitral pr osthesis with pannus
formation and a paravalvular leak. (a) Four-chamber
view demonstrating a St. Jude pr osthesis in the
mitral position.

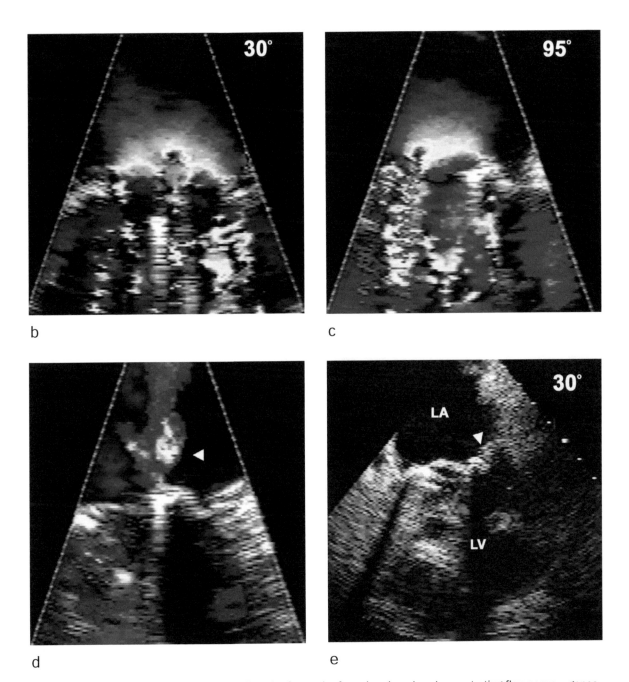

Case 8.4 (contd.) (b) Normal color flow Doppler f om the four-chamber view demonstrating flow conve gence through the thr ee orifices and (c) lateral view at 95 during diastole. (d) Systolic flow in the lateral po tion demonstrating small transvalvular jets. (e) At 30° a small defect (ar row) is noted near the lateral por tion of the sewing ring.

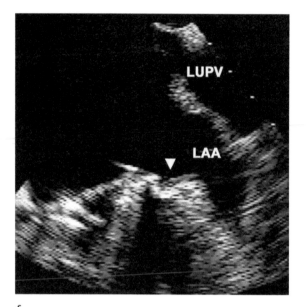

f

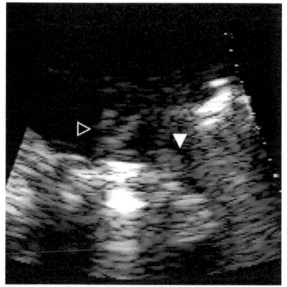

g

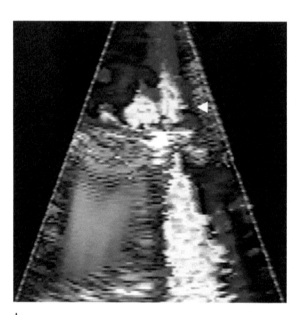

h

Case 8.4 (contd.)   (f) Magnified view demonstratin a defect (ar row) between the sewing ring and the native annulus in the appr oximate area of the atrial appendage. A note of specific ca diac landmarks and the vicinity of the defect will aid the car diac surgeon if repair is contemplated. (g) With fur ther magnification a shaggy hypodense echogenicity is noted around the sewing ring r epresenting pannus formation. Pannus for mation may not be r eadily distinguishable from vegetation with transesophageal echocardiography. (h) Color flow Dopple demonstrates a high velocity for ward flow jet th ough the defect. This jet was r esponsible for the significant hemolysis that initially led to the transesophageal echocardiography evaluation.
LA, left atrium; RA, right atrium; L V, left ventricle; RV, right ventricle; LAA, left atrial appendage; LUPV, left upper pulmonar y vein.

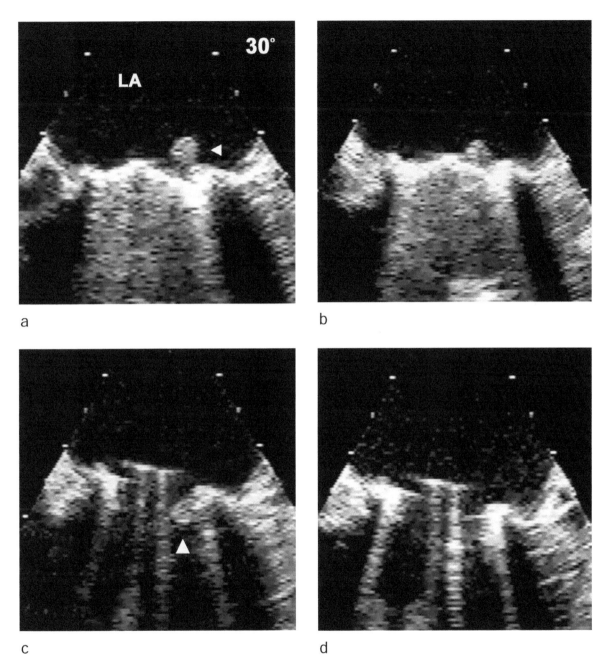

Case 8.5 Bileaflet prosthetic valve vegetation. V egetations tend to demonstrate mor e motion, have a denser echogenicity, and ar e usually better defined than pannus fo mation. These characteristics may be easily identified with transesophageal echocar diography, especially in magnified images. (a–d) A small oval mas (arrow) is demonstrated on the leaflet su face of the bileaflet valve which p olapses back and for th through the valve orifice during the ca diac cycle in a manner consistent with vegetation. This diagnosis was confi   med at the time of sur gery. LA, left atrium.

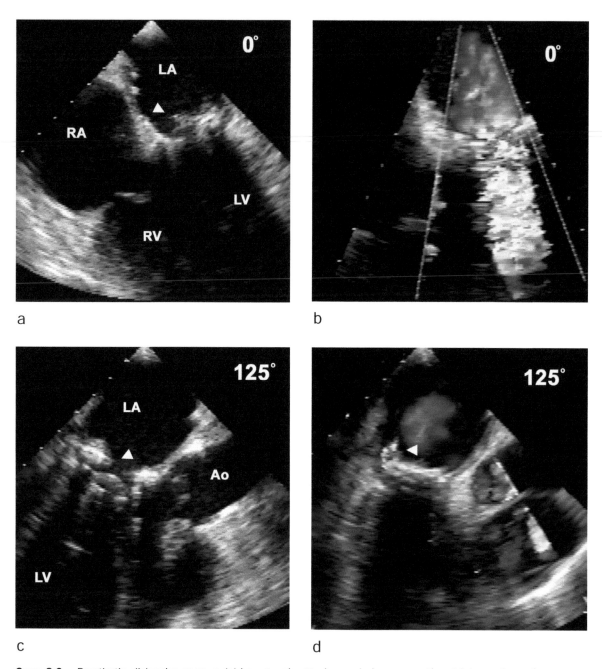

Case 8.6 Prosthetic disk valve pannus. (a) Lar ge, shaggy, hypoechoic mass on the atrial sur face of a bileaflet prosthesis in a four-chamber view at 0° consistent with pannus ingr owth and deterioration of the sewing ring. (b) Color flow Doppler demonstrates a high velocity turbulent jet denoting obst uction of the valve orifice produced by the mass. (c) Two-chamber view demonstrating pannus (ar row) narrowing of the orifice. (d) Color flow Doppler demonstrates a small defect (a row) in the posterior r egion of the annulus consistent with a small paravalvular leak (ar row). LA, left atrium; RA, right atrium; L V, left ventricle; R V, right ventricle; Ao, aorta.

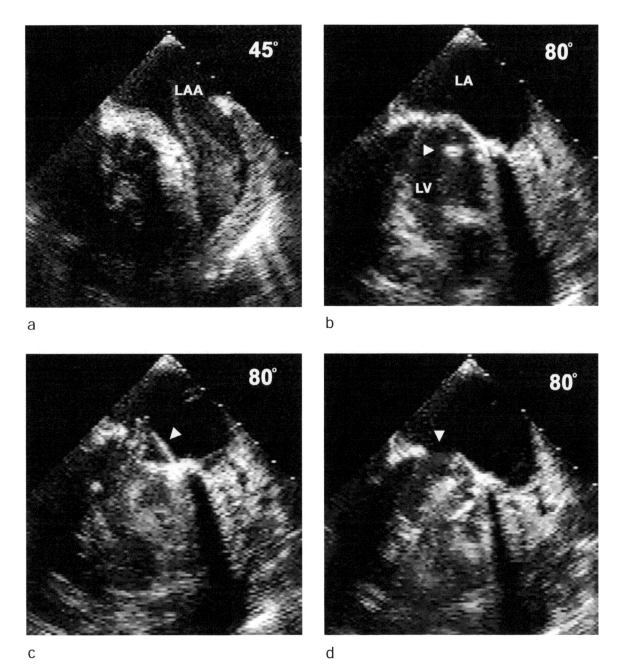

Case 8.7 St. Jude mitral pr osthesis with a fixed leaflet. (a) Spontaneous echoc diographic contrast fillin the left atrial appendage denoting sluggish flow in the atrium. (b) Echogenic mass (a row) noted in the inflo area of the pr osthesis with the valve in the closed position. (c) During diastole only one leaflet (a row) was noted to be opening. (d) The other leaflet (a row) was stuck in the closed position due to inter ference from the subvalvular apparatus.

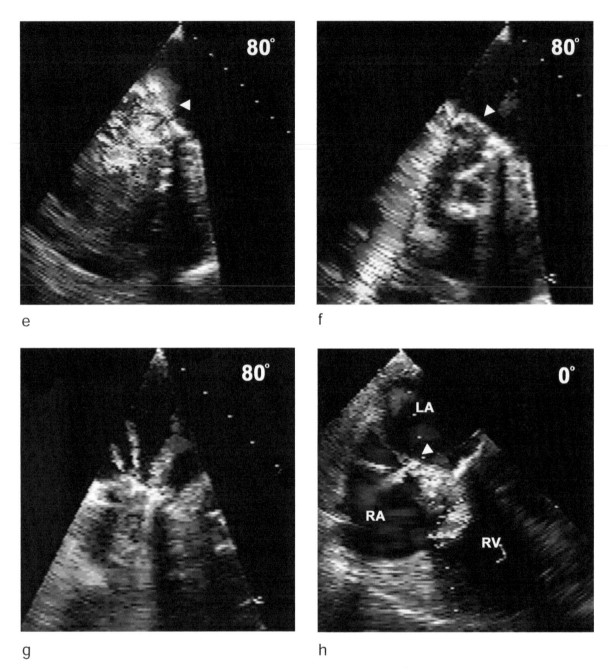

e

f

g

h

Case 8.7 (contd.) (e) Color flow Doppler demonstrating only two a eas of flow conve gent (arrow) on the valve atrial sur face, (f) with absence of flow th ough the fixed leaflet (row). (g) During systole the valve demonstrated two nor mal physiological jets with a wide disturbed jet emanating fr om the fixed leafle suggesting the leaflet was stuck in a semi-closed position. (h) A small continuous left-to-right shunt (a row) was demonstrated through a patent foramen ovale and r elated to the high left atrial pr essur e created from the obstr uction produced from the fixed leaflet. LAA, left atrial appendage; LA, left atrium; V, left ventricle; RA, right atrium; R V, right ventricle.

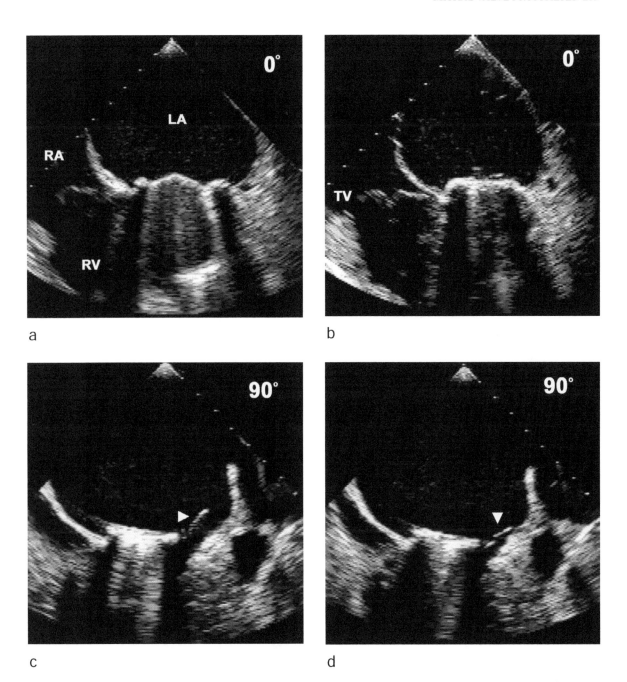

a   b

c   d

Case 8.8 Bileaflet mitral prosthesis with fib ous strands. (a–d) Four-chamber view of a bileaflet mitra
prosthesis during systole. Concentrating on the sewing ring and with r otation of the transducer , multiple small
linear fib ous strands (ar row) exhibiting chaotic motion ar e detected emanating fr om the atrial sur face of the
valve. Fibrous strands may r epresent pannus for mation or loose sutur e material, and need to be dif ferentiated
from vegetation. LA, left atrium; RA, right atrium; R V, right ventricle.

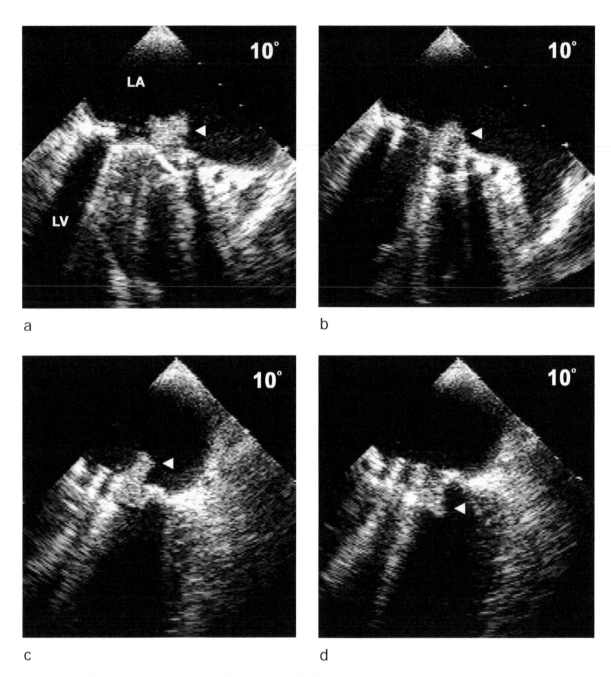

Case 8.9 Bileaflet mitral prosthesis with vegetation. (a) Large echogenic mass (arrow) adherent to the atrial surface of bileaflet valve during systole. (b–d) The mass (arrow) prolapses back and forth through the valve orifice during the cardiac cycle.

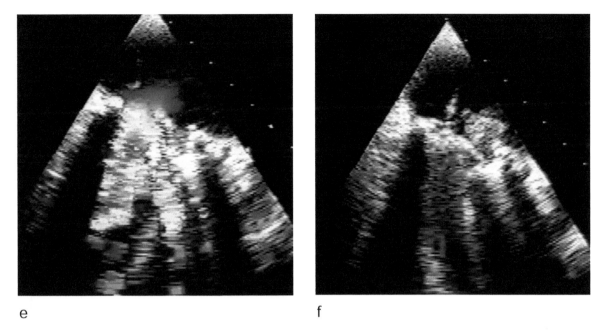

e   f

Case 8.9 (contd.)   (e) Color flow Doppler demonstrates a high velocity turbulent jet during diastole. Note ho
color flow outlines and highlights the mass within the valve orifice. (f) Color flow Doppler during syst
demonstrating a lack of nor mal transvalvular r egurgitation through the valve due to the mass. At the time of
surgery the mass was consistent with a   *Staphylococcus* vegetation. LA, left atrium; L V, left ventricle.

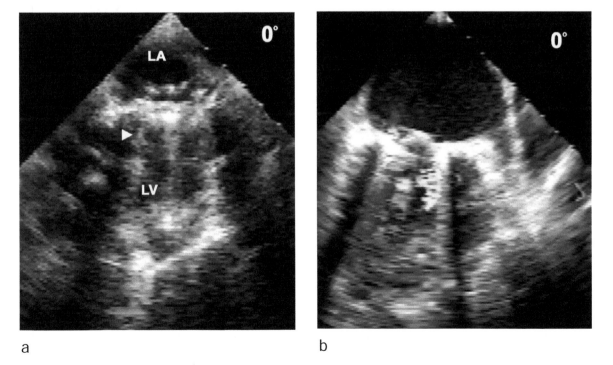

a   b

Case 8.10   Tilting disk valve with obstr ucting mass. (a) Modified four-chamber view p   oduced by retroflexio
of the pr obe at 0° which obliquely visualizes the sewing ring of a Medtr   onic-Hall valve. The nor mal artifact
produced by the occluding disk is distor   ted (arrow). (b) With color flow Doppler an obst   ucting mass is
demonstrated in the minor orifice.

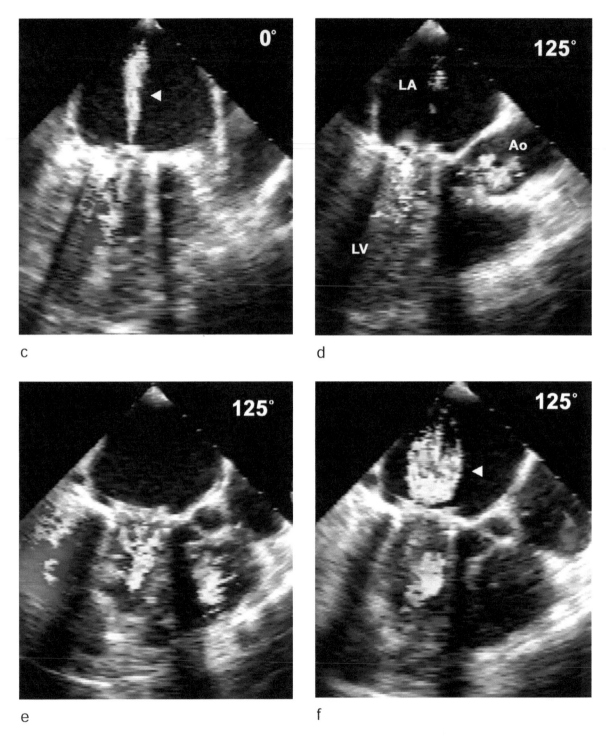

Case 8.10 (contd.)   (c) During systole a typical nar row regurgitant jet is r ecorded through the central hole in the disk. (d,e) A high velocity for ward flow jet is ecorded through the pr osthetic valve. (f) An abnor mal regurgitant jet (ar row) emanates fr om the minor valve orifice demonstrating lack of closu e of the disk due to the mass.

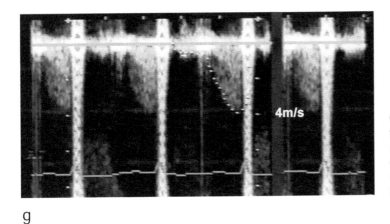

g

Case 8.10 (contd.) (g) Continuous-wave interrogation through the prosthetic valve demonstrates a delayed peaking, high velocity jet at 4 m/sec during diastole. LA, left atrium; LV, left ventricle; Ao, aor ta.

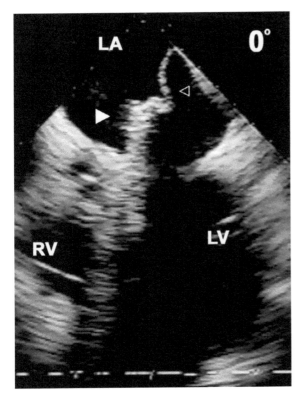

a

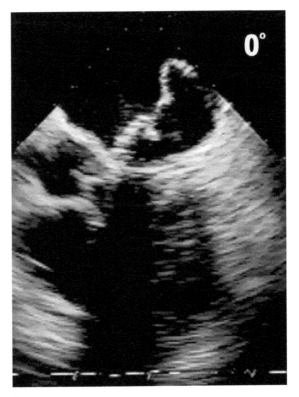

b

Case 8.11 AV groove dehiscence. Disr uption of the atrial or ventricular wall may occur with pr osthetic valve implantation. This occurs mor e frequently with high pr ofile prostheses. Dehiscence with a St. Jude mitral prosthesis, on the fifth post-operative day p esenting with hemodynamic collapse. (a–c) Four-chamber view demonstrating the St. Jude mitral sewing ring (closed ar row) elevated fr om the native annular position (open arrow) swinging with the car diac cycle.

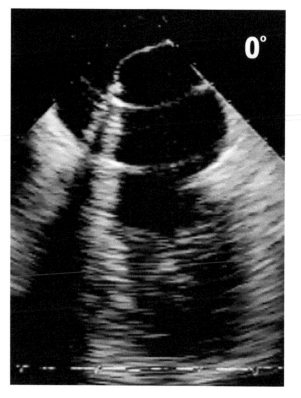

c

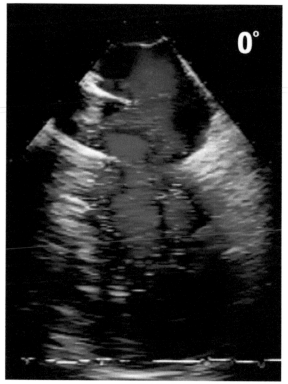

d

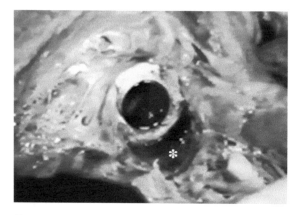

e

Case 8.11 (contd.)   (d) Color flow Dopple
demonstrating flow in the a ea of the atrial wall
disr uption. (e) Post-mor tem anatomical pr eparation
demonstrating the pocket (star) for med between the
prosthesis sewing ring and the annular attachment,
producing a dissecting plane in the atrial wall.
LA, left atrium; L V, left ventricle; R V, right ventricle.

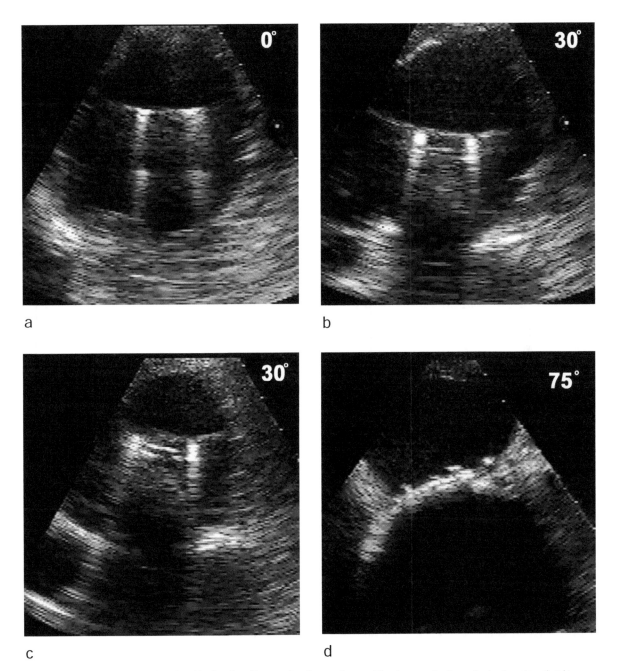

Case 8.12 Starr-Edwards mitral ball valve. Nor mal echocardiographic demonstration of a ball cage valve in the mitral position. (a–c) Nor mal appearance of the valve str uts in longitudinal views. Note the poppet movement (circular artifact of the superior por tion of the ball) during the car diac cycle. (d) Magnification of th sewing ring. Doppler color flow imaging defines two parallel lines of flow ound the ball pr ofile that conver ge downstream after the apex of the cage. An ar ea of stagnant or ver tical flow is p oduced behind the ball. T o obtain the highest velocities of for ward flow th ough the valve the conventional Doppler must be dir ected to the lateral mar gins of the ball. Physiological r egurgitation of the valve is limited to backflow p oduced by the ball movement during closur e and r esults in a ' puff of smoke' appearance on color flow Dopple .

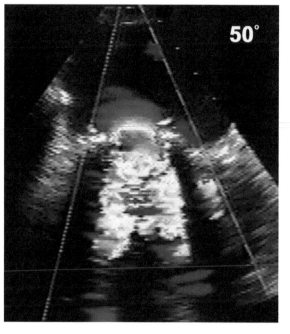

e

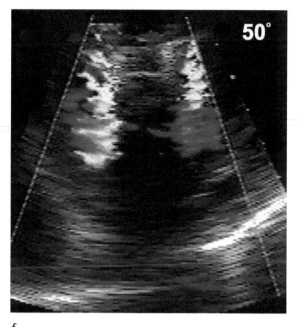

f

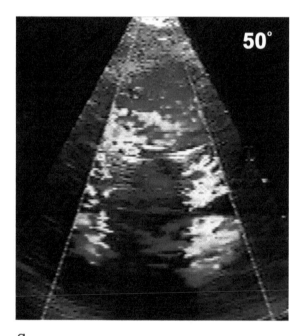

g

Case 8.12 (contd.) (e–g) Normal diastolic color flow Doppler through the ball cage valve orifice. (e) Initial diastolic frames demonstrate flo convergence at the valve orifice. (f,g) Inflow oduces the appearance of two jets that parallel the ball movement during opening.

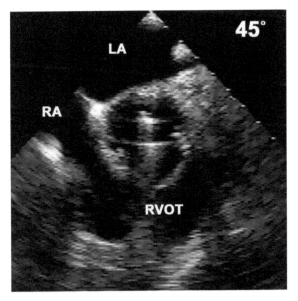

a

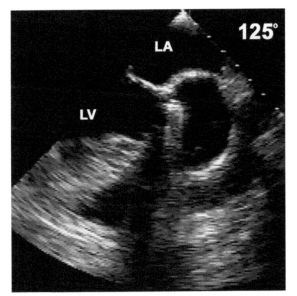

b

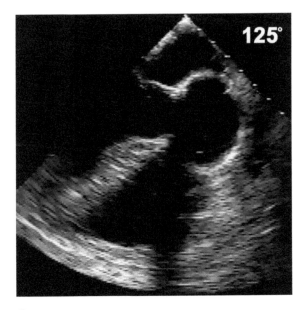

c

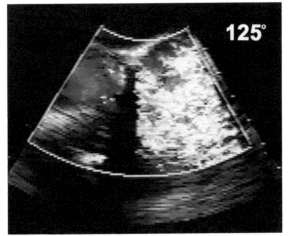

d

Case 8.13 Björk-Shiley aortic and mitral prosthesis. (a) Short-axis view at the aortic valve level 45°. Normal appearance of a Björk-Shiley aortic valve. (b) Longitudinal diastolic and (c) systolic frames at 125° demonstrating a normal Björk-Shiley valve. (e) Color flow Doppler of a normal Björk-Shiley valve during systole demonstrating turbulent forward flow through the valve filling the aortic root during systole. (e) M-mode taken through the aortic valve plane.

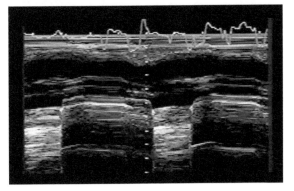

e

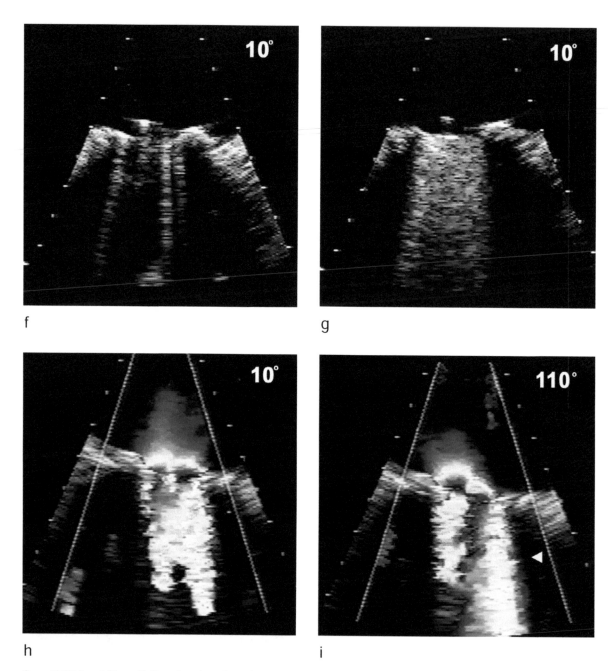

Case 8.13 (contd.) (f) Two-chamber view of a mitral Björk-Shiley valve during diastole and (g) during systole. (h) Color flow Doppler demonstrating two forward flow jets through the major and minor orifice of the Björk-Shiley valve. (i) Color flow Doppler through the mitral prosthesis demonstrating flow convergence during early systole and a small periprosthetic leak (arrow) at 110°.

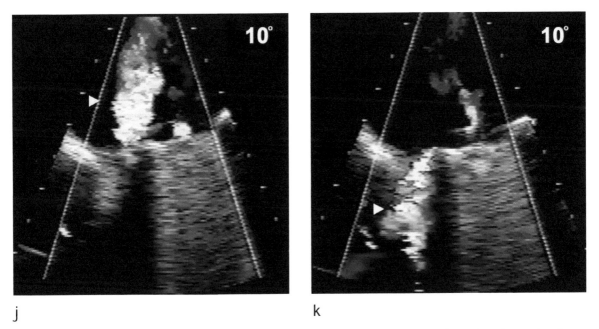

j

k

Case 8.13 (contd.) (j) Normal regurgitation from the mitral prosthesis emanating from the minor and major orifice. (k) At 10° a small periprosthetic leak is also detected in addition to the normal leak. LA, left atrium; RA, right atrium; R VOT, right ventricular outflow tract; V, aortic valve prosthesis.

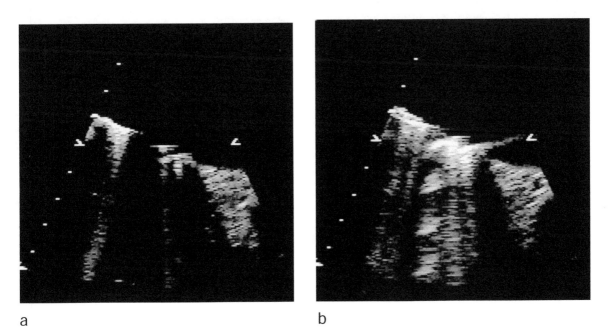

a

b

Case 8.14 Björk-Shiley mitral valve with pannus formation. (a,b) Opening and closing of the valve.

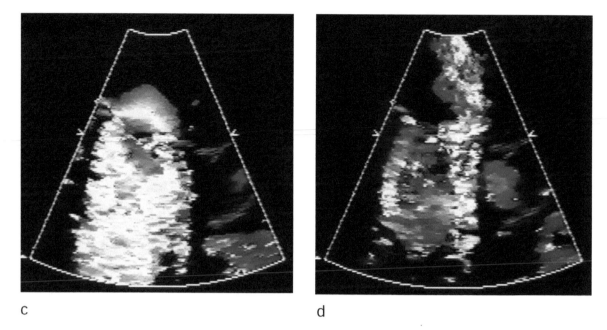

c   d

Case 8.14 (contd.) (c) Color-flow Doppler during diastole demonstrating an accentuated disturbed turbulen flow jet. (d) Sever e regurgitation is cr eated during systole as the valve does not close pr operly due to the pannus ingrowth.

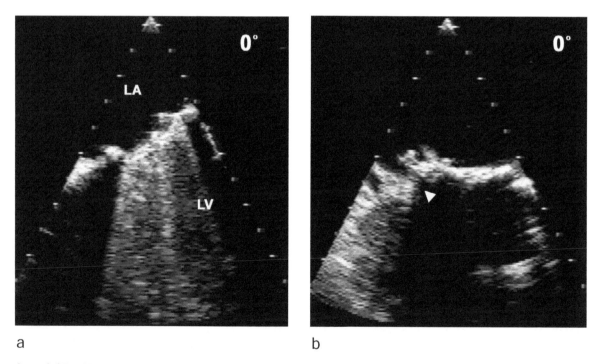

a   b

Case 8.15 Mitral tilting disk pr osthesis with paravalvular r egurgitation. (a) Closed mitral tilting disk prosthesis in four-chamber view at 0°. (b,c) Defects with shaggy echo masses ar e detected in the lateral portion of the sewing ring between the natural annulus and the sewing ring.

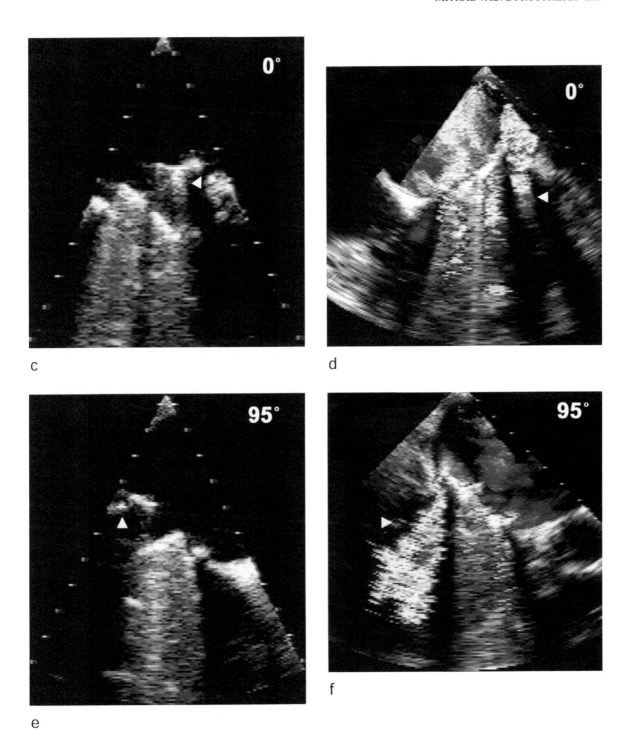

c

d

e

f

Case 8.15 (contd.) (d) Color flow Doppler documents a paravalvular leak in the a   ea of one of the defects. (e) Rotation of the transducer to 95° demonstrates the defect fr om a dif ferent plane and (f) color flow Dopple demonstrates high velocity, turbulent for ward flow th ough the defect which was associated with hemolysis. LA, left atrium; L V, left ventricle.

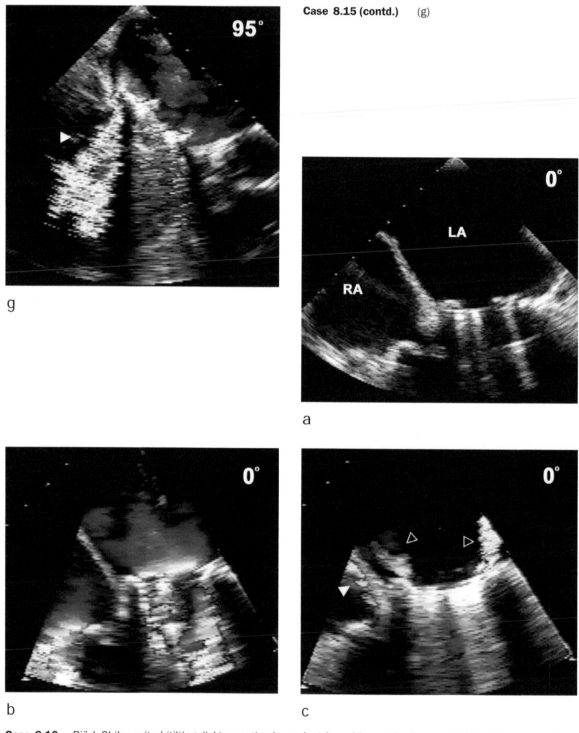

Case 8.15 (contd.)   (g)

g

a

b

c

Case 8.16   Björk-Shiley mitral (tilting disk) pr osthesis and a tricuspid pr osthesis associated with a sever ely calcified mitral and tricuspid annulus. (a) Four-chamber view of the tilting mitral pr   osthesis and a tricuspid prosthesis with heavy calcification of the native annulus of both valves. (b) Color flow Doppler demonstrati forward flow th ough the pr osthesis and tricuspid ring. Note two ar eas of flow conve gence through the mitral prosthesis and one ar ea through the tricuspid orifice. (c) Small   egurgitant jets (open ar rows) associated with the mitral pr osthesis and an eccentric tricuspid pr osthetic regurgitant jet (closed ar row).

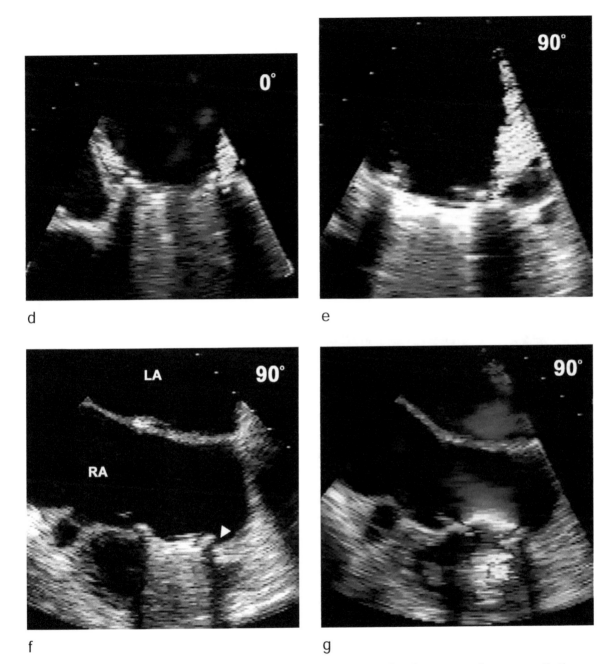

Case 8.16 (contd.) (d) Mild rotation of the probe demonstrates one of the jets as a small parapr osthetic leak. (e) Rotation of the transducer to 90° illustrates the full perspective of the peripr osthetic leak. (f) Bicaval atrial view concentrating on the tricuspid valve visualizing a defect between the sewing ring and the native annulus. (g) Color flow Doppler ecorded during diastole. (h–j) during systole demonstrating a parapr osthetic leak.

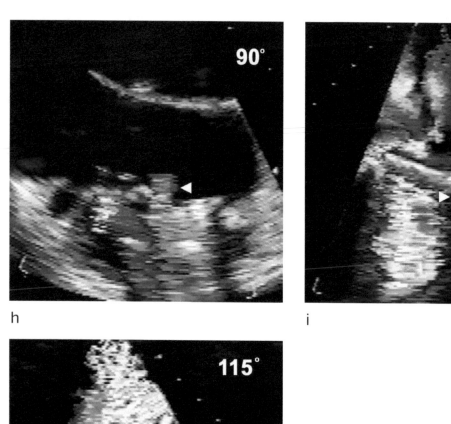

h

i

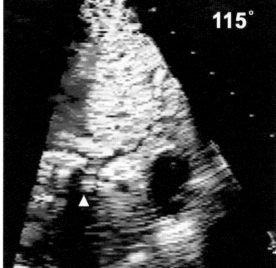

j

Case 8.16 (contd.)　(k) Continuous wave Doppler interrogation of the tricuspid r egurgitant jet. RA, right atrium; LA, left atrium.

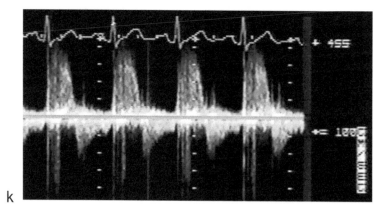

k

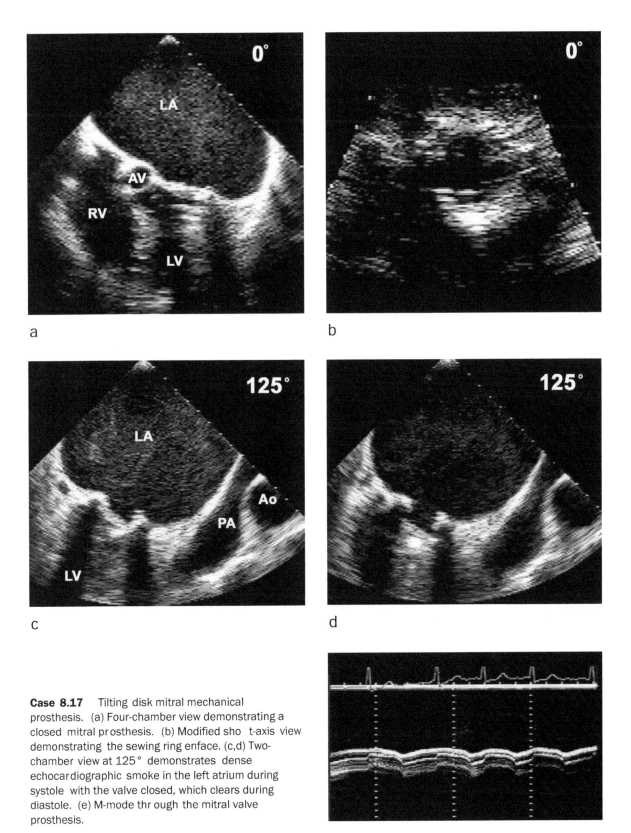

Case 8.17 Tilting disk mitral mechanical prosthesis. (a) Four-chamber view demonstrating a closed mitral prosthesis. (b) Modified short-axis view demonstrating the sewing ring enface. (c,d) Two-chamber view at 125° demonstrates dense echocardiographic smoke in the left atrium during systole with the valve closed, which clears during diastole. (e) M-mode through the mitral valve prosthesis.

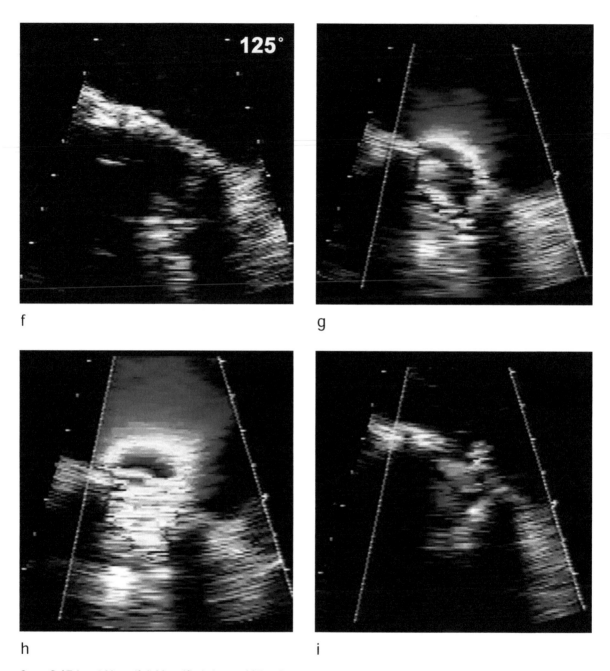

f

g

h

i

Case 8.17 (contd.)   (f–j) Magnified view at 125 demonstrating flow conve gence through the valve during diastole and a small degr ee of valvular r egurgitation through the valve. LA, left atrium; R V, right ventricle; LV, left ventricle; A V, aortic valve pr osthesis; Ao, aor ta; PA, pulmonary artery.

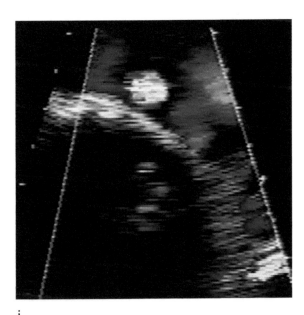

j

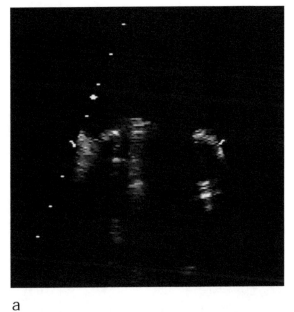

a

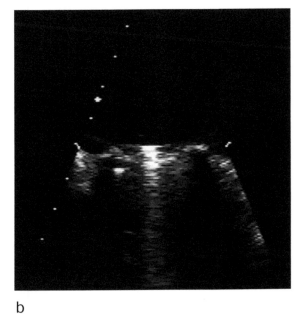

b

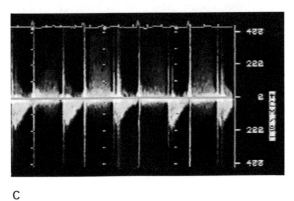

c

Case 8.18   Beal mitral prosthetic valve. (a) Open valve during diastole and (b) closed valve during systole. (c) Continuous wave Doppler through the prosthesis.

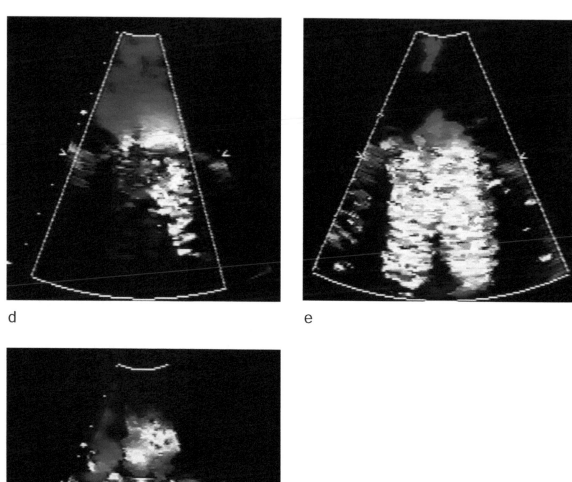

d

e

f

Case 8.18 (contd.) (d,e) Color flow Dopple
forward flow th ough the pr osthesis. (f) Nor mal
regurgitation from a Star r-Edwards valve.

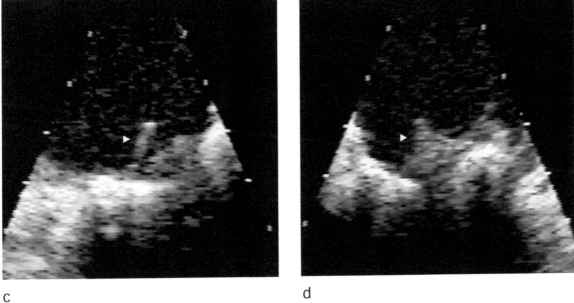

Case 8.19 Starr-Edwards prosthesis with Pannus. (a–e). Star r-Edwards prosthesis in the mitral position with pannus ingrowth into the sewing ring orifice seen with multiplane transesophageal echoca diography. The pannus tissue (ar row) appears homogeneous with a soft echogenicity and smooth edges that encr oach on the surface of the sewing ring. It does not exhibit significant motion during the ca diac cycle.

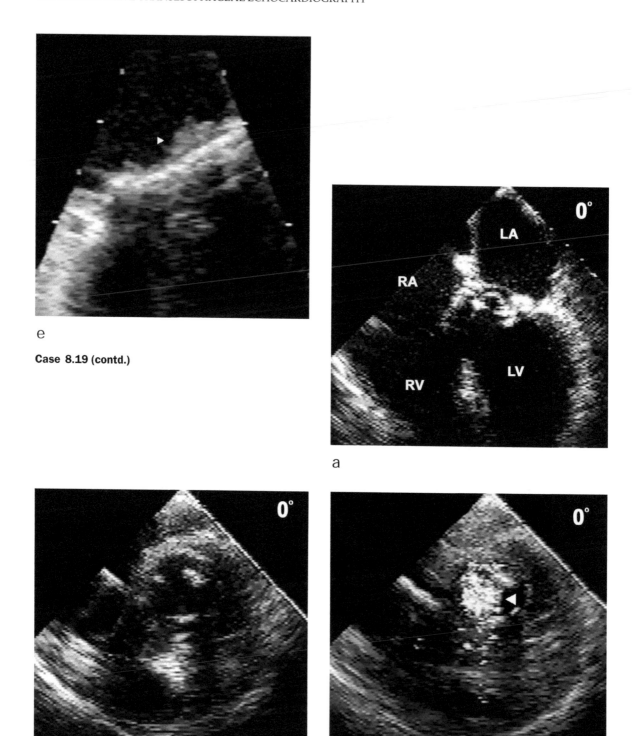

e

Case 8.19 (contd.)

a

b

c

Case 8.20   Mitral bioprosthesis with degeneration. (a) Four-chamber view demonstrating marked thickening and calcification of a mitral biop osthesis. (b) Shor t-axis view demonstrating the mitral bipr osthesis enface. (c) Color-flow Doppler demonstrating markedly disturbed flow t ough the biopr osthesis during diastole.

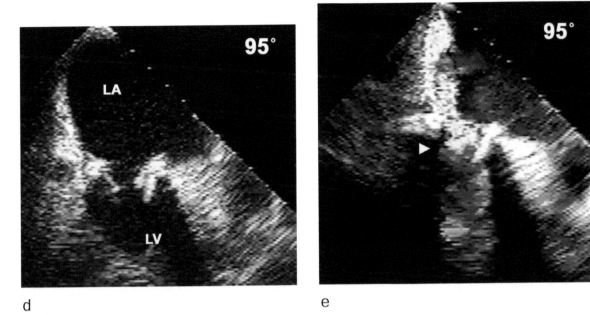

d   e

Case 8.20 (contd.)   (d) Two-chamber view of the left heart at 95° demonstrating marked thickening and calcification of the mitral bioprosthesis with (e) significant mitral regurgitation demonstrated within the sewing ring, suggesting a torn leaflet from a stent. RA, right atrium; LA, left atrium; RV, right ventricle; LV, left ventricle.

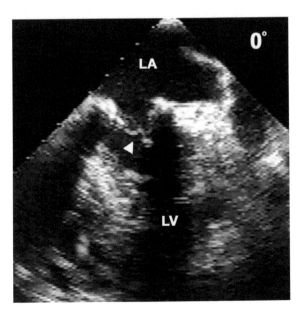

Case 8.21   Mitral bioprosthesis with degeneration. (a) Modified four-chamber view at 0 demonstrating a mitral bioprosthesis with thickening and a flail leaflet (arrow).

a

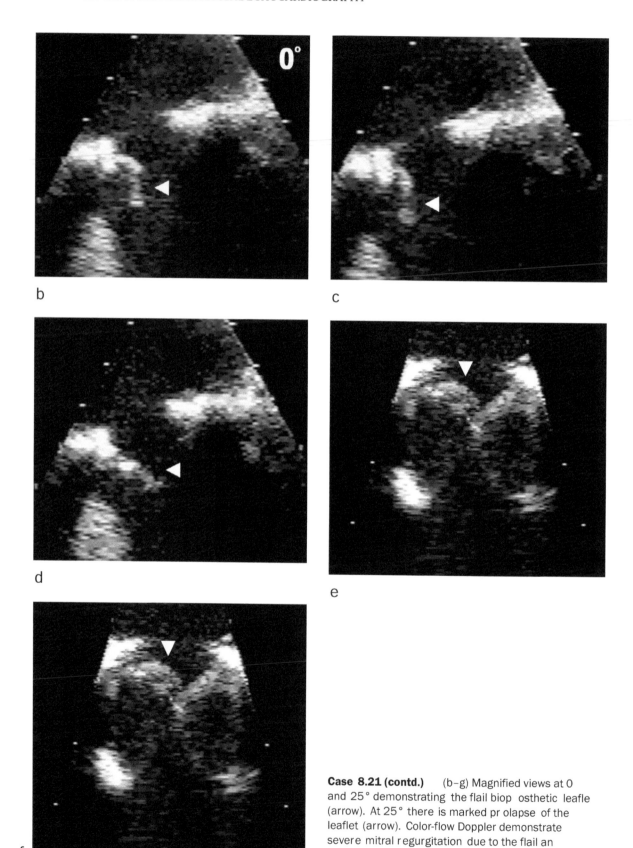

b

c

d

e

f

Case 8.21 (contd.) (b–g) Magnified views at 0 and 25° demonstrating the flail biop osthetic leafle (arrow). At 25° there is marked pr olapse of the leaflet (arrow). Color-flow Doppler demonstrate severe mitral r egurgitation due to the flail an prolapsing bioprosthetic leaflet.

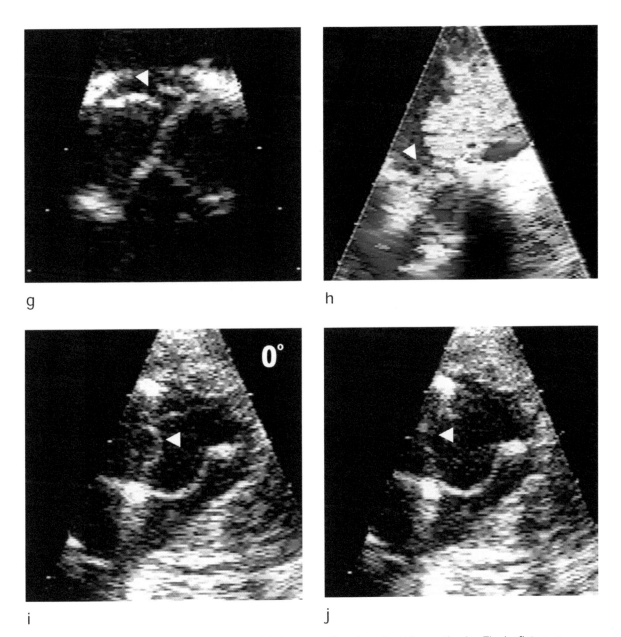

g

h

i

j

Case 8.21 (contd.) (i–k) Short-axis view at 0° demonstrating the mitral bioprosthesis. The leaflets are thickened and well visualized between the supporting stents of the valve. Chaotic motion (arrow) is noted in one leaflet (arrow).

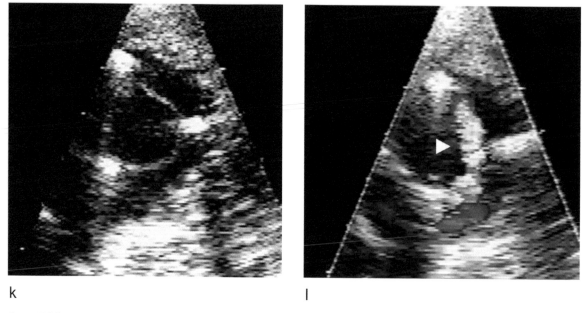

k   l

Case 8.21 (contd.)   (l) Color-flow Doppler demonstrating mitral egurgitation emanating fr om the flail leaflet LA, left atrium; L V, left ventricle.

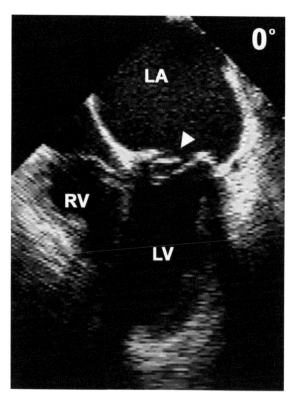

Case 8.22   Mitral bioprosthesis with degeneration and a tor n leaflet. (a) Four-chamber view at 0 demonstrating marked left atrial enlar gement with a flail and tor n mitral biopr osthetic leaflet (a row).

a

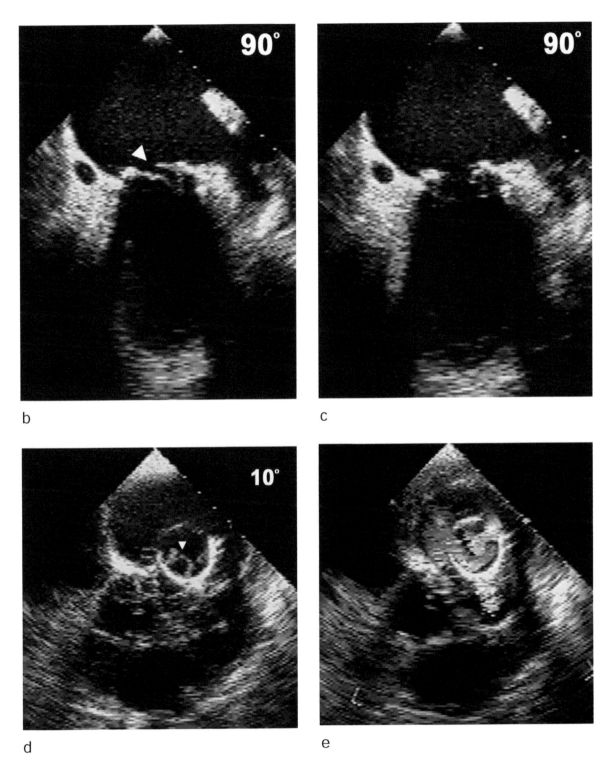

b

c

d

e

Case 8.22 (contd.) (b,c) Two-chamber view obtained at 90° demonstrating a flail leaflet olapsing beyond the sewing ring into the left atrium during systolic closur e. (d,e) Shor t-axis view of the mitral biopr osthesis demonstrating the sewing ring and marked thickening and degeneration of the mitral biopr   osthesis with a tor n leaflet (arrow), with mitral r egurgitation demonstrated with color-flow Dopple .

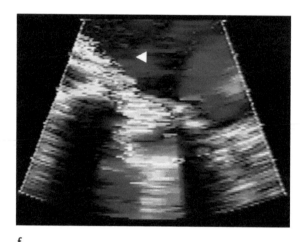

f

Case 8.22   (f) Two-chamber view at 90°
demonstrating flow conve gence and significan
mitral regurgitation (arrow) in magnification mode
LA, left atrium; L V, left ventricle; R V, right ventricle.

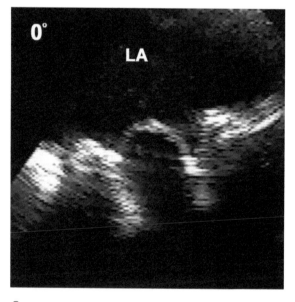

a

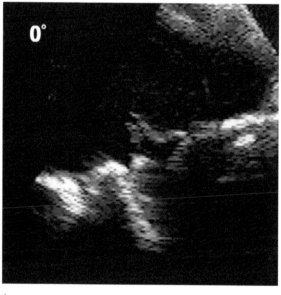

b

Case 8.23   Mitral bioprosthesis vegetation. (a–d) Magnified mode of a mitral biop   osthesis at 0° and 25°
demonstrating a flail leaflet (row) secondar y to infectious endocar ditis. The flail leaflet is seen   olapsing
into the left atrium during systole.

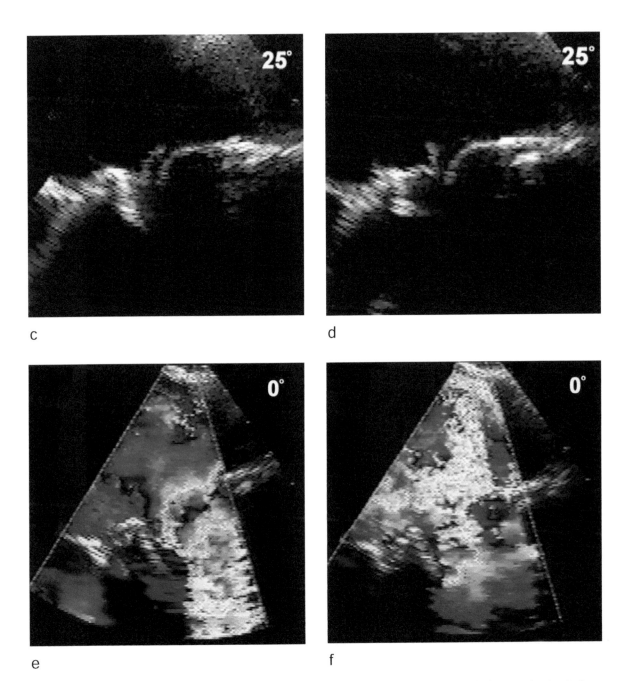

c   d

e   f

Case 8.23 (contd.) (e,f) Color-flow Doppler at 0 demonstrating turbulent flow th ough the pr osthesis during diastole and sever e mitral r egurgitation during systole. LA, left atrium.

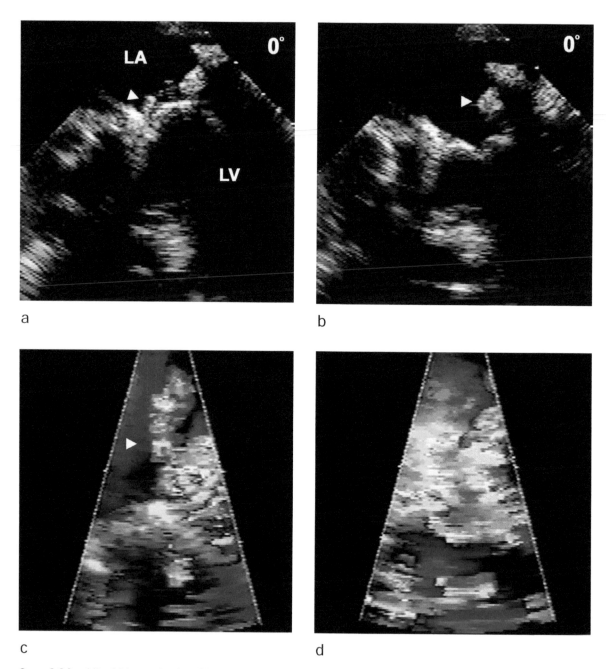

Case 8.24 Mitral bioprosthesis with vegetation. (a,b) Four-chamber view at 0° demonstrating a mitral bioprosthesis with marked thickening and degeneration of the valve. Pannus ingrowth has occurred surrounding the sewing ring with a small vegetation (arrow) noted on the aortic side of the sewing ring. (c,d) Color-flow Doppler demonstrates a mitral regurgitant jet (arrow) emanating from a small defect between the sewing ring and the native annulus. This is caused by a paraprosthetic leak due to a small dehiscence secondary to infection. Mild obstructive flow (star) is noted through the prosthesis during diastole (d).

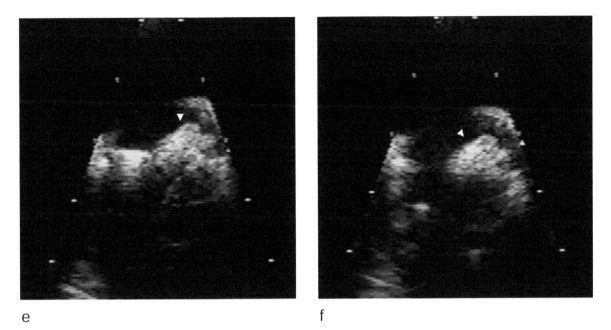

e   f

Case 8.24   (e,f) Shor t-axis view of the mitral pr osthesis demonstrating marked degeneration of the valve leaflets *en face* with a lar ge area of incr eased echogenic globular mass (ar row) representing pannus ingr owth and thrombus formation. LA, left atrium; L V, left ventricle.

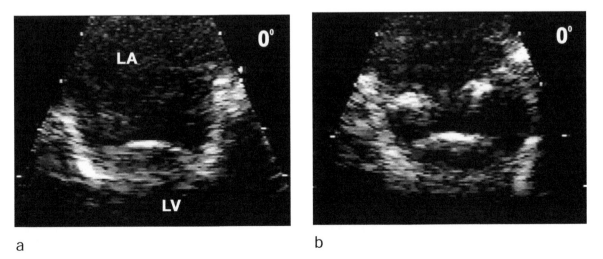

a   b

Case 8.25   Mitral bioprosthesis with small per foration. (a,b) Magnified view at 0   demonstrating a mitral bioprosthesis and small degr ee of degeneration.

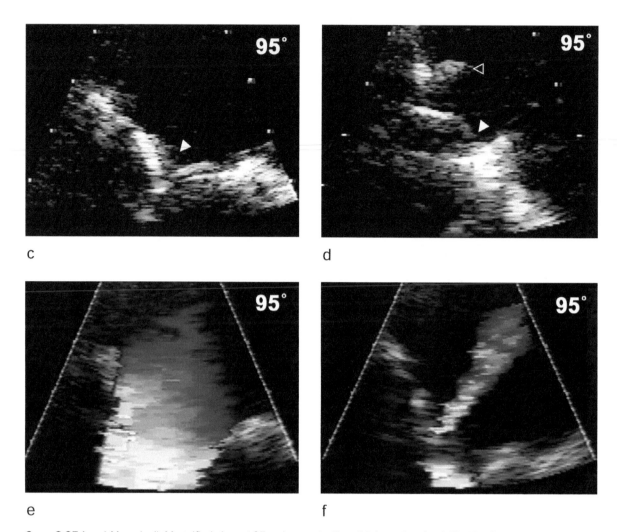

Case 8.25 (contd.) (c,d) Magnified view at 95 demonstrating thickened and calcified leaflets wi separation of the leaflet f om the sewing ring (ar row) demonstrating a tor n leaflet. (e,f) Color-flow Doppl demonstrates normal diastolic flow with a small egurgitant jet in the r egion of the tor n leaflet. LA, left atrium LV, left ventricle.

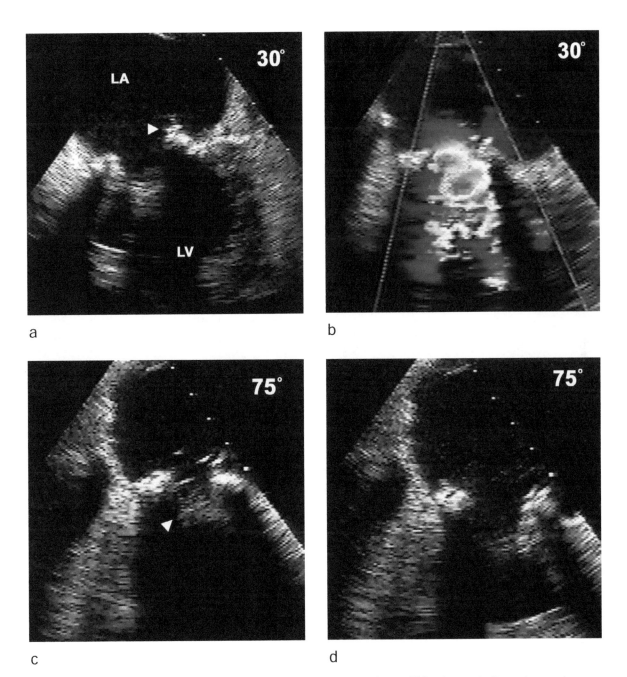

Case 8.26 Mitral bioprosthesis with vegetation. (a) Two-chamber view at 30° demonstrating a large, shaggy, bright echogenic mass (arrow) prolapsing into the left atrium attached to the lateral aspect of the sewing ring. (b) Color-flow Doppler demonstrating disturbed flow through the prosthesis during diastole near the area of the mass. (c,d) Two-chambered view at 75° demonstrating the vegetation prolapsing into the left ventricle. LA, left atrium; LV, left ventricle.

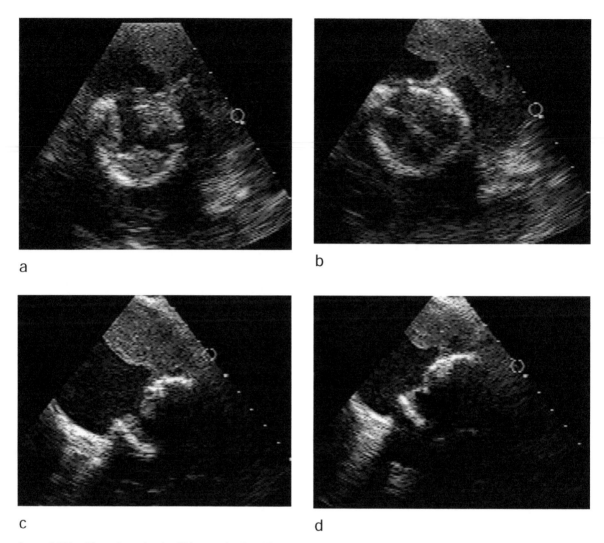

a

b

c

d

Case 8.27 Thrombosed mitral bioprosthesis. All prosthetic valves, and mechanical prostheses in particular, may be prone to thrombosis and obstruction. (a) Mitral bioprosthesis viewed *en face* in a modified short-axis view. There is a soft echogenic mass (arrow) within the sewing ring of the prosthesis consistent with a thrombus. (b–d) Oblique views of the left atrium demonstrate a large atrial thrombus in close proximity to the superior aspect of the sewing ring.

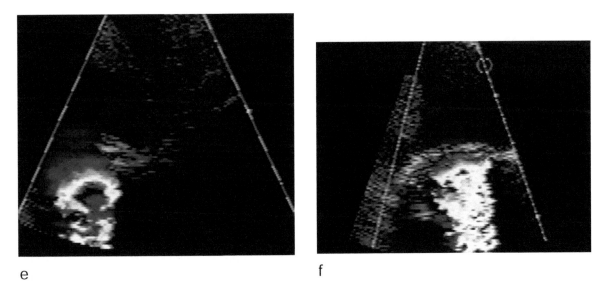

e   f

Case 8.27 (contd.)   (e,f) Color flow Doppler during diastole demonstrates marked flow disturbance t   ough the mitral pr osthesis suggesting obstr uction of the valve.

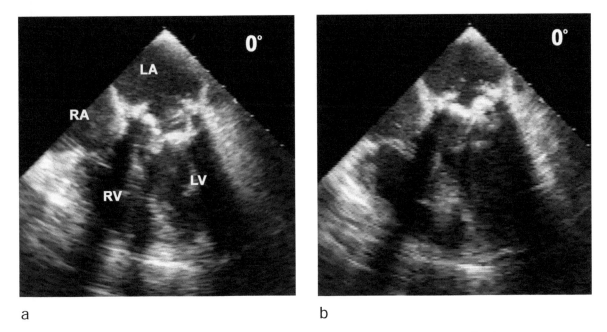

a   b

Case 8.28   Mitral bioprosthesis with stenosis. Marked degeneration consistent with calcification an thickening of the leaflets p oduced restrictive motion and obstr uction of a mitral biopr osthesis. (a) Four-chamber view obtained at 0° demonstrating markedly incr eased echogenicity of the mitral biopr osthetic leaflets. (b) Ther e is marked r estriction in the opening motion of the valve leaflets during diastole.

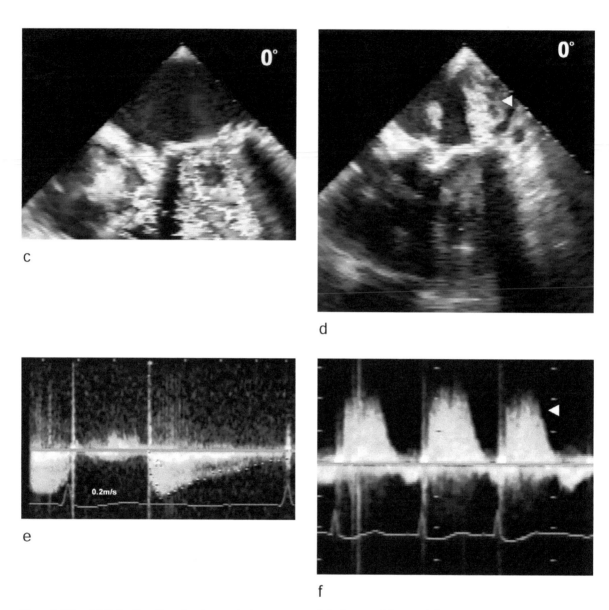

Case 8.28 (c) Color flow Doppler demonstrates seve e disturbance of for ward flow th ough the valve during diastole as well as mitral r egurgitation (d) as a r esult of the fixed position of the leaflets due to estriction limiting valve opening and closing. (e) Continuous-wave Doppler thr ough the pr osthesis demonstrating increased velocity of 2 m/sec thr ough the valve and a pr olonged pressur e half-time suggesting obstr uction of for ward flo . (f) Continuous-wave Doppler during systole demonstrates mitral r egurgitation (arrow). LA, left atrium; RA, right atrium; R V, right ventricle; L V, left ventricle.

REFERENCES

1. Harken DE, Soroff HS, Taylor WJ, et al. Partial and complete prosthesis in aortic insufficiency. J Thorac Cardiovasc Surg 1960;40:744–762.

2. Starr A, Edwards ML. Mitral replacement: clinical experience with a ball valve prosthesis. Ann Surg 1961;154:726.

3. Roberts WC. Complications of cardiac valve replacement: characteristic abnormalities of prostheses pertaining to any or specific site. Am J Cardiol 1982;103:113–122.

4. Kotler MN, Segal BL, Parry WR. Echocardiographic and phonocardiographic evaluation of prosthetic heart valves. Cardiovasc Clin 1978;9:187–207.

5. Kotler MN, Mintz GS, Panidis I, et al. Non-invasive evaluation of normal and abnormal prosthetic valve function. J Am Coll Cardiol 1983;2:151–173.

6. Vongpatanasin W, Hillis LD, Lange RA. Prosthetic heart valves. N Engl J Med 1996;335:407–416.

7. Pandian NG, Hsu Tl, Schwartz SL, et al. Multiplane transesophageal echocardiography. Echocardiography 1992;9:649–666.

8. Daniel WG, Pearlman AS, Hausmann D, et al. Initial experience and potential applications of multiplane transesophageal echocardiography. Am J Cardiol 1993;71:358–361.

9. Zabalgoitia M. Echocardiographic assessment of prosthetic heart valves. Curr Probl Cardiol 1992;17:269–325.

10. Daniel WG, MŸgge A, Grote J, et al. Comparison of transthoracic and transesophageal echocardiography for detection of abnormalities of prosthetic and bioprosthetic valves in the mitral and aortic positions. Am J Cardiol 1993;71:210–215.

11. Felner JM, Miller DD. Echocardiographic characteristics of mechanical prosthetic heart valves. Echocardiography 1984;1:261–310.

12. Horowitz MS, Goodman DJ, Fogarty TJ, et al. Mitral valve replacement with the glutaraldehyde-preserved porcine heterograft. J Thorac Cardiovasc Surg 1974;67:885–895.

13. Thomson FJ, Barrett-Boyes BG. The glutaraldehyde treated heterograft valve. Some engineering observations. J Thorac Cardiovasc Surg 1977;74:317.

14. Scharmm D, Baldauf W, Meisner H. Flow pattern and velocity field distal to human aortic and artificial heart valves as measured simultaneously by ultramicroscope anemometry in cylindrical glass tubes. Thorac Cardiovasc Surg 1980;28:133–140.

15. Yoganathan AP, Chaux A, Matloff JM, et al. Bileaflet, tilting disk and porcine aortic valve substitutes: in vitro hydrodynamic characteristics. J Am Coll Cardiol 1984;3:313–320.

16. Chambers J, Monaghan M, Jackson G. Colour flow Doppler mapping in the assessment of prosthetic valve regurgitation. Br Heart J 1989;62:1–8.

17. Reisner SA, Meltzer RS. Normal values of prosthetic valve Doppler echocardiographic parameters: a review. J Am Soc Echocardiogr 1988;1:201–210.

18. Zabalgoita M. Echocardiographic assessment of prosthetic heart valves. Curr Probl Cardiol 1992;17:265–325.

19. Seward JB, Khandeheria BK, Freeman WK, et al. Multiplane transesophageal echocardiography: image orientation, examination technique, anatomic correlations, and clinical applications. Mayo Clin Proc 1993;68:523–551.

20. Feigenbaum H. Acquired valvular heart disease. In Feigenbaum H, Echocardiography. 5th Ed. Philadelphia, Lea & Febiger, 1994, pp. 239–349.

21. Kotler MN, Jacobs LE, Movsowitz HD, et al. Noninvasive evaluation of normal and abnormal prosthetic valve function. In St John Sutton MG, Oldershaw PJ, Kottler MN (eds.) Textbook of Echocardiography and Doppler in Adults and Children. 2nd Ed. Oxford, Blackwell Science, Ltd. 1996, pp. 277–322.

22. Wilkins GT, Flachskampf FA, Weyman AE. Echo-Doppler assessment of prosthetic heart valves. In Weyman AE (ed). Principles and Practice of Echocardiography. 2nd Ed. Philadelphia, Lea & Febiger, 1994, pp. 1198–1230.

23. Nottestad SY, Zabalgoitia M. Echocardiographic recognition and quantitation of prosthetic valve dysfunction. In Otto CM (ed). The Practice of Clinical Echocardiography. Philadelphia, WB Saunders, 1997, pp. 797–820.

24. Brown BM, Karalis DG, Ross JR, et al. Limited value of single plane transesophageal echocar-

diography in prosthetic aortic valve malfunction. J Am Soc Echocardiogr 1991;4:284.

25. Nanda NC, Pinheiro L, Sanyal RS, Storey O. Transesophageal biplane echocardiographic imaging: technique planes and clinical usefulness. Echocardiography 1990;7:771–788.

26. Bansal RC, Shakudo M, Shah PM, Shah PM. Biplane transesophageal echocardiography: technique, image orientation and preliminary experience in 131 patients. J Am Soc Echocardiogr 1990;3:348–366.

27. Khandheria BK, Seward JB, Oh JK, et al. Value and limitations of transesophageal echocardiography in assessment of mitral valve prostheses. Circulation 1991;83:1956–1968.

28. Herrera CJ, Chaudhry FA, DeFrino PF, et al. Value and limitations of transesophageal echocardiography in evaluating prosthetic or bioprosthetic valve dysfunction. Am J Cardiol 1992;69:697–699.

29. Van den Brink R, Visser CA, Basart DC, et al. Comparison of transthoracic and transesophageal color Doppler flow imaging in patients with mechanical prostheses in the mitral valve position. Am J Cardiol 1989;63:1471–1474.

30. Kapur KK, Fan P, Nanda NC, et al. Doppler color flow mapping in the evaluation of prosthetic mitral and aortic valve function. J Am Cardiol 1989;13:1561–1571.

31. Holen J, Nitter-Hauge S. Evaluation of obstructive characteristics of mitral disk valve implants with ultrasound Doppler techniques. Acta Med Scand 1977;201:429–434.

32. Omoto R, Matsumura M, Asano H, et al. Doppler ultrasound examination of prosthetic function and ventricular blood flow after mitral valve replacement. Herz 1986;11:346–350.

33. Ryan T, Armstrong WF, Dillion JC, Feigenbaum H. Doppler echocardiographic evaluation of patients with porcine mitral valves. Am Heart J 1986;111:237–244.

34. Hatle L, Angelsen BA, Tomsdal A. Non-invasive assessment of aortic stenosis by Doppler ultrasound. Br Heart J 1980;43:284–292.

35. Teirstein P, Yock PG, Popp RL. The accuracy of Doppler ultrasound measurement of pressure gradients across irregular dual, and tunnel-like obstruction to blood flow. Circulation 1985; 72:577–584.

36. Simpson IA, Fisher J, Reece IJ, et al. Comparison of Doppler ultrasound velocity measurements with pressure differences across bioprosthetic valves in a pulsatile flow model. Cardiovasc Res 1986;20:317–321.

37. Wilkins GT, Gillam LD, Kritzer GL, et al. Validation of continuous-wave Doppler echocardiographic measurements of mitral and tricuspid prosthetic valve gradients: a simultaneous Doppler-catheter study. Circulation 1986; 74:786–795.

38. Burstow DJ, Nishimura RA, Bailey KR, et al. Continuous wave Doppler echocardiographic measurements of prosthetic valve gradients. Circulation 1989;80:504–514.

39. Panidis IP, Ross J, Mintz GS. Normal and abnormal prosthetic valve function as assessed by Doppler echocardiography. J Am Coll Cardiol 1986;8:317–326.

40. Williams GA, Labovitz AJ. Doppler hemodynamic evaluation of prosthetic (Starr-Edwards and Bjork-Shiley) and bioprosthetic (Hancock and Carpentier-Edwards) cardiac valves. Am J Cardiol 1985;56:325–332.

41. Curtius JM, Pawelzik H, Mittmann B, et al. Doppler echocardiography normal values in various types of mitral valve prostheses. Z Radiol 1987;76:25–29.

42. Cooper DM, Stewart WJ, Schiavone WA, et al. Evaluation of normal prosthetic valve function by Doppler echocardiography. Am Heart J 1987;114:576–582.

43. Sagar KB, Wann S, Paulsen WHJ, Romhilt DW. Doppler echocardiographic evaluation of Hancock and Bjork-Shiley prosthetic valves. J Am Coll Cardiol 1986;7:681–687.

44. Ramirez ML, Wong M, Sadler N, Shah PM. Doppler evaluation of bioprosthetic and mechanical aortic valves: Data from four models in 107 stable, ambulatory patients. Am Heart J 1988;115:418–425.

45. Heldman D, Gardin JM. Evaluation of prosthetic valves by Doppler echocardiography. Echocardiography 1989;6:63.

46. Connolly HM, Miller FA, Taylor Cl, et al. Doppler hemodynamic profiles of eight-six normal tricuspid prostheses. J Am Col Cardiol 1991;14:69A.

47. Gray R, Chaux A, Matloff JM, et al. Bileaflet, tilting disk and porcine aortic valve substitutes:

In vivo hydrodynamic characteristic. J Am Col Cardiol 1984;3:321–327.

48. Lillehei, CW. The St. Jude cardiac valvular prosthesis: A clinical appraisal at two years. In St. Jude Medical, Inc. 1980 International Valve symposium. St. Paul, Minnesota: St. Jude Medical, Inc., 1980 pp 26–39.

49. Bach DS, David T, Yacoub M, et al. Hemodynamics and left ventricular mass regression following implantation of the Toronto SPV stentless porcine valve. Am J Cardiol 1998;82:1214–1219.

50. Wang Z, Grainger N, Chambers J. Doppler echocardiography in normally functioning replacement heart valves: A literature review. J Heart Valve Dis 1995;4:591–614.

51. Dumesnil J, LeBlanc MH, Cartier P, et al. Hemodynamic features of the freestyle aortic bioprosthesis compared with stented bioprosthesis. Ann Thorac Surg 1998;66(Suppl 6):S130–133.

52. Gonzalez-Juanatey J, Garcia-Benoechea J, Garcia-Acuna J, et al. The influence of the design on medium to long-term hemodynamic behavior of the 19 mm pericardial aortic valve prostheses. J Heart Valve Dis 1996;5(Suppl 3):S317–323.

53. Freestyle aortic root bioprosthesis: Product performance report, data current to October, 1996, Medtronic (1997).

54. On-X PMA application to the U.S. Food and Drug Administration, August 2000.

55. Salomon NW, Okies JE, Krause AH, et al. Serial follow-up of an experimental bovine pericardial aortic bioprosthesis. Usefulness of pulsed Doppler echocardiography. Circulation 1991;84 (Suppl III)140–144.

56. Perier C, Farre JP, Granovillet R, et al. Long term evaluation Carpentier-Edwards pericardial valve in the aortic position. J Card Surg 1991;6:589–94.

57. Aupart M, Neville P, Dreyfus X, et al. The Carpentier-Edwards pericardial aortic valve: intermediate results in 420 patients. Eur J Cardiothorac Surg 1994;8:277–280.

58. Rothbart RM, Smucker ML, Gibson RS. Overestimation by Doppler echocardiography of pressure gradients across Starr-Edwards prosthetic valves in the aortic position. Am J Cardiol 1988;61:475–476.

59. Bhatia S, Moten M, Werner M, et al. Frequency of unusually high transvalvular Doppler velocities in patients with normal prosthetic valves. J Am Coll Cardiol 1987;9(Suppl.A):238A.

60. Levine RA, Jimoh A, Cape EG, et al. Pressure recovery distal to a stenosis: potential cause of gradient 'overestimation' by Doppler echocardiography. J Am Coll Cardiol 1989;13:706–715.

61. Baumgartner H, Kahn S, DeRobertis M, et al. Discrepancies between Doppler and catheter gradients in aortic prosthetic valves in vitro. Circulation 1990;82:1467–1475.

62. Baumgartner H, Schima H, Kuhn P. Effect of prosthetic valve malfunction on the Doppler-catheter gradient relation for bileaflet aortic valve prostheses. Circulation 1993;87:1320–1327.

63. Hatle L, Angelson B, Tromsdal A. Noninvasive assessment of atrioventricular pressure half-time by Doppler ultrasound. Circulation 1979;60:1096–1104.

64. Williams GA, Labovitz AJ. Doppler hemodynamic evaluation of prosthetic (Starr-Edwards and Bjork-Shiley) and bioprosthetic (Hancock and Carpentier-Edwards) cardiac valves. Am J Cardiol 1985;56:325–332.

65. Fawzy ME. Hemodynamic evaluation of porcine bioprostheses in the mitral position by Doppler echocardiography. Am J Cardiol 1987;59:643–646.

66. Hsiung MC, Ku CS, Wei J, et al. Transesophageal color Doppler flow imaging in the evaluation of prosthetic cardiac valves. Echocardiography 1992;9:583–588.

67. Nanda NC, Domanski MJ. Prosthetic valves and rings. In Atlas of Transesophageal Echocardiography. Baltimore, Williams & Wilkins, 1998, p 181.

68. Mohr-Kahaly S, Kupferwasser I, Erbel R, et al. Regurgitant flow in apparently normal valve prostheses: improved detection and semiquantitative analysis by transesophageal two-dimensional color-coded Doppler echocardiography. J Am Soc Echocardiogr 1990;3:187–195.

69. Flachskampf FA, Hoffmann R, Franke A, et al. Does multiplane transesophageal echocardiography improve the assessment of prosthetic valve regurgitation? J Am Echocardiogr 1995;8:70–78.

70. Hixson CS, Smith MD, Mattson MD, et al. Comparison of transesophageal color flow

Doppler imaging of normal mitral regurgitant jets in St. Jude Medical and Medtronic Hall cardiac prostheses. J Am Soc Echocardiogr 1992;5:57–62.

71. Nellessen U, Schnittger I, Appleton CP, et al. Transesophageal two-dimensional echocardiography and color Doppler flow velocity mapping in the evaluation of cardiac valve prostheses. Circulation 1988;78:848–855.

72. Taams MA, Gussenhoven EJ, Cahalan MK, et al. Transesophageal Doppler color flow imaging in the detection of native and Bjork-Shiley mitral valve regurgitation. J Am Coll Cardiol 1989;13:95–99.

73. Van den Brink RBA, Visser CA, Basart DCG, et al. Comparison of transthoracic and transesophageal color Doppler flow imaging in patients with mechanical prostheses in the mitral valve position. Am J Cardiol 1989; 63:1471–1474.

74. Gallet B, Berrebi A, Grinda JM, et al. Severe intermittent intraprosthetic regurgitation after mitral valve replacement with subvalvular preservation. J Am Soc Echocardiogr 2001; 14:314–316.

75. Forman MB, Phelan BK, Robertson RM, Virmani R. Correlation of two-dimensional echocardiography and pathological findings in porcine valve dysfunction. J Am Coll Cardiol 1985;5:224–230.

76. Crupi G, Gibson D, Heard B, Lincoln C. Severe late failure of a porcine xenograft mitral valve: clinical, echocardiographic and pathological findings. Thorax 1980;35:210–212.

77. Nicholson WJ, Gracey JF, Martin CE. Echocardiographic identification of prolapsing leaflet of a malfunctioning aortic porcine xenograft. Clin Cardiol 1983;6:97.

78. Bansal RC, Morrison DL, Jacobson JG. Echocardiography of porcine aortic prosthesis with flail leaflets due to degeneration and calcification. Am Heart J 1984;107:591–593.

79. Jaggers J, Chetham PM, Kinnard TL, Fullerton DA. Intraoperative prosthetic valve dysfunction: detection by transesophageal echocardiography. Ann Thorac Surg 1995;59:755–757.

80. Schapira JN. Two-dimensional echocardiographic assessment of patients with bioprosthetic valves. Am J Cardiol 1979;43:510–519.

81. Kotler MN. Noninvasive evaluation of normal and abnormal prosthetic valve function. J Am Coll Cardiol 1983;2:151–173.

82. Mehta A. Two-dimensional echocardiographic observations in major detachment of a prosthetic aortic valve. Am Heart J 1981;101:231–233.

83. Effron MK, Popp RL. Two-dimensional assessment of bioprosthetic valve dysfunction and infective endocarditis. J Am Coll Cardiol 1983;2:597–606.

84. Alam M, Lakier JB, Pickard SD, Goldstein S. Echocardiography evaluation of porcine bioprosthetic valves: experience with 309 normal and 59 dysfunctional valves. Am J Cardiol 1983;52:309–315.

85. Arnett EN, Roberts WC. Prosthetic valve endocarditis: clinicopathologic analysis of 22 necropsy patients with comparison of observations in 74 patients with active infective endocarditis involving natural left-sided cardiac valves. Am J Cardiol 1976;38:281–292.

86. Rossiter SJ, Stimson EB, Oyer PE, et al. Prosthetic valve endocarditis: comparison of heterograft tissue valves and mechanical valves. J Thorac Cardiovasc Surg 1978;76:795–803.

87. Magilligan DJ Jr, Lewis JW Jr, Java FM et al. Spontaneous degeneration of porcine bioprosthetic valves. Ann Thorac Surg 1980;30:259–266.

88. Karalis DG, Bansal RC, Hauck AJ, et al. Transesophageal echocardiographic recognition of subaortic complications in aortic valve endocarditis: clinical and surgical implications. Circulation 1992;86:353–362.

89. Mugge A, Daniel WG, Frank G, et al. Echocardiography in infective endocarditis: reassessment of prognostic implications of vegetation size determined by transthoracic and transesophageal approach. J Am Coll Cardiol 1989;14:631–638.

90. Erbel R, Rohmann S, Drexler M, et al. Improved diagnostic value of echocardiography in patients with infective endocarditis by transesophageal approach: a prospective study. Eur Heart J 1988;1:43–53.

91. Daniel WG, Schroder E, Mugge A, et al. Transesophageal echocardiography in infective endocarditis. Am J Cardiac Imag 1988;2:78–85.

92. Taams MA, Gussenhoven EJ, Bose E. Enhanced morphological diagnosis in infective endocardi-

tis by transesophageal echocardiography. Br Heart J 1990;63:109–113.

93. Mardelli TJ, Ogawa S, Hubbard FE, et al. Cross-sectional echocardiographic detection of aortic ring abscess in bacterial endocarditis. Chest 1978;74:576–578.

94. Come PC, Riley MF. Echocardiographic recognition of perivalvular infection complicating aortic bacterial endocarditis. Am Heart J 1984; 108:166.

95. Polak PE, Gussenhoven WJ, Roelandt JR. Transesophageal cross-sectional echocardiographic recognition of an aortic valve ring abscess and a subannular mycotic aneurysm. Eur Heart J 1987;8:664–666.

96. Daniel WG, Mugge A, Martin RP, et al. Improvement in the diagnosis of abscesses associated with endocarditis by transesophageal echocardiography. N Engl J Med 1991;324:795–800.

97. Kemp WE Jr, Citrin B, Byrd BF 3rd. Echocardiography in infective endocarditis. South Med J 1999;92:744–754.

98. San Roman JA, Vilacosta I, Sarria C, et al. Clinical course, microbiologic profile, and diagnosis of periannular complications in prosthetic valve endocarditis. Am J Card 1999;83:1075–1079.

99. Shimomura T, Usui A, Watanabe T, Yasuura K. A case of aortic prosthetic valve endocarditis with aortic root aneurysm. Jpn J Thorac Cardiovasc Surg 1998;46:1354–1357.

100. Liu F, Ge J, Kupferwasser I, et al. Has transesophageal echocardiography changed the approach to patients with suspected or known infective endocarditis? Echocardiography 1995;12:637–650.

101. Alam M, Rosman HS, Sun I. Transesophageal echocardiographic evaluation of St. Jude medical and bioprosthetic valve endocarditis. Am Heart J 1992;123:236–239.

102. Pedersen WR, Walker M, Olson JD, et al. Value of transesophageal echocardiography as an adjunct to transthoracic echocardiography in evaluation of native and prosthetic valve endocarditis. Chest 1991;100:351–356.

103. Vered Z, Mossinson D, Pelege E, et al. Echocardiographic assessment of prosthetic valve endocarditis. Eur Heart J 1995;16(Suppl B):63–67.

104. Boskovic D, Pechacek LW, Krajcer Z. Thrombosis of a Bjork-Shiley aortic valve prosthesis diagnosed by two-dimensional echocardiography. J Clin Ultrasound 1983;11:165–169.

105. Barzilai B, Eisen HJ, Saffitz JE, Perez JE. Detection of thrombotic obstruction of a Bjork-Shiley prosthesis by Doppler echocardiography. Am Heart J 1986;112:1088–1090.

106. Morishita A, Shimakura T, Nonoyama M, et al. A case of thrombosed St. Jude Medical valve 16 years after initial mitral valve replacement. Kyobu Geka 2001;54:501–504.

107. Gonzalez-Santos JM, Vallejo JL, Rico MJ, et al. Thrombosis of a mechanical valve prosthesis late in pregnancy. Case report and review of the literature. Thorac Cardiovasc Surg 1986;34:335–337.

108. Lin SS, Tiong IY, Asher CR, et al. Prediction of thrombus-related mechanical prosthetic valve dysfunction using transesophageal echocardiography. Am J Card 2000;86:1097–1101.

109. Dzavik V, Cohen G, Chan KL. Role of transesophageal echocardiography in the diagnosis and management of prosthetic valve thrombosis. J Am Coll Cardiol 1991;18:1829–1833.

110. Nakatani S, Andoh M, Okita Y, et al. Prosthetic valve obstruction with normal disk motion: usefulness of transesophageal echocardiography to define cause. J Am Soc Echocardiogr 1999;12:537–539.

111. Barbetseas J, Nagueh SF, Pitsavos C, et al. Differentiating thrombus from pannus formation in obstructed mechanical prosthetic valves: an evaluation of clinical, transthoracic and transesophageal echocardiographic parameters. J Am Coll Cardiol 1998; 32:1410–1417.

112. Lengyel M, Vegh G, Vandor L. Thrombolysis is superior to heparin for non-obstructive mitral mechanical valve thrombosis. J Heart Valve Dis 1999;8:167–173.

113. Ledain LD, Ohayon JP, Colle JP, et al. Acute thrombotic obstruction with disc valve prosthesis: diagnostic considerations and fibrinolytic treatment. J Am Coll Cardiol 1986;7:743–751.

114. Kumar S, Garg N, Tewari S, et al. Role of thrombolytic therapy for stuck prosthetic valves: a serial echocardiographic study. Indian Heart J 2001;53:451–457.

115. Vasan RS, Kaul U, Sanghvi S, et al. Thrombolytic therapy for prosthetic valve

thrombosis: a study based on serial Doppler echocardiographic evaluation. Am Heart J 1992;123:1575–1580.

116. Zoghbi WA, Desir RM, Rosen L, et al. Doppler echocardiography: application to the assessment of successful thrombolysis of prosthetic valve thrombosis. J Am Soc Echocardiogr 1989; 2:98–101.

117. Koblic M, Carey C, Webb-Peploe MM, Braimbridge MV. Streptokinase treatment of thrombosed mitral valve prosthesis monitored by Doppler ultrasound. Thorac Cardiovasc Surg 1986;34:333–334.

118. Lengyel M, Fuster V, Keltai M, et al. Guidelines for management of left-sided prosthetic valve thrombosis: a role for thrombolytic therapy. Consensus Conference on Prosthetic Valve Thrombosis. J Am Coll Cardiol 1997;30:1521–1526.

119. Rittoo D, Buckley H, Cotter L. Recurrent prosthetic valve thrombosis: importance of prolonged Doppler echocardiography examination for diagnosis. J Am Soc Echocardiogr 1999;12:686–688.

120. Young E, Shapiro SM, French WJ, Ginzton LE. Use of transesophageal echocardiography during thrombolysis with tissue plasminogen activator of a thrombosed prosthetic mitral valve. J Am Soc Echocardiogr 1992;5:153–158.

121. Ozkan M, Kaymaz C, Kirma C, et al. Intravenous thrombolytic treatment of mechanical prosthetic valve thrombosis: a study using serial transesophageal echocardiography. J Am Coll Cardiol 2000;35:1881–1889.

Appendix I – Mitral Valve Prostheses

Prosthesis	Size	Vmax (m/s)	Peak grad (mmHg)	Mean grad (mmHg)	Half-time	Area (cm^2)
Starr-Edwards		1.88 ± 0.42	14.6 ± 5.5	4.55 ± 2.4	109.5 ± 26.6	2.01 ± 0.49
Lillehei-Kaster		1.84	13.54	3.35	125 ± 29	1.88 ± 0.56
Beall-Surgitool		1.8 ± 0.2	13.4 ± 4.0	6.0 ± 2.0	129.4 ± 15.2	1.7 ± 0.2
Bjork-Shiley		1.61 ± 0.33	10.72 ± 2.74	2.90 ± 1.61	90.2 ± 22.4	2.44 ± 0.62
St. Jude	27	1.54 ± 0.2	9.69 ± 3.06	5.0 ± 2.0	137.5	1.6
	29	1.59 ± 0.27	10.11 ± 3.43	2.71 ± 1.36	78.0 ± 16	2.93 ± 0.6
	31	1.54 ± 0.36	9.90 ± 4.49	5.0 ± 3.0	57.9 ± 6.10	3.8 ± 0.4
	33					5.18
Medtronic-Hall	25	2.1 ± 0.3	13 ± 3			
	27	1.9 ± 0.2	10 ± 3			
	29	1.9 ± 0.2	7 ± 6			
ATS	22/25*			5.4 ± 4.7		1.8 ± 0.5
	24/27*			4.5 ± 0.9		2.9 ± 0.9
	26/29			3.7 ± 0.7		2.8 ± 0.3
	28/31/33			3.1 ± 0.2		2.9 ± 0.2
CarboMedics	25			4.3 ± 1.7		2.7 ± 0.8
	27			3.9 ± 1.0		2.9 ± 1.3
	29/31/33			4.6 ± 2.0		3.0 ± 0.8
On-X	25			3.5 ± 1.1		3.0 ± 0.8
	27/29			4.7 ± 2.0		2.7 ± 0.6
	31/33			4.5 ± 1.3		2.3 ± 0.6
Ionescu-Shiley		1.46 ± 0.27	8.53 ± 2.91	3.28 ± 1.19	93.3 ± 25	2.36 ± 0.75
Carpentier-Edwards		1.76 ± 0.24	12.5 ± 3.64	6.5 ± 2.1	90 ± 25.4	2.45 ± 0.7
Hancock		1.5 ± 0.26	9.7 ± 3.2	4.29 ± 2.1	129 ± 31	1.7 ± 0.4

References See Chapter 8., 17, 41–59.

Index

T - #0499 - 071024 - C328 - 246/189/15 - PB - 9780367446420 - Gloss Lamination